Psychosocial Interventions in the Home

Housecalls

Nancy A. Newton, PhD, a clinical psychologist, is an Associate Professor at The Chicago School of Professional Psychology. A practicing clinician for 20 years, Dr. Newton served as partner and CEO of Dana Home Care, Inc. from 1991 to 1997. At Dana, she developed innovative in-home psychosocial intervention programs for psychiatric clients, the elderly, and women with postpartum depression. These programs integrated the treatment efforts of paraprofessional and professional mental health staff. Dr. Newton has published and presented at national professional conferences on a number of topics, including psychotherapy with the elderly, mentoring and professional development, psychology of women, and meditation and psychotherapy.

Kadi Sprengle, PhD, has worked both as a paraprofessional and as a clinical psychologist in the homes of mentally ill children and adults. Twenty years ago she began as a mental health worker in a demonstration project led by the Illinois Alliance for the Mentally Ill. She later received her doctorate in Clinical Psychology from Northwestern University's School of Medicine. Since then she has worked in a variety of inpatient and community settings. Currently in private practice, she serves as a consultant to child welfare agencies and works with adults and children who face trauma or major mental illness. She also teaches assessment at the Illinois School of Professional Psychology—O'Hare.

Psychosocial Interventions in the Home

Housecalls

Nancy A. Newton, PhD

Kadi Sprengle, PhD

Editors

 SPRINGER PUBLISHING COMPANY

Springer Publishing Company, Inc.
536 Broadway
New York, NY 10012-3955

Acquisitions Editor: Bill Tucker
Production Editor: Pamela Lankas
Cover design by James Scotto-Lavino

00 01 02 03 04 / 5 4 3 2 1

Library of Congress Cataloging-in-Publication Data

Psychosocial interventions in the home: housecalls / Nancy A. Newton
 and Kadi Sprengle, editors.
  p. cm.
 Includes bibliographical references and index.
 ISBN 0-8261-1339-7
 1. Home-based mental health services.   I. Newton, Nancy A.
 II. Sprengle, Kadi.
 RC439.57 .G84 2000
 362.2'4—dc21

                                                    99-087587

Printed in the United States of America

With gratitude and respect, we dedicate this book to Paul Sanders, PhD and Dolores M. Newton.

Contents

Acknowledgments

W e gratefully acknowledge the contributions of many people to this book. It reflects what we have learned from many colleagues and clients. We wish to thank the administrative staff and caregivers of Dana Home Care, and especially William Brauer, President, who worked with dedication and enthusiasm to create a unique example of the best in home care. The caseworkers and investigators of the Glen Ellyn office of the Department of Children and Family Services make the tough calls regarding the safety of children, and fight to expand services for families under their guardianship. Elizabeth Edgar of the National Alliance for the Mentally Ill introduced us to others working in the field.

We learned invaluable lessons, personally and professionally, from clients who welcomed us into their homes, shared their lives, and believed in our ability to help. We thank the residents and staff of the 7720 House (funded by the Illinois Alliance for the Mentally Ill) for inspiration.

We thank Phyllis Kupperman, M. J. Werthman, Mary Beth Napier, Ann Overton, David Starr, Stephanie Hamilton, and the people who willingly and very ably wrote of their experiences in the chapters of this book. Peg White, librarian of the Chicago School of Professional Psychology, cheerfully found the time in an already busy schedule to research the widely diverging literatures we reviewed. Linda Cirillo volunteered her time and talents as copyeditor and we are grateful.

Without the inspiration and patient support of Bill Tucker, Managing Editor of Springer Publishing Company, this book would never have been conceived. The efforts of Emily Epstein and Production Editor Pamela Lankas helped bring it to fruition. In taking on the daunting task of actually writing a book, Linda Edelstein has served as our model and inspiration. The Sunday Night Writing Group—Margit Kir Stimon, Kathleen Slomski, and Linda Edelstein—has been an ongoing source of encouragement. And, on a more personal note, Nancy expresses heart-felt gratitude to her husband of 25 years, Ed Nagel, whose unwavering support in too many ways to publicly elaborate, has made this book (and the career it reflects) possible.

Preface

At the Annual Meeting of the American Psychological Association in 1997, we organized a symposium on in-home psychosocial models of care. The symposium focused on the care models being developed for psychiatric clients by staff of Dana Home Care. The presentation constituted such an unusual offering for a psychological convention that it caught the attention of a senior editor, Bill Tucker, from Springer Publishing Company. Thus, the process that culminated in this book began.

As psychologists, each of our careers had taken unusual turns, leading us into working with clients in their homes. As coowner of Dana Home Care, Nancy had been actively involved in developing and implementing a model for treating acutely and severely disturbed adult psychiatric clients. The model was designed to be an alternative to hospitalization and a strategy for shortening hospital stays. This work was fueled by idealism about creating innovative treatment models based on Buddhist perspectives for cultivating mind–body synchronicity as a path to psychological healing. It was grounded in appreciation for the uniquely useful therapeutic role that carefully selected, trained, and supervised paraprofessional home care workers can provide through ordinary interactions with severely disturbed people.

Starting as a paraprofessional (with no training or credentials) in a home-based experimental program run by the Alliance for the Mentally Ill, Kadi returned to working with alternative programs after completing her doctorate in clinical psychology. She was involved in the development of two alternatives to hospitalization programs before joining a county health department. There, her position involved making emergency house calls to screen children in crisis. She assessed whether they were appropriate for one of the emergency, community-based programs the county had developed or whether hospitalization was necessary. Currently, as part of a general private practice, she provides home-based therapy and assessment to children who have been neglected or abused.

In doing the research for this book, we discovered that the observations we had made about working with clients in their homes were far from atypical. Like us, the vast majority of clinicians who enter their clients' homes have never been trained in, or even exposed to, the unique aspects of developing a therapeutic relationship, conducting psychosocial assessments, and doing therapy on the client's turf—an arena in which the clinician no longer has home court advantage. Over time and through trial and error, each of us had developed a solid understanding of the particular arena of in-home services in which we practiced; we knew virtually nothing about the experiences of other home-based mental health professionals working with other populations in other service delivery systems. We discovered that clinicians working with different age groups, in different settings, and with different issues often reach similar conclusions about their work, struggle with similar issues, and hit similar obstacles. Like us, they rarely seem to know about each other's perspectives.

We also learned (often from heated discussions with each other and with colleagues) that the idea of home-based treatment can prompt strong feelings and opinions. Not the least of the issues is defining what constitutes in-home treatment. Is it limited to services provided to maintain a client with his or her biological family? Does therapeutic care provided for a patient in someone else's home constitute home-based service?

Clinicians and clients alike are divided over the question of what makes a home. In this book, you will come across a variety of answers to that question. For example, can a real home for children who have been abused be built away from the family? Is a foster home a real home?

Parents of chronically ill adult children face a similar dilemma. If their children cannot live in complete independence, can they find help in creating the best home possible outside the home of their parents? In discussing this book project with members of the National Alliance for the Mentally Ill, we found that many parents report sharp criticism from social service agencies when they decide to ask their adult children to move out. These agencies argued that group homes or independent living programs were no place to create a home.

Other issues arise when cost, quality of care, and optimal location for treatment are blended. Too often the argument that "home is better" has been a rationalization for policymakers' real (and unacknowledged) agenda of saving money and avoiding responsibility for providing services. Families of adult chronic psychiatric patients, of children with severe emotional disturbance, and of the elderly have become suspicious of mental health systems that argue for home-based services. All too often they have found themselves coping with overwhelming demands without guidance and support.

For clinicians who have been well socialized to attend to legal and ethical standards, a multitude of concerns arise regarding the rights of the client and safeguards for the therapist when the therapist knocks on the client's door.

We also discovered that our hard-won knowledge of the financial realities of home-based interventions was not unusual. Kadi knew all too well the consequences of community-based programs that have been assigned very ambitious goals by government policies supporting "less restrictive care" and "community services" but with far too little money than could possibly allow them to deliver what was promised.

Dana Home Care was a for-profit company with a 17-year history of providing personal care services to the elderly. As Medicare and private insurance do not cover those services for people with chronic medical or psychiatric diagnoses, such as Alzheimer's disease, our clients were private payors. HomePsych, the program we developed for younger adult psychiatric clients, was targeted for managed care and private-pay clients. HomePsych actually got its initial impetus from inquiries about services from those organizations. The inconsistency of referrals, the many delays in getting paid, and the unending demands of hiring quality staff in an increasingly competitive job market, however, led Nancy and her business partner to close Dana in 1997 between submission of the proposal for the APA symposium and its actual delivery. A cautionary note for home-based clinicians tired of the difficulties associated with public funding and excited about potential managed care market opportunities. After closing Dana, we collected virtually 100% of our receivables from private-pay clients. The only significant receivable that remained uncollectable (despite all the formal and informal pressure we could bring to bear) was $20,000 from a large, nationwide managed-care company. The bill was for care they had requested, certified, and carefully case managed for a client whose treatment had, from everyone's perspective, been an unqualified success.

In the process of reading the literature on in-home services, discussions with people we encountered along the way, and our own dialogue, our goals for this book became clear. They are twofold: (a) to introduce clinicians working in home-based psychosocial services to each other, and (b) to introduce people who have never done this work to the challenges and opportunities inherent within it.

To achieve these goals, we have included an overview of in-home psychosocial services in the United States. We've included chapters on crucial pragmatic and clinical issues, such as legal matters, managed behavioral health care perspectives, training, and in-home assessment strategies. In addition to providing information, we wanted to convey what it is really like to work with clients in their homes. Thus, we've included chapters that describe people's experiences and tell their stories: mental health professionals working with challenging children and families, a respite care worker, a therapeutic foster mom, doulas who care for women with postpartum depression, and a client.

We hope that this information challenges your thinking not only about the possibilities that entering a different treatment environment can provide but also the implications of this work for interventions with clients in any setting.

Contributors

Charles Barringer, PsyD
Staff Psychologist
Uptown Primary Care Center
Chicago Department of
    Public Health
Chicago, Illinois

Mark Epstein, JD
Epstein & Epstein
Chicago, Illinois

Alice Farrell, MS, ED
St. Charles, Illinois

Nancy Flowers, LCSW
Long-Term Care Ombudsman
City of Evanston
Evanston, Illinois

Diane L. Gould, LCSW
Cooper Foundation Childhood
    Disability and Family Support
    Specialist
Jewish Children's Bureau of
    Metropolitan Chicago
Northbrook, Illinois

Julia M. Klco, PsyD
Prairie Path Clinical Services, PC
Wheaton, Illinois

Karen Laing
President
Birthways
Chicago, Illinois

Charlene Rivette, LCSW
Assistant Director of Foster Care
    and Adoptions
Little City Foundation
Palatine, Illinois

David Stark
Board Member
Windhorse Associates
Northhampton, Massachusetts

Diane Stephenson, PhD, CEAP
Corporate Consultant on Research,
    Design and Implementation
Value Options, Inc.
EAP/Clinical Consultant
Federal Occupational Health
Chicago, Illinois

PART ONE

Introduction

Current Landscape of Home-Based Programs

Nancy A. Newton

The first three chapters serve as an overview of the field of home-based services. First, Nancy Newton describes the variety of programs offering home- and community-based mental health services. She presents us with the diversity of rapidly changing programs, many isolated from each other, some in conflict with each other. Drawing from this diversity, she then highlights problems and issues shared by all programs that attempt to deliver services at the client's door.

This chapter provides an overview of current approaches to home-based psychosocial services for clients experiencing or at risk for some form of significant psychological distress. Programs are included that provide a significant component of treatment in the client's home or in an alternative home-like setting. The chapter covers programs that serve a wide range of populations—elderly, adults, adolescents, and children with severe psychiatric symptoms, families either experiencing or at risk for crisis, and children with developmental disabilities and their families. These programs have different historical roots, arising out of independent efforts to meet the needs of specific populations. They draw upon a variety of theories, treatment models, and specific interventions. Service providers range from highly educated mental health professionals to volunteers with minimal training and supervision. Mental health professionals who developed these programs have different professional allegiances, although nursing and social work are the most often represented specializations. As a result, there has often been little sharing of information among home-based clinicians who work with different populations. It is this chapter's lofty goal to open that dialogue.

This chapter is not intended to provide a comprehensive review of the often-extensive literature that exists on some of these approaches to home-based treatment. Instead, it provides an overview of the different ways in which mental health professionals currently conceptualize and provide in-home psychiatric services. Historical roots, treatment philosophy, interventions, staffing patterns, and empirical data on program effectiveness are briefly summarized. Reviewing these varied treatment approaches allows identification of the shared problems and issues that characterize in-home psychiatric services and that differentiate them from services provided in more traditional inpatient and outpatient settings. It lays the groundwork for systematic thinking about the home environment as a context for treatment.

For the purposes of this review, programs have been organized by the age group that they serve, from infants in high-risk families to the elderly. Within some age groups, different types of home-based programs are identified.

FAMILY VISITS: PREVENTION AND EARLY-INTERVENTION PROGRAMS

Healthy Start in Hawaii is a well-known and widely replicated example of programs designed to identify and support high-risk families through in-home services (Hawaii Department of Health, 1992). During their hospital birth admission, all new mothers in Hawaii are interviewed and screened for risk of child abuse based on factors such as single-parent status, low self-esteem, and history of maltreatment as a child. Based on these criteria, potentially at-risk mothers begin receiving home visits by paid paraprofessional staff within three months after the child's birth. During the child's first year, the visits occur weekly for approximately one hour each. Home visitors may teach infant care skills, model parenting skills, provide emotional support, and/or monitor the mother's and baby's health and well-being. They then continue on a schedule consistent with the family's needs until the child reaches age five. Child development specialists also periodically visit the home to assess the child's cognitive development and parent–child interaction patterns.

In 1990, over 4,000 early-intervention programs in the United States provided home visiting services (Roberts & Wasik, 1990). In her 1995 review of home visiting programs in the United States and Europe, Karen McCurdy identified four common objectives: prevent child abuse and neglect, enhance the health and safety of the child, facilitate the child's development and functioning, and improve parental caregiving skills. Although programs may target families with children of any age, they often focus on families with children under age three. Target families may be identified and services initiated prenatally or immediately after birth.

McCurdy (1995) outlined the rationale for home visiting services. Research suggests that social isolation places families at higher risk for maltreating their children and makes them less likely to seek out support through either informal social networks or formal social service programs. Other lines of research suggest that social support inhibits harmful behavior and enhances nurturing behavior in at-risk mothers. Thus, home visiting programs strive to prevent abuse and neglect by providing potentially powerful social support and guidance to families at risk for child-rearing problems before problems arise.

Structurally, home visiting programs vary along a number of dimensions (McCurdy, 1995):

when services are initiated: during early to late pregnancy to immediately after birth
how long services continue: from as little as 18 weeks to up to 5 years
intensity: home visits may be weekly, biweekly, monthly
staff: nurses, social workers, developmental psychologists, paraprofessionals
participant selection: examples of selection criteria include mother's age (i.e., adolescent mothers), factors correlated with high risk for child abuse, first time mothers in rural areas, pregnant women at risk for poor birth outcomes, families of low birth weight infants

A 1990 Government Accounting Office (GAO) Report identified four elements critical to the success of home visiting services: clear program objectives, structured programs delivered by skilled home visitors, comprehensive focus with strong community ties, and secure funding over time (McCurdy, 1995). Based on her review of the empirical literature and her personal study of 48 programs, McCurdy adds four additional critical elements:

• Intense level of services. Programs that provide weekly visits have greater impact while programs with monthly visits may have little to no impact. "Intensity of service has the most consistent relationship with positive outcomes" (p. 30).

- Early intervention, either prenatally or at birth. Particularly first-time mothers may be more receptive to guidance and support before the birth; initiating services prenatally also allows the client to establish a relationship with home visiting staff prior to the baby's arrival.
- Long-term services. Programs that provide visits for 1 to 3 years seem to have the most effect; programs of 6 months or less rarely have an impact.
- Include a focus on child health care and safety issues.

It is also likely that home visiting programs are most effective with mothers who are both at risk *and* possess a sufficiently high level of psychological functioning to benefit from the assistance. "The family must be functioning with some minimum of coherence and healthy adaptiveness in order to profit from the support of a home visitor" (Halpern, 1984, p. 41).

CHILDREN–FAMILY-PRESERVATION PROGRAMS

Family-preservation programs were developed to prevent out-of-home placement for children in troubled families. In the early 1970s, critics became increasingly vocal about the large numbers of children, particularly ethnic minority children, being placed outside of their homes (Pecora, 1991). At that time, widespread attitudes favored placement rather than parental involvement in addressing the needs of distressed children or families in crisis. Federal funding encouraged foster care placement over preventive or restorative services. In response, critics expressed concern about curbing the high financial costs entailed in out-of-home placement and developing programs that might more favorably impact on the child's long-term development. Social activists argued that society should be willing to invest as many resources in preserving families as in providing substitute family care services (Pecora, Fraser, & Haspala, 1989).

Wells (1995) traced the historical roots of family-preservation programs to the "friendly visitors" of the late 1800s. Hired by charity organizations to identify worthy cases and distribute funds, friendly visitors were "expected to be combination detectives and moral influences. They were to ascertain the reason for the applicants' need and to help them overcome it" (Bremner, 1971, p. 52; quoted in Wells, 1995). The Family Centered Project of St. Paul in the early 1950s is the more recent source of many of the ideas at the heart of family-preservation programs (Wells, 1995). Homebuilders, which was established in

Tacoma, Washington, in 1974 (Kinney et al., 1990), remains a prototype for many current programs.

Homebuilders was designed to provide intensive, flexible, goal-oriented, short-term services to families in crisis. Families were referred when either (a) one or more children was in jeopardy of being removed from the home by local child protective agencies or (b) family conflict was so intense that either the parents could no longer care for the child or the child was threatening to run away. Presenting problems included one (and often more) of the following: child abuse and neglect, family violence, or developmental disabilities or mental illness in a parent or child (Kinney et al., 1990). Generally, these were multi-problemed families in whom emotional and psychological distress was inextricably interwoven with poverty and limited access to employment and other resources.

In Homebuilders, an assigned staff person works intensely with the family in its home to defuse the precipitating crisis and prepare the family to handle future crises more effectively. Specific services vary according to the family's needs—counseling, education in parenting and homemaking skills, assistance in meeting basic needs for clothing, shelter, transportation, or food. Limiting their caseloads to one or two families means that staff can work intensely with each family on a flexible schedule, individualized to meet the family's needs. For the 4- to 6-week duration of the intervention, the staff person is available to the family on an emergency basis 24 hours a day.

Initial studies suggested that the Homebuilders model was successful in diminishing use of hospitalization. For example, 12-month follow-up data on 3,497 cases seen between 1974 and 1987 showed that 88% had avoided state-funded placement in foster care, group care, or psychiatric institutions (Kinney et al., 1990). The early success of Homebuilders encouraged the provision of funding for family-oriented support programs through the Adoption Assistance and Child Welfare Reform Act of 1980. After an initial decrease in frequency and length of child placement, however, the positive trends had reversed by the mid-1980s (McKenzie, Mikkelsen, Stelk, Bereika, & Monack, 1995). By the late 1980s, the increasing number of children needing placement combined with decreasing availability of foster families once again highlighted the need for intensive support services for at-risk families (Minuchin, 1995). The 1993 federal Family Preservation and Family Support Initiative addressed this need.

During the 1990s, these programs have grown from small-scale demonstration projects to a widely accepted component of most child welfare services. Wells (1995) attributes their expansion to a number of factors. They are consistent with current social values that support children growing up within their own families. Current public policy encourages permanency planning, treatment in the least restrictive setting, and community-based programs in the child welfare, mental health and juvenile justice system. The financial support of several prominent American foundations has significantly underwritten their growth.

Intensive family-preservation services tend to replicate either the Homebuilders programs or models based on family systems theory (Henggeler, Schoenwald, Pickrel, Brondun, Borduin, & Hall, 1994). Specific programs, however, vary greatly in terms of goals, clinical methods, duration of treatment, size of caseload, and nature and number of concrete services provided. Target populations also have expanded to include families coping with varied problems that threaten their stability, adoptive and foster families in crises, families preparing for reunification following external child placement, and adolescent juvenile offenders (Butts & Barton, 1995; Pecora, 1991).

Despite their variability, family-preservation programs share three core beliefs: the problems of individual children are best addressed through enhancing family functioning; working with families in their homes increases the potential impact of services; and effective interventions are time-limited and integrate concrete and psychosocial services (Wells, 1995). According to Pecora (1991), family-preservation programs are characterized by 14 attributes. Among the most defining characteristics are that they are short term (less than 90 days), intense (two or more interventions a week for 1–4 hours each), and home based. Staff are available for crisis intervention 24 hours a day, 7 days a week; and staff believe in family empowerment and keeping children in their own homes.

A major research study of the 1980s on family-preservation programs followed 453 families in Washington (a nonprofit agency) and Utah (a child welfare agency) (Pecora et al., 1989). The results demonstrated significant improvements in child and family functioning; 69% of children remained in their homes throughout service delivery and during the 12-month follow-up. The services families received were both intense and varied (Lewis, 1991). Therapists reported an average of 37 hours of direct client contact during the 4–6 weeks of intervention, with high usage levels of a range of psychotherapy, educational, and social learning services. An average of 31.8 different clinical services were provided to each family. About three fourths of families received some type of concrete service (most commonly transportation).

Although the research on family-preservation programs is extensive, variability among programs limits the extent to which results of specific studies can be generalized. In addition, research is hampered by poor research design, limited measures of functioning, inadequate analysis, small samples, and lack of control groups.

In their review of the research, Pecora et al. (1989) concluded that "on balance the data indicate that [home-based services], and [family preservation service] programs in particular, are successful in preventing placement in 40% to 90% of cases referred to them" (p. 333). In reviewing studies with rigorous controls, Wells (1995) concludes that "family preservation services may reduce child placement in the short run but their effectiveness diminishes over time." The level of success appears to directly relate to the breadth and depth of services provided. Spaid, Lewis, and Pecora (1991) analyzed the existent research in an effort to identify the factors responsible for treatment success. Although tentative, they suggest that the following variables correlate with success: greater attainment of specific treatment goals, lack of alternative outside social support for the family, and greater provision of concrete services, such as housing, transportation, and employment. Success is less likely when there has been prior child placement in foster, group, or institutional care and when a significant amount of time lapses between the crisis and therapist's response.

CHILDREN WITH SEVERE EMOTIONAL DISTURBANCE

Criticism of mental health services for children and adolescents with severe emotional disturbance (SED) is long-standing, dating back at least to the 1909 White House Conference on Children (Wells, 1995). More recently, the report of the 1969 Joint Commission on the Mental Health of Children, *Crisis in Child Mental Health* (1970), magnetized the nation's awareness of the poor quality of inpatient psychiatric care for children: "There are a few superb institutions in the country, many are marginal; however, most are disgraceful and intolerable" (p. 42). Other problems were the absence of community resources and lack of clear lines of responsibility and accountability for meeting the needs of children (Kuperminc & Cohen, 1995).

A 1979 class action lawsuit brought on behalf of children housed in state training schools and psychiatric institutions in North Carolina brought things to a head. After a year of gathering evidence that supported the plaintiffs' claims that these children had significant, unmet treatment and educational needs, North Carolina negotiated a settlement. One of the settlement agreements was that the four plaintiffs and other similar children receive treatment in less restrictive and intrusive settings. The resulting service model involved: a wide continuum of services within the community; a system of case managers to develop and oversee implementation of individual habilitation plans; and a management system to keep the continuum flexible and responsive (Behar, 1986). Funding was also made available so that highly individualized, often quite nontraditional services could be "wrapped around" the child at the discretion of case managers.

> Examples might be the purchase of supervision and on-the-job training that allows a youngster to work in a barbershop and learn a marketable skill; the development of supervised apartment living for a young mother and her new baby to provide her psychological support and training in care of the newborn; or the purchase of piano lessons to enhance a musical talent and, consequently, enhance a child's self-esteem. (Behar, 1986, p. 19)

Despite the skepticism of mental health professionals that children with such severe behavior problems, including aggression and assault, could be treated while living at home, the "Fort Bragg Managed Care Experiment" which tested the model in North Carolina demonstrated that children could be treated effectively with less hospital care (Burchard, 1996). In 1984, the federal government created the Child and Adolescent Service System Program (CASSP) to provide states with the needed technical assistance and financial aid to restructure their systems of care from reliance on inpatient and residential programs to community-based services.

Integrated systems of community-based services for severe emotionally disturbed children became known as "wraparound" models (Stroul & Friedman, 1988). They attempt to solve problems of discontinuity and lack of coordination in care, transfer of the child from provider to provider, and obstacles to family involvement in care planning (McKelvey, 1988). According to VanDenBerg and Grealish (1996), eight elements define the model:

(a) Wraparound efforts must be based in the community.
(b) Services and supports must be individualized to meet the needs of the children and families and not designed to reflect the priorities of the service systems.
(c) The process must be culturally competent and build on the unique values, strengths, and social and racial make-up of children and families.
(d) Parents must be included in every level of development of the process.
(e) Agencies must have access to flexible, noncategorized funding.
(f) The process must be implemented on an interagency basis and be owned by the larger community.
(g) Services must be unconditional. If the needs of the child and family change, the child and family are not to be rejected from services. Instead, the services must be changed.

(h) Outcomes must be measured. If they are not, the wraparound process is merely an interesting fad. (p. 9)

Over the last two decades, wraparound programs have evolved a unique, community-based, service delivery model (VanDenBerg & Grealish, 1996). Key is an oversight team composed of agency and school representatives, clergy, business leaders, parents, and community advocates. Generally, subcommittees of the oversight team actually oversee the wraparound process. They identify potential clients and contract with "broker" agencies who assume responsibility for coordinating care, managing the funds available for flexible services, and overseeing program implementation. VanDenBerg and Grealish emphasize that rather than a "model" to be implemented, wraparound is a process to be molded to meet the needs of individual communities. They point to eight lessons that have been learned about what makes the system work:

1. If the adults disagree, the child fails.
2. The wraparound process requires system collaboration.
3. Managed care can hurt or help the wraparound process.
4. The more complex the needs of the child and family, the more individualized the plan needs to be.
5. Flexible funds are necessary and must be managed carefully.
6. The wraparound process cannot be implemented with either just a "top down" or "grassroots up" approach.
7. Confidentiality and liability issues can be effectively resolved.
8. Parent advocacy and parent-professional partnerships are crucial. (pp. 18–19)

Family-Centered Intensive Case Management (FCICM), one of the first community-based programs implemented by the New York State Office of Mental Health, is an example of a wraparound program (Evans et al., 1994). It was designed to provide families caring for SED children at home with the same services that families serving as treatment foster families were receiving. FCICM consists of four key service elements: case management/case coordination, wraparound services, flexibility of funding and services, and interagency collaboration (Evans et al., 1994, p. 229). The family is viewed as the child's primary resource and thus as having the central role in accomplishing treatment goals for the child. A team consisting of a case manager and a parent advocate who has had the experience of raising a child with SED do "whatever it takes" to support a group of eight families caring for their children. "Whatever it takes" includes services such as behavior management and self-help skills development, parent and family support groups, planned and emergency respite care, sibling recreational groups, and expenditure of flexible service dollars for items such as home repair and recreational opportunities. A 1993 study compared the effectiveness of the FCICM program with therapeutic foster care. Thirty-nine children were randomly assigned either to FCICM or therapeutic foster care. The majority of children had major/persistent disruption in their behavior toward others and in their moods and emotions, and age-appropriate role performance. Evans et al. conclude that "given intensive and individualized supports, children with SED can be cared for effectively in their own homes" (p. 237).

Other research studies have demonstrated that wraparound programs can positively impact the quality of children's lives by decreasing rates of foster placement or, once placed, frequency of moves and behavioral problems (runaway days or involvement with the juvenile justice system) (Clark, Lee, Prange, & McDonald, 1996). Little difference is generally found, however, in degree of improvement in emotional/ behavioral adjustment between children involved in wraparound programs and control groups (Clark et al., 1996).

The Yale Intensive In-home Child and Adolescent Psychiatry Services (YICAPS) is an example of efforts to integrate wraparound, community-based services with inpatient models of care (Woolston, Berkowitz, Schaefer, & Adnopoz, 1998). YICAPS brought together two existing programs: the Family Support Service at the Yale Child Study Center, a grant-funded family-preservation program, and the Children's Psychiatric Inpatient Service at Yale-New Haven Hospital. This relationship allows for the integration of inpatient psychiatric treatment, when needed, with the extension of evaluation and treatment into the home setting. A two-person clinical team provides home-based evaluation (including the physical home and neighborhood environment), develops a treatment plan with the family, and provides treatment of the identified problems in the child and family. Services include individual and family therapy, parent training, behavior management, and medication management. Intensive case management links the child and family to appropriate services, coordinates services, and empowers the family to become their own advocates. Crisis intervention services are available 24 hours a day, 7 days a week. Funding for YICAPS includes commercial insurance, managed care, Medicaid, case-specific funding from state agencies, and out-of-pocket family funding.

THERAPEUTIC FOSTER CARE

A long-standing remedy for troubled families has been brief or lengthy out-of-home placement of children with other families who are paid to provide care. These "foster families" are expected to provide safe, nurturant respite until the family can be reunited. Building on this basic model, "therapeutic foster families" are designed to treat children and adolescents with severe emotional disturbance in the community. They provide "residential therapy within a family setting" (Fine, 1993). Treatment foster parents try to provide a healthy home environment and relationships that promote development and provide corrective and/or compensatory social and emotional experiences. They receive additional training, support, and pay; they are considered integral members of a treatment team within a program that defines itself as serving clients who would otherwise be in nonfamily institutional care (Eckstein, 1995). Farrell (chapter 10, this volume) describes her experiences as a therapeutic foster mom for a severely disturbed child. Rivetle (chapter 9, this volume) provides an in-depth description of therapeutic foster care.

Continuum Advocate Home Network exemplifies this model (Eckstein, 1995). It is a long-term therapeutic, community-based family foster care program established in 1978 to served troubled children and adolescents. The treatment foster home is one component of a network of services, including emergency shelter, residential treatment, transitional and independent living, youth corrections, and family outreach services. Foster parents or "advocates" are viewed as professional caregivers who work closely with a social worker to provide therapeutic services to the child. Interventions include behavior modification, crisis intervention, case management, social support, advocacy, mediation, and education and process groups. Training for "advocates" includes an initial 18-hour program, weekly team meetings, and a minimum of 40 hours a year of continuing education.

Another model is the Family Based Treatment (FBT) program in New York State (Evans et al., 1994). It includes a family specialist, a cluster of five treatment families and one respite family. The family specialist provides support and training to the treatment and respite families, advocates for the child, and prepares the biological families for reunification. The treatment and respite families are involved in all aspects of treatment planning, implementation, and evaluation, including implementing structure, behavior management plans, and working with the children to attain goals.

Continuum and Family Based Treatment are examples of programs in which foster parents are seen as full-fledged professional members of the mental health team. In these programs, treatment foster parents are highly trained and their efforts are integrated into a program of psychotherapy, medication, crisis management, special educational services, and targeted family interventions (Rosenfeld, Altman, &

Kaufman, 1997). The expectation is that children will eventually return to their families or regular foster families. The extent to which a "therapeutic" foster home differs from traditional foster homes, however, varies across programs. Often, the differences are minor. The foster parent may receive somewhat more training and support and the child receives mental health services. As the child's functioning improves, these services diminish but the child remains with the foster family with the same time restrictions and expectations as other foster care services.

Mentor Clinical Care (MCC) combines elements of therapeutic foster care and hospitalization to treat acutely disturbed children, adolescents, and adults (McKenzie, Mikkelsen, Stelk, Bereika, & Monack, 1995). Drawing upon its experience serving public sector clients, MCC developed the "Mentor Hospital Diversion Program" to meet the needs of third-party payors (health maintenance organizations, insurance companies and others). The program's goals are similar to those generally met in hospital settings—diagnostic assessment, pharmacologic intervention, case management, and intensive psychotherapy for the child and family (McKenzie et al., 1995). Rather than admitting the child to an inpatient facility, however, the child enters the home of a mental health technician known as a mentor. Considered a member of the professional treatment team, the mentor takes primary responsibility for monitoring patient status, overseeing the child's schoolwork, implementing behavioral management programs, life skills training, and therapeutic activities. The mentor's role is integrated into an intensive and comprehensive psychiatric treatment program. Program duration is expected to be less than 30 days. The outcome data gathered on 89 children compares favorably to data on inpatient treatment. At discharge, 72.3% returned home to a biological family member; 15.7% were discharged to a less restrictive setting such as foster care or a group home; 4.8% were discharged to a more restrictive treatment setting, such as an inpatient psychiatric unit (McKenzie et al., 1995). At 6-month follow-up, 48.4% were living with their parents, a relative, family friend, or adoptive home; 13.4% were in foster care or group homes.

FAMILY TRAINING AND SUPPORT PROGRAMS

These programs provide specific training to enhance the ability of primary family caregivers to meet the needs of the impaired family member, generally a child. Mental health professionals or paraprofessionals assess and train the family in specific skills. These programs tend to be small-scale, locally-focused, innovative, stand-alone efforts. They are often a direct result of family initiatives. An example of such a program is Families for Early Autism Treatment (Huff, 1996). This program was jointly organized by families and professionals to provide a variety of support services to families with young autistic children, aged 18 to 60 months. As is often true of these programs, a wide variety of services are provided, including counseling, in-home and workshop training, advocacy, and so on. Another example is a program developed to assist young children who are deaf-blind to develop communication skills (Watkins, Clark, Strong, & Barringer, 1994). Using Helen Keller as a model, paraprofessionals (called "interveners") spend two hours each day providing direct and meaningful interaction with the child in his or her home. Techniques used include tactile and/or other appropriate communication forms, massage, daily care, and mobility training.

ADULT PSYCHIATRIC CLIENTS—COMMUNITY SUPPORT PROGRAMS FOR SEVERELY DISTURBED CLIENTS

Historically, whether severely disturbed psychiatric clients received care primarily in community or institutional settings reflected society's cultural values, public policy, and economic priorities. Recent trends in the United States are no exception to this pattern. Following decades of emphasis on institutional care, the de-institutionalization movement of the 1950s to 1970s led to the discharge of thousands of patients from long-term, often lifelong, hospitalizations in large, publicly funded psychiatric institutions. Between 1955 and 1985–1986, the number of episodes of hospitalization (residents plus admissions) dropped from 818,000 to 445,181 (Singer, 1996). The clients being discharged were diagnosed with schizophrenia, psychosis, depression and manic-depression, paranoia, and severe personality disorders. Their symptoms significantly impaired their ability to care for themselves, disrupted their reality-based connection with the people and world around them, and made them vulnerable to injury from self and others. Introduction of neuroleptic medications provided the rationale for discharging long-institutionalized patients and shortening stays for newly admitted patients. Even with more effective neuroleptic medications, however, mental health professionals were concerned about the capacity of many of these clients to adapt to community living on an ongoing basis and to be treated in the community in times of crisis.

In response, a number of carefully designed demonstration projects were conducted during the 1960s and 1970s to investigate the effectiveness of home and community-based services in helping clients adapt to and maintain community living (Fenton, Tessier, Struening,

Smith, & Benoit, 1982; Kiesler, 1982; Pasamanick, Scarpitti, & Dinitz, 1967). The hope was that, with sufficient training and support, clients could better adapt in the community and learn the skills required to sustain independent living, thus reducing the likelihood of future hospitalizations. Sprengle (chapter 3, this volume) briefly describes such a program. While specific programs varied in terms of care models and treatment interventions, they were generally based in a case management model that emphasized coordination between service providers, the client, and the client's support systems. Home visits were integrated into all of the programs, primarily as a means of insuring follow-up and monitoring of clients who were often unreliable in following through with outpatient treatment.

One of the initial studies, The Louisville Homecare Project (Pasamanick et al., 1967) addressed the question of whether clients in crisis could safely and effectively be treated in their homes rather than in the hospital. Investigators selected 152 schizophrenic patients when they applied for admission to Central State Hospital in Louisville. They were randomly assigned to one of three groups: a group of 54 patients that remained in the hospital and two groups totaling 98 patients who returned home, 57 with appropriate antipsychotic medication and 41 with placebo medication. All of the patients who returned home were visited weekly by specially trained public health nurses for three months, then every other week for three months, then monthly for up to 30 months. Clients were also seen in an outpatient clinic by a psychiatrist; social workers provided assistance when needed. Study results indicated that 77% of the patients who returned home on antipsychotic medication and 34% of those on placebo medication were safely treated at home. Patients treated at home scored higher on measures of mental status, domestic functioning, and social participation than those who were admitted to the hospital. Once services were discontinued, however, so did their positive benefits. Five years following discontinuation of the home visits, there were no differences between the three groups in rates of hospitalization or on ratings on psychosocial measures.

Other studies replicated the findings of the Louisville Homecare Project. Summarizing the results of eight major English and American research studies of community-based care models for chronic psychiatric patients, Fenton et al. (1982) concluded that "sufficient evidence is available now to consider implementing community-based treatment more widely" (p. 17). Their review found that community-based treatment was a less expensive, clinically effective alternative for a significant proportion of individuals requesting inpatient treatment; family involvement is not an essential prerequisite for community-based treatment; and the main differences between community- and hospital-based programs lie in the locale and continuity of treatment and flexibility in the roles of treatment staff.

In the early 1970s, staff of Mendota Mental Health Institute in Madison, Wisconsin developed one of the most widely studied and replicated community-based models for providing support and monitoring to adults with chronic psychiatric disorders (Meisler & Santos, 1997). Known as Training in Community Living (TCL) or Program for Assertive Community Treatment (PACT), the program's core was a treatment team who assumed full clinical responsibility for the client in the community. The program's goals were to reduce psychiatric symptoms, improve quality of life and psychosocial functioning, and reduce need for hospitalization. Services included "close psychiatric monitoring, including the taking of medications; facilitating the acquisition of basic resources (housing, entitlements, and general health care); support in dealing with life's daily problems, which can easily overwhelm clients; teaching and reinforcing essential skills in the natural environment (e.g., homemaking, financial management, communication, and employment); modifying pathological dependency relationships; and developing a supportive network among family and significant others; thus decreasing their stress and frustration in relating to the client" (Meisler & Santos, 1997, p. 175). Staff essentially did whatever needed to be done to support the client's adjustment and independence. Services were available 24 hours a day and 7 days a week.

The initial research study compared 21 patients assigned to the Mendota TCL program to 20 patients who received standard inpatient treatment and 20 patients assigned to a research unit designed to prepare them for discharge (Meisler & Santos, 1997). The pilot study lasted five months. While there were no differences between the groups in psychiatric diagnosis and symptoms, the TCL subjects spent an average of 6 days in the hospital compared to an average of 100 days in the two control groups. After five months of involvement in the TCL program, patients were much more likely to be living independently and working. While the experimental and control groups differed significantly in their ability to manage independent living, there were no posttreatment differences between the groups in levels of psychiatric symptoms or self-esteem. A second study in 1972 (Meisler & Santos, 1997) followed patients for 14 months after they had been discharged from the experimental program and returned to more traditional outpatient care. Similar to the results of the Louisville Homecare Project, experimental subjects no longer showed most of the independent living gains they had made while involved in the TCL program.

Since the 1970s, comprehensive case management programs have become an accepted strategy to support severely disturbed clients in their communities. Organizational structure, orientation, intensity of service, and availability of services varies widely between specific programs (Meisler & Santos, 1997). Two primary organizational structures are that of the individual case manager working within a community mental health center or freestanding agency and that of the treatment team responsible for the care of multiple patients. Case managers may define their roles as service brokers, rehabilitation agents, or clinicians. Their services generally include outreach, linkage to community programs and services, monitoring of client functioning, and advocacy. In their 1997 review of the empirical literature on TCL programs, Meisler and Santos identify the traits that seem to characterize effective programs:

- They are based on ecological models—the belief that understanding and treatment of psychopathology requires attention to both the client and the broad social and environmental context in which the client exists.
- Treatment is pragmatic, emphasizing action-oriented, clearly defined interventions.
- Interventions occur in the client's natural environment.
- Treatment planning and implementation is flexible, continually changing in response to the client's needs and circumstances.
- There is a high degree of accountability of treatment team members, with ongoing systematic monitoring of treatment effectiveness.

How these basic principles are implemented may be a function of the realities of the community context: mobility, accessibility, community resources, communications, cultural values, and economic realities. Often, the roles and interventions of the home-based mental health worker seem far removed from the traditional world of mental health services. A description of efforts to support Mr. M, an adult schizophrenic client who lived with his family on a rural coastal island in South Carolina, exemplifies the flexibility, practicality, and comprehensiveness of the assistance these programs offer in their efforts to improve the quality of life of their clients (Lachance, Deci, Santos, Halewood, & Westfall, 1997). Prior to intervention, neighbors reported that Mr. M had not been seen by neighbors for several years. He had barricaded himself in the family home, using a hole in the floor as a toilet and only allowing food and water to be given to him through a slot in the door. He had not bathed or changed clothes for years.

The ROADS (Rural Outreach, Advocacy and Direct Services) team slowly developed a relationship with Mr. M and his family. ROADS visited him at least once a week and administered his injections (psychotropic medication) monthly. The ROADS psychiatrist visited him at home because he still refused to travel. ROADS focused on improving his environment and hygiene, arranging through other social services and volunteer agencies for running water in the house, an outhouse, a refrigerator, mattresses, roof repairs, and window screens. ROADS helped him obtain Medicaid and a disability income. They worked with his family on basic hygiene and food preparation, including convincing the family to not let their chickens run free in the house. Mr. M's environment was clearly pathological for him, particularly in view of the fact that his alcoholic father had attempted to kill him on four occasions because of his frustration with Mr. M and his unwillingness to work. Mr. M strongly resisted efforts to be relocated, however, even with other family members who lived nearby because he said, "This is home and it is the only home I've ever known." Mr. M still lives with his family. He now sits out with his family in the living room and walks around in the yard. He eats with the family and takes baths about weekly, although he still prefers to wear layers of clothes. (Lachance et al., 1997, pp. 242–243)

One consistent finding across studies is that the benefits of community-based services do not extend after discontinuation of services (Meisler & Santos, 1997). One explanation is that these programs become their clients' primary source of social support (Mandiberg, 1995). Often the nature of their symptoms impairs the ability of severely disturbed clients to create and maintain viable social support networks apart from their treatment team. The less formal and more extensive personal connections that naturally evolve between staff and clients in community settings can make the interweaving of social and treatment support much more evident than in hospital settings. Discontinuation of treatment is then inevitably accompanied by loss of the informal social support the team has provided, further increasing the client's vulnerability. Several programs have directly addressed this issue by creating community social support systems that extend beyond the treatment team. In the Santa Clara County Clustered Apartment project, staff worked with clients to establish "three non-clinical-nonrehabilitation model patient communities based on mutual support and interdependence among patients" (Mandiberg, 1995, p. 193). Clients' homes were clustered within 5 minutes walking distance of each other, and community organizers helped clients establish a mutually supportive and interdependent community. With support and effort, clients were able to establish supportive communities in which they helped stabilize each other and sometimes managed crisis without resorting to hospitalization.

Other programs have addressed this issue by embedding formal treatment within a broader supportive community context. For example, Windhorse Associates has developed a community of clients, staff, family, and friends who want to create a genuinely respectful and healing community that extends beyond formal treatment plans and interventions (Fortuna, 1995; Stark, chapter 15, this volume). Frequent social gatherings celebrate the seasons, birthdays, and personal achievements. Shared interests—writing, the arts, gardening—create other opportunities for relationships. Thus, even when treatment ends, community connections can persist.

ADULTS: CLIENTS IN ACUTE CRISIS

The general expectation in the mental health field is that clients who are in severe states of crisis will not be treated on an outpatient basis but will be hospitalized. Several innovative programs, however, have taken on the challenge of creating home-based programs for clients in acute crisis.

CRISIS HOMES

In 1972, the Southwest Denver Community Mental Health Center extended the concept of community-based care to a new level. Polak, Kirby, and Deitchman (1995) found that, even with a well-developed network of home visits and community supports, it was inevitable that some clients would need separation from their natural home environments in times of acute distress. They concluded that when there is imminent or threatened danger to self or others, crises that overwhelm clients' natural support systems, extreme isolation or withdrawal that exacerbates psychiatric symptoms, or involvement in dysfunctional relationships, entry into a different, "safer" environment may be necessary. To provide that environment outside of the hospital, Polak et al. (1995) developed the model of "crisis homes."

The Southwest Denver Community Mental Health Center contracted with six families who agreed to take up to two acutely disturbed clients at a time into their homes. The families agreed to provide room, board, and patient care for a daily fee. Clinical staff who visited the patient daily provided formal treatment; psychiatric nurses and psychiatrists were always on call. By design, the homes varied in terms of ethnicity and language, intensity of available support, and the extent to which "sponsoring" families actively participated in formal treatment plans. Despite the variability, commonalities did emerge:

The family sponsors tended quite naturally to treat patients in their homes as guests. They oriented themselves more to the strengths and positive features of patients than to their pathology, and they were much less likely than mental health professionals to view all patient behavior in an illness framework. Home sponsors were warm, outgoing, healthy people who were rich in life experience. We provided little formal mental health training, but focused on encouraging sponsor families to use their already existing skills. (Polak et al., 1995, p. 218)

Polak et al. (1995) summarize the benefits of crisis homes over hospitalization:

- A number of specifically different community environments provides a more individually tailored and responsive system than the larger, less diversified environment of the psychiatric hospital.
- Sponsor families provide a clear model of healthy individual and family behavior that can be generalized to the patient's real-life setting more easily than the learning that takes place in the artificial psychiatric hospital environment.
- In this "medium is the message" age, admission to a normal home rather than a hospital makes an immediate, clear statement to the patient and his or her family. The patient is expected to have higher self-esteem, feel less stigma, and assume greater responsibility for his or her own behavior than if he or she were hospitalized. (p. 219)

Unfortunately, the family sponsor program ended in 1987. The experiences of this program exemplifies the lifespan of many innovative, community-based programs developed to treat people with psychiatric problems. As leadership and staff of the Southwest Denver CMHC changed and evolved, program priorities also shifted. Interest in developing the family sponsor homes and knowledge of how to effectively treat clients within this model waned. The final blow to the program was the consolidation of the CMHC with the larger Denver Mental Health Corporation. As Polak et al. note, "It is quite clear that alternatives to acute psychiatric hospitalization cannot survive without continued commitment to the concept by the leadership of the mental health structure in which they operate and both commitment and skill on the part of the clinical staff" (p. 223).

As the Denver crisis home program was ending, a similar program was instituted in Madison, Wisconsin (Bennett, 1995). Dane County maintains from one to six crisis home families who provide temporary places of respite for people in crisis. As in the Denver program, crisis home providers are ordinary people who openly welcome clients into their homes, recognize when they need to call for help, and acknowledge their clients' difficulties without minimizing their strengths. The program is a component of the emergency services unit, ensuring that 24-hour support is available for both families and clients. Clients are involved in outpatient mental health services. In 1992, the program had 140 separate crisis home admissions, with an average length of stay of 3 days. Clients were admitted as an alternative to hospitalization, when transitioning out of the hospital or, less frequently, as a result of a housing issue or "precrisis" situation. Similar to Polak et al., Bennett suggests that clients respond positively to being a guest in the home of someone providing a safe and supportive environment. He suggests that many clients feel honored to be welcomed into a pleasant living environment; even severely disturbed people are able to rise to the occasion of being a "guest."

POSITIVE ALTERNATIVES TO HOSPITALIZATION

Positive Alternatives to Hospitalization (PATH) contracts with managed care companies to provide an alternative to hospitalization for clients whose distress is so significant that it warrants inpatient admission (Moy & Pigott, 1997). A multidisciplinary team (psychologists, psychiatrists, social workers, and nurses) provides intensive in-home crisis intervention services. Within an hour of referral, the crisis worker meets with the client and his/her family at their home. This initial meeting may last a number of hours. Its goals are to establish a strong therapeutic alliance, complete a careful assessment, defuse strong feelings and crises, and develop a mutually agreed upon treatment plan. Crisis intervention services continue to be accessible 24 hours a day; interventions continue at an intense rate, often with multiple contacts per week. A wide range of individual, family, and group treatment modalities are used, with the priority given to problem-focused interventions. A key strategy is the involvement of the client's support system.

Pigott & Trott (1993) studied 600 clients treated by PATH over a 2-year period. Their results supported the program's effectiveness. Need for hospitalization was averted for 81% of referred clients; PATH clients had 400% lower psychiatric rehospitalization rate than comparable non-PATH clients; and there was a 50% decrease in psychiatric inpatient days. Pigott & Trott suggest four factors are essential to the success of such a program: treating patients in the least restrictive environment; easily accessed care; flexible, multimodal treatment approaches; and presence of a strong client support system.

WINDHORSE

Windhorse Associates was developed in Boulder, Colorado in the 1970s by faculty and students of Naropa Institute; it has expanded to

Nova Scotia and Massachusetts (Fortuna, 1995). The objective is to treat psychologically disturbed adults in their home environments, using a treatment model that emphasizes the possibility of significant recovery (Podvoll, 1990). Viewing psychosis as a disruption in the balance of the body-mind-environment system, treatment strategies focus on using ordinary interests and activities of daily life to create balance. The program's core is the "therapeutic household" consisting of the client and live-in housemate(s). Housemates help the client to bring order into his/her life by establishing daily structure and routine. Other staff supplement the efforts of the housemate(s) by involving the client in other activities, such as sports or discussions of politics. The client is also involved in intensive psychotherapy. Team meetings include the client, his/her housemate(s), and sometimes family members. Stark (chapter 15, this volume) describes his experiences as a Windhorse client.

Fortuna (1995) describes a typical schedule for one Windhorse client, Jonah. Jonah was diagnosed as having chronic schizophrenia and had entered Windhorse following 3 years of little progress in a European residential treatment center:

8 A.M.: Awakened by housemate or alarm; Jonah tried to dress and to attend to hygiene.

9 A.M. to Noon: Team therapist helped Jonah with dressing and hygiene, if needed, and to tidy the bedroom; prepared breakfast, ate together, and cleaned up; took medication; reviewed daily checklist for morning routine; did preassigned house chores together; remained at home or engaged in an outside activity such as walking, shopping, or going to the library, a café, or a class; rode bus alone to IP (intensive psychotherapy) appointment.

12–12:50 P.M.: IP session.

1–1:30 P.M.: Rode bus or walked home alone.

1:30–3:30 P.M.: Attended language tutorial or session with acupuncture and massage therapist, or rested at home alone.

3:30–6:30 P.M. (less structured than morning shift): Engaged in an outside activity with team therapist; remained at home and conversed, read, or listened to music; prepared dinner, ate, and cleaned up together, with housemate; took medication.

Evening: Spent time with housemate or alone; went to bed after dinner or stayed up later (regular bedtime encouraged). (pp. 177–178)

DANA HOME CARE

Dana Home Care was founded in Boulder, Colorado in the 1970s to provide in-home assistance to frail, elderly people. It shared many of Windhorse's attitudes and strategies for working with people in their homes. Even while providing concrete personal care and housekeeping services, priority was given to creating a home environment and caregiver-client relationships that maximized clients' sense of well-being and self-esteem. Hiring procedures screened for staff who naturally conveyed these attitudes; orientation and training programs taught them how to express those attitudes through the practical tasks of caregiving (Newton & Brauer, 1989). As a result, elderly and even younger adult clients were often referred because psychological problems interfered with their ability to live independently or to accept home care.

Although philosophically similar to Windhorse, structurally Dana developed as a private pay, personal care services agency. By the early 1990s, it had a twenty year history of providing in-home services (personal care, light housekeeping, meals, errands, companionship) to adults and older adults with a variety of psychological and physical problems. Caregivers included certified nursing assistants and other paraprofessional level caregivers, graduate and undergraduates students in the social sciences, and artists. Care programs ranged from 4 hours once a week to 24 hours, 7 days a week. A team of three or four caregivers staffed programs involving extensive amounts of time. In the early 1990s, Dana staff developed HomePsych to provide managed care funded in-home support to psychiatric clients as an alternative to hospitalization or as a transition following hospitalization. Services included personal care and housekeeping as well as in-home treatment interventions designed to complement the work of the client's own mental health professionals. Newton and Brauer (chapter 11, this volume) and Barringer (chapter 12, this volume) provide case examples of HomePsych services and care models.

ADULT PSYCHIATRIC CLIENTS—ALTERNATIVE RESIDENTIAL PROGRAMS

A variety of supportive living arrangements have been developed for severely disturbed psychiatric patients that combine home-style living with built-in support. Models include living with a roommate who also serves as a designated provider and households in which several patients reside with a support person. While promising concepts, the availability of such programs is limited.

Adult foster care is a long-standing model for providing home-based care to chronic psychiatric patients (Deci & Mattix, 1997). Similar to child foster care, paid providers take one or two adult patients into their homes. These patients become members of the household. The trained foster care provider takes an active role in teaching independent living skills and managing medication regimes. Often, the efforts of the foster care provider is supplemented by "assisting neighbors" who involve clients in community activities or "companions" who assist consumers in planning and carrying out leisure activities.

The extent of adult foster care programs in the United States is unknown (Deci & Mattix, 1997) although a 1989 study identified 5,214 adults with psychiatric diagnoses in foster care. Research on its effectiveness is rare. Deci and Mattix (1997) report only one systematic research study—a 1977 study which evaluated the relationship between social functioning and foster-care home characteristics. In the 210 male veterans studied, social functioning increased after four months in homes that had only one or two clients, children present in the home, and a total of less than 10 people in the household.

It is estimated that 65% of adult psychiatric patients are discharged to their families and 35%–40% live with their families on an ongoing basis (Lefley, 1996). Often the decision to live with their families reflects economic necessity and lack of alternatives as much as choice. In view of the frequency with which adult clients reside with their families, the lack of attention in the literature to respite care and support for these families is striking. To the extent that programs do exist, they often emerge out of the grass-roots efforts of the families themselves and tend to base their interventions on competency-based models which emphasize helping families cope with the stress of living with someone with a disabling chronic illness (Falloon, Boyd, & McGill, 1984; Falloon & Fadden, 1992).

OLDER ADULTS—HOME HEALTH CARE

Although home health care in the United States traces its roots to the 1880s, introduction of Medicare funding in 1965 spawned the birth and development of the home health care industry as it exists today. By the end of 1996, there were over 20,000 home care agencies in the United States (National Association for Home Care, 1997). The Association estimates that 7.4 million people received home care services in 1997 at a cost of over $40 billion. In 1995, Medicare funded approximately 50% of home health care services. The other 50% was almost equally divided between Medicaid funding and out-of-pocket private payment. Private insurance only covered about 4% of the costs of home health care.

A variety of organizations provide home health care services. The majority are Medicare-certified home health care agencies. These agencies may be free standing or affiliated with hospitals, rehabilitation facilities, or skilled nursing facilities. Other organizations include Medicare-certified hospice programs and a variety of non-Medicare certified agencies, such as personal care agencies. Personal care agencies often provide services that are not eligible for Medicare funding, such as long-term care for clients with chronic illness. In contrast to Medicare funded agencies, these agencies experience little to no government regulation.

Consistent with Medicare guidelines, home health care agencies focus on delivering restorative medical care to acutely ill, homebound elderly. To qualify for Medicare coverage, care needs must be intermittent. Generally, services are initiated following hospital discharge in order to facilitate a transition to home or they may provide an alternative to hospitalization. Ongoing support for patients with chronic disorders, such as Alzheimer's disease or schizophrenia, is not covered. Patient care, agency, and program administration are generally under the direction of registered nurses. Registered nurses conduct assessments, develop and oversee care plans, implement medical interventions, carry out patient teaching and training activities, and coordinate and supervise patient care. Often, however, care involves a multidisciplinary team, including social workers, occupational therapists, physical therapists, and/or home health aides. Medicare also funds personal care, housekeeping, and meal preparation services provided by home health aides on a short-term basis and when identified in the care plan.

From its inception, the focus of the home care industry has been elderly patients with primary medical diagnoses. Only 29% of 4003 home health care agencies surveyed in 1983 indicated they had the capability to treat patients with psychiatric disorders (Harper, 1989). Recognition of the high frequency of psychiatric symptoms in the elderly and the likely occurrence of psychological symptoms secondary to physical illness, however, has sensitized home health care professionals to the importance of attending to psychiatric symptoms in their elderly patients (Harper, 1992). In a 1988 study, home health workers estimated that more than 50% of their elderly patients had behavioral and mental disorders (Harper, 1989). Commonly seen behaviors included "confusion or delirium; wandering, pacing, or restlessness; cognitive impairment; depression, sadness, self-depreciation; feelings of hopelessness; agitation or aggressiveness; alcohol abuse; hostility; behavioral or emotional problems associated with the presence of physical illness or drug–drug interactions or side effects; confusion following stroke, hip surgery, and falls; and lithium-induced diabetes" (Harper, 1992, p. 127).

Increasing interest in providing services to home-care clients with primary psychiatric diagnoses followed recognition of the need

(Kozlak & Thobaben, 1992; Richie & Lusky, 1987). Changes in Medicare funding and newly evolving opportunities for alliances with managed care organizations also contributed to greater enthusiasm in home health care agencies. Psychiatric patients, however, continue to be a minor part of the population they serve. In 1994, only 2.2% of patients who received home and hospice care had a primary mental diagnosis (National Association for Home Care, 1997).

Medicare maintains strict, although evolving, criteria for funding in-home psychiatric care. Interpretation and application of these criteria are at the discretion of the agency administering Medicare benefits for a particular state or geographical region. There is strong emphasis on documentation, diagnosis-driven care plans, and clear delineation of professional roles and responsibilities. To be covered by Medicare, psychiatric services must be provided by an agency that does not primarily care for clients with psychiatric problems. Agency staff must include a registered nurse with specialized psychiatric training and experience. The plan of care must be developed and reviewed by a physician (not necessarily a psychiatrist). The patient must have an Axis I, *Diagnostic and Statistical Manual of Mental Disorders* (DSM-IV; American Psychiatric Association, 1994) diagnosis and a care plan which describes the treatment goals and related services. Care plans often include interventions such as assessment of mental health status, monitoring treatment response, medication management, collection of lab specimens and monitoring of results, health-related education and support of the client and client's family, community referrals, and case management (Horton-Deutsch, Farran, Loukissa, & Fogg, 1997). To qualify for Medicare coverage, the client must be homebound, due to either physical limitations or refusal to leave the home secondary to psychiatric problems. Homebound status can be granted even if the client leaves his/her home for medical care or brief trips outside the home, but generally not if the client leaves home for more extensive services, such as to attend a partial hospitalization program.

A psychiatric nurse's care for a 74-year-old married woman experiencing severe symptoms of major depression illustrates this model (Proehl & Berila, 1997). The client's psychiatrist recommended home care when he ascertained that the client was not responding to outpatient therapy and refused electroconvulsive therapy. On her first visit, the nurse discovered a disheveled, sad, anxious, and exhausted woman who reported feelings of guilt, helplessness, and hopelessness. The client's husband reported that her current presentation was very uncharacteristic of his previously active and attractive wife. The nurse worked with the psychiatrist to adjust the client's medication. She initiated a behavioral plan which encouraged the client's husband to set limits on his wife's self-defeating behavior and to stop taking responsibility for things she needed to do.

> I also used supportive psychotherapy by allowing the client to vent feelings and thoughts, but set limits on how much I would listen to her negate and shame herself. The patient was initially so depressed that her thinking was often distorted. I gently helped her reframe unrealistic thoughts and reorient to reality. Medication and illness teaching for both the patient and her husband was important. Reinforcing the concept of depression as a treatable illness seemed to give this woman relief from her guilt and hopelessness. Helping the family understand the time frame in which antidepressant medications work also aided in building hope. . . . The client's recovery was dramatic over the 2.5 month period I worked with her. Her anxiety lessened with the help of new relaxation techniques and medication. This allowed her to focus on the behavioral plan with success and gave her the patience to stay on her antidepressant medicine. (Proehl & Berila, 1997, p. 165)

Horton-Deutsch et al. (1997) conducted a descriptive study of clients treated for depression by a home health care agency. They examined a sample of 107 adults over 65 with a primary or secondary diagnosis of depression. Medicare was the primary payor for their care. They ranged in age from 66 to 102, with a mean age of 79 years. Eighty-seven percent were female. An inpatient geropsychiatric unit was the largest referral source, referring 34% of the clients. Average length of care was 7.7 months. Cared tended to be multidisciplinary, including registered nurses, occupational therapists, social workers, and home health aides. Thirty-two percent of the clients were discharged because their treatment goals were met; 26% were hospitalized or entered nursing homes; 16% refused service; 9% died.

RESPITE CARE PROGRAMS

Respite care is "care provided on a short-term basis to a dependent person living in the community to relieve the primary caregiver of responsibility for the constant care of that person. Respite care is defined by the function it serves, as a substitute for an unpaid caregiver who may perform many caregiving tasks" (Abrahams, Bishop, & Hernandez, 1991). Although the disabled or impaired person is the direct recipient of the care, its objective is to relieve primary family caregivers either for periods of time or of tasks on an ongoing basis that are particularly demanding or onerous. The dependent person is generally someone who requires intense levels of personal care and attention over extended periods of time. He or she may be a physically frail or mentally impaired elderly person (Abrahams et al., 1991; Klein, 1987), a handicapped adult, or a developmentally disabled child (Stalker & Robinson, 1994).

The negative psychological and physical impact of long-term, intense caregiving is well documented (Lefley, 1996; Singer, 1996). By providing temporary relief for family caregivers, respite programs support caregivers' ability to provide ongoing primary care, maintain the identified client in the home, avoid hospitalization and institution-alization, and enhance their caregiving effectiveness. It gives full-time family caregivers the opportunity to engage in activities necessary for their own self-care and psychological and physical well-being (Oazwa, 1993). Care intensity ranges from a few hours daily, several days a week over a long period of time to intensive, 24-hour care on a short-term basis. Barringer (chapter 12, this volume) describes his experiences as a respite care worker for a child with SED.

Respite services are often one component of a continuum of community-based caregiver education and support services. Because respite care is defined by the function it serves, it may be provided within a variety of settings. Day care centers, nursing homes, institutional settings, and foster families also provide respite care. However, family members generally state preferences for in-home respite services (Abrahams et al., 1991). In-home care avoids the need to physically transport frail or bed-dependent clients; it minimizes demands on the care recipient to adjust to unfamiliar surroundings. Families who have made sacrifices to keep dependent family members out of institutions may resist respite care when it is provided in those same institutions (Starkey & Sarli, 1989). Different settings, however, may be important in order to meet different respite care needs (Brody, Saperstein, & Lawton, 1989).

The background, training, and supervision of people who provide respite care vary widely. Often, volunteers are used. A number of respite programs for caregivers of frail elderly have attempted care sharing models with disappointing results (Petchers, Biegel, & Snyder, 1991; Stone, 1986). Missouri had more success in their program in which respite care volunteers earned service credits for their volunteer hours (Oazwa, 1993). Service credits could be redeemed for respite care by the volunteers themselves or family members over age 60. Oazwa found, however, that, while attracting volunteers, few service credits were actually exchanged.

Despite the obvious value that respite care programs would seem to have for overburdened caregivers, these programs are not as widely available or, when available, as enthusiastically embraced by families as one would expect (Brody et al., 1989; Starkey & Sarli, 1989). This lack of enthusiasm reflects a number of issues. The design and development of respite care programs may not be in line with family needs. Families may be discouraged by the hassle of arranging service and orienting workers. If services fail to meet their exact needs, having respite may seem more cumbersome than doing without. While caregivers may prefer the convenience of in-home respite, concerns about loss of privacy and trusting an unknown worker often discourage them from actually using services. Needed auxiliary services, such as transportation, may not be included, making services impractical to use. Family members sometimes expect that they should be able to handle caregiving on their own, have difficulty trusting someone else to give sensitive care, or fear criticism or interference from respite workers. Thus, although respite care programs seem like a good idea, families often decide to go without or make their own informal arrangements for caregiving breaks.

CONCLUSIONS

In recent decades, mental health professionals have been visiting their clients' home for a variety of reasons: to serve people who are unlikely or unwilling to seek out and maintain regular contact with providers in more traditional settings, to provide cost-effective alternatives to inpatient care, and to institute comprehensive, integrated treatment approaches for clients with multidimensional needs. Vulnerable and frail populations, generally with severe psychiatric symptoms, multiple needs, and few resources are most likely to be the focus of home-based services.

The literature describes both sophisticated care models, such as the Program for Assertive Community Treatment, family preservation services, and wraparound models for children with SED, that have been developed and refined over several decades. It hints at the variety of small-scale, innovative programs that have been tried. These include models for acutely disturbed clients (such as crisis homes) and small-scale programs that serve families managing a particular problem, such as a child with autism. Currently, they include a variety of innovative programs such as PATH, YICAPS (Yale Intensive In-home Child & Adolescent Psychiatry Services), and Mentor Community Care designed to appeal to behavioral managed health care organizations. The literature describing in-home treatment programs over the last two decades suggests that these programs have often been enthusiastically instituted and then disappeared as funding, vision, and staff interest waned. They may grow out of a particular professional need or interest; they also find their roots in grass-roots efforts.

Whatever the population or the specific nature of their distress, clinical observation and empirical research supports the potential effectiveness of home-based services. With appropriate interventions of sufficient intensity, individual clients and families in crisis can often be stabilized in their own homes without requiring hospitalization or institutional placement. When out-of-home treatment is unavoidable, brief-stay crisis homes and longer-term therapeutic foster homes are innovative alternatives to hospitalization. Research studies have also consistently shown that clients—whether they are individuals or families—who face the multiple problems of poverty, few social supports, severe psychiatric disturbance, social stigma and prejudice, and limited access to employment, housing, and other resources often need ongoing support to sustain crisis-free living. For the most vulnerable clients, intense, short-term, home-based programs have no greater long-term effects than short-term hospitalization.

Despite their variety, commonalities do emerge that differentiate these programs from psychiatric models developed based on clinic-, office-, or hospital-based practice. Moy and Pigott (1997) suggest several of these commonalities:

- They work with clients in their natural environments, thus reducing barriers to access and engaging clients and their families who might not otherwise pursue psychiatric treatment.
- Programs tend to be goal-oriented, often incorporating intensive crisis-intervention models into treatment.
- They incorporate a significant amount of case management services, including coordination between mental health providers and services, concrete services (i.e., transportation, housing, financial management), client advocacy, resource networking, and vocational assistance.

In contrast to clinic and inpatient mental health models, which are often under the direction and supervision of doctoral level professionals, M.A. level social workers (and more recently in the home health arena, registered nurses) are likely to have conceptualized the program, developed and monitored the treatment plan, and provided supervision and training. There is a heavy reliance on paraprofessionals with, at most, college degrees to deliver services. Doctoral level mental health professionals—whether PhDs or MDs—if included at all are more likely to be behind-the-scene clinical supervisors and program planners.

Over time, clinicians who work in the homes of their clients tend to express certain similarities in their orientation toward treatment that differentiates them from their office- and hospital-based peers. Whatever their attitude before first knocking on a client's door, it seems predictable that over time, these clinicians become more focused on clients' strengths as a basis for treatment planning. They are more likely to view clients from a holistic perspective that includes not only their immediate family but also their physical environment and broader community and the economic, political, social realities of their lives. Without minimizing the importance of therapeutic relationships that emerge in the home setting, they become more inclined to also incorporate concrete, pragmatic interventions into the treatment plan.

One of the concerns raised by mental health professionals more accustomed to outpatient practice and to the hospital as the only safe and secure environment for very troubled people is the extent to which home-based programs can serve very severely disturbed clients. Research suggests that these clients can be treated at home. In the early research on community-based services with chronic psychiatric clients, clients were often randomly assigned to either intensive community services or inpatient treatment when they sought hospital admission. In their comparison of children receiving partial hospitalization, outpatient, and home-based services, Dore, Wilkinson, and Sonis (1992) found that children in home-based treatment were more likely to have experienced abuse and neglect and to have parents with psychiatric or substance abuse histories. They were as likely as children in partial hospitalization programs to have made suicide threats or gestures and were viewed as more dysfunctional in activities of daily living. Home-based family therapy programs have been found to be an effective alternative for juvenile delinquents who might otherwise be incarcerated (Santos, Henggeler, Burns, Arana, & Meisler, 1995).

In his review of innovative community-based programs, such as Windhorse and Crisis Homes, that serve very disturbed adults in acute crisis, Warner (1995) directly addresses safety concerns. He noted that these programs accept clients who are uncooperative or who manifest "agitation and disruptiveness, threatening behavior, or imminent risk of violence or self-harm" (p. 237). To adequately treat this population, they have developed strategies for quickly defusing potentially volatile behavior and ensuring the safety of everyone. One of their observations is that an understated, low-key response that does not draw attention to the behavior and increase the drama is often very effective. When initiated in a timely manner and without aggression, strategies, such as accompanying a client for a walk or sitting and talking, defuse tension while avoiding the power struggles that often escalate the problem. A noninstitutional environment makes this type of response much more likely and workable.

Despite their promise, integration of home-based services into mainstream mental health services is only beginning. Many areas of the country do not provide adequate community-based care and obstacles to its implementation are difficult to overcome. The effectiveness of in-home services challenges many long-cherished assumptions about psychiatric treatment. As Santos et al. (1995) suggest, "a powerful inertia of clinicians wedded to hospital- and office-based practice, coupled with the fee-for-service financing that rewards such practice, has maintained the status quo in the mental health service delivery system" (p. 1121). For home-based programs to develop, they must "co-opt and surmount the inevitable opposition to the restructuring of the existing prevailing systems of inpatient and outpatient treatment that is necessary for financing large-scale development of new program models" (p. 1121). It involves changing attitudes at all levels of the multiple funding sources that underwrite mental health care. Equally important will be reaching the point where education of mental health professionals routinely introduces them to the home as a legitimate location for providing mental health services and prepares them for the unique aspects of working with clients in their homes. Clients and clinicians alike have been socialized to expect the hospital as a safe haven in times of crisis, whether or not hospitalization is the most effective intervention. They have assumed that motivation and ability to get to the clinician's office is a basic criterion for getting help. The programs described in this chapter fundamentally challenge these and many other assumptions about mental health treatment.

REFERENCES

Abrahams, R., Bishop, C., & Hernandez, W. (1991). Respite service delivery: Learning from current programs. *Pride Institute Journal of Long Term Home Health Care, 10,* 16–28.

Allness, D., & Knoedler, W. (1998). *The PACT model of community-based treatment for persons with severe and persistent mental illness: A manual for PACT start-up.* Arlington, VA: NAMI Campaign to End Discrimination.

American Psychiatric Association. (1994). *Diagnostic and statistical manual of mental disorders* (4th ed.). Washington, DC: American Psychiatric Press.

Behar, L. (1986). A state model for child mental health services: The North Carolina experience. *Children Today, 15,* 16–21.

Bennett, R. (1995). The crisis home program of Dane County. In R. Warner (Ed.), *Alternatives to the hospital for acute psychiatric treatment* (pp. 227–236). Washington, DC: American Psychiatric Press.

Brody, E. M., Saperstein, A. R., & Lawton, M. P. 1989. A multi-service respite program for caregivers of Alzheimer's patients. *Journal of Gerontological Social Work, 14,* 41–74.

Burchard, J. D. (1996). Evaluation of the Fort Bragg Managed Care Experiment. *Journal of Child and Family Studies, 5,* 173–176.

Butts, J. A., & Barton, W. H. (1995). In-home programs for juvenile delinquents. In I. M. Schwartz & P. AuClaire (Eds.), *Home-based services for troubled children* (pp. 131–155). Lincoln: University of Nebraska Press.

Clark, H. B., Lee, B., Prange, M. F., & McDonald, B. A. (1996). Children lost within the foster care system: Can wraparound service strategies improve placement outcomes? *Journal of Child and Family Studies, 5,* 39–54.

Deci, P. A., & Mattix, G. N. (1997). Adult foster care: The forgotten alternative. In S. W. Henggeler & A. B. Santos (Eds.), *Innovative approaches to difficult-to-treat populations* (pp. 253–362). Washington, DC: American Psychiatric Press.

Dore, M. M., Wilkinson, A. N., & Sonis, W. A. (1992). Exploring the relationship between a continuum of care and intrusiveness of children's mental health services. *Hospital and Community Psychiatry, 43,* 44–48.

Eckstein, M. A. (1995). Foster family clusters: Continuum advocate home network. In L. Combrinck-Graham (Ed.), *Children in families at risk: Maintaining the connections* (pp. 275–298). New York: Guilford.

Evans, M. E., Armstrong, M. I., Dollard, N., Kuppinger, A. D., Huz, S., & Wood, V. (1994). Development and evaluation of treatment foster care and family-centered intensive case management in New York. *Journal of Emotional and Behavioral Disorders, 2,* 228–239.

Falloon, I. R. H., Boyd, J. L., & McGill, C. W. (1984). *Family care of schizophrenia.* New York: Guilford.

Falloon, I. R. H., & Fadden, G. (1992). *Integrated mental health care.* Cambridge: Cambridge University Press.

Fenton, F. R., Tessier, L., Struening, E. L., Smith, F. A., & Benoit, C. (1982). *Home and hospital psychiatric treatment.* Pittsburgh, PA: University of Pittsburgh Press.

Fortuna, J. (1995). The Windhorse Program for Recovery. In R. Warner (Ed.), *Alternatives to the hospital for acute psychiatric treatment* (pp. 171–192). Washington, DC: American Psychiatric Press.

Government Accounting Office (1990). *Home visiting: A promising early intervention strategy for at-risk families.* (GAO/HRD-90-83). Washington, DC: Author.

Government Accounting Office. (1992). *Child abuse: Prevention programs need greater emphasis.* (GAO/HRD-92-99). Washington, DC: Author.

Halpern, R. (1984). Lack of effects for home-based early intervention? Some possible explanations. *American Journal of Orthopsychiatry, 54,* 33–42.

Harper, M. S. (1989). Behavioral, social and mental health aspects of home care for older Americans. *Home Health Care Services Quarterly, 9,* 61–124.

Harper, M. S. (1992). Home- and community-based mental health services for the elderly. In K. C. Buckwalter (Ed.), *Geriatric mental health nursing: Current and future challenges* (pp. 122–136). Thorofare, NJ: Slack.

Hawaii Department of Health. (1992). *Healthy start.* Honolulu, HI: Department of Health, Maternal and Child Health Branch.

Henggeler, S. W., & Borduin, C. M. (1990). *Family therapy and beyond: A multisystemic approach to treating the behavior problems of children and adolescents.* Pacific Grove, CA: Brooks/Cole.

Henggeler, S. W., Schoenwald, S. K., Pickrel, C. S., Brondun, M. J., Borduin, C. M., & Hall, J. A. (1994). *Treatment manual for family preservation using multisystemic therapy.* Columbia, SC: Health and Human Service Finance Commission.

Horton-Deutsch, S. L., Farran, C. J., Loukissa, D., & Fogg, L. (1997). Who are these patients and what services do they receive? *Home Healthcare Nurse, 15,* 847–854.

Huff, R. (1996). Community-based early intervention for children with autism. In C. Maurice, G. Green, & S. C. Luce (Eds.), *Behavioral intervention for young children with autism: A manual for parents and professionals* (pp. 211–266). Austin, TX: Pro-Ed.

Joint Commission on Mental Health for Children. (1970). *Crisis in child mental health: Challenge of the 1970s.* New York: Harper & Row.

Kiesler, C. A. (1982). Mental hospitals and alternative care: Noninstitutionalization as potential public policy for mental patients. *American Psychologist, 37,* 349–360.

Kinney, J., Haapala, D., Booth, C., & Leavitt, S. (1990). The homebuilders model. In J. K. Whittaker, J. Kinney, E. M. Tracy, & C. Booth (Eds.), *Reaching high-risk families: Intensive family preservation in human services* (pp. 31–64). New York: Aldine de Gruyter.

Klein, S. M. (Ed). (1987). *In-home respite care for older adults: A practical guide for program planners, administrators, and clinicians.* Springfield, IL: Charles C. Thomas.

Kozlak, J., & Thobaben, M. (1992). Treating the elderly mentally ill at home. *Perspectives in Psychiatric Care, 28,* 31–35.

Lachance, K. R., Deci, P. A., Santos, A. B., Halewood, N. M., & Westfall, J. M. (1997). Rural assertive community treatment: Taking mental health services on the road. In S. W. Henggeler & A. B. Santos (Eds.), *Innovative approaches to difficult-to-treat populations* (pp. 239–252). Washington, DC: American Psychiatric Press.

Lefley, H. P. (1996). *Family caregiving in mental illness.* Thousand Oaks, CA: Sage.

Lesseig, D. Z. (1987, October). Home care of psych problems. *American Journal of Nursing,* pp. 1317–1326.

Lewis, R. E. (1991). What are the characteristics of intensive family preservation services? In M. W. Fraser, P. J. Pecora, & D. A. Haapala (Eds.), *Families in crisis: The impact of intensive family preservation services* (pp. 93–108). New York: Aldine De Gruyter.

Mandiberg. J. (1995). Can interdependent mutual support function as an alternative to hospitalization? The Santa Clara County Clustered Apartment Project. In R. Warner (Ed.), *Alternatives to the hospital for acute psychiatric treatment* (pp. 193–212). Washington, DC: American Psychiatric Press.

McCurdy, K. (1995). *Home visiting.* (Working Paper Number 866). Chicago: National Committee to Prevent Child Abuse.

McKenzie, J., Mikkelsen, E. J., Stelk, W., Bereika, G., & Monack, D. (1995). The role of a home-based mentor program in the psychiatric continuum of care for children and adolescents. In L. Combrinck-Graham (Ed.), *Children in families at risk: Maintaining the connections* (pp. 209–227). New York: Guilford.

Meisler, N., & Santos, A. B. (1997). From the hospital to the community: The great American paradigm shift. In S. W. Henggeler & A. B. Santos (Eds.), *Innovative approaches to difficult-to-treat populations* (pp. 167–238). Washington, DC: American Psychiatric Press.

Miller, L. S. (1994). Primary prevention of conduct disorder. *Psychiatric Quarterly, 65,* 273–285.

Minuchin, P. (1995). Foster and natural families: Forming a cooperative network. In L. Combrinck-Graham (Ed.), *Children in families at risk: Maintaining the connections* (pp. 251–274). New York: Guilford.

Morris, M. (1996). Patients' perceptions of psychiatric home care. *Archives of Psychiatric Nursing, 10,* 176–183.

Moy, S., & Pigott, H. E. (1997). Home-based services. In R. K. Schreter, S. S. Sharfstein, & C. A. Schreter (Eds.), *Managing care, not dollars* (pp. 27–41). Washington, DC: American Psychiatric Press.

National Association of Home Care. (1997). *Basic statistics about home care* 1997 [on-line]. Available: http://www.nahc.org/consumer/hcstats.html

Newton, N. A., & Brauer, W. F. (1989, June). In-home mental health services. *Caring,* pp. 16–19.

Oazwa, M. N. (1993). Missouri service credit system for respite care: An exploratory study. *Journal of Gerontological Social Work, 21,* 147–160.

Pasamanick, B., Scarpitti, F. B., & Dinitz, S. (1967). *Schizophrenics and the community.* New York: Appleton-Century-Crofts.

Pecora, P. J. (1991). Family-based and intensive family preservation services: A select literature review. In M. W. Fraser, P. J. Pecora, & D. A. Haapala (Eds.), *Families in crisis: The impact of intensive family preservation services* (pp. 17–47). New York: Aldine De Gruyter.

Pecora, P. J., Fraser, M. W., & Haapala, D. A. (1989). Intensive home-based family treatment: client outcomes and issues for program design. In J. Hudson & B. Galaway (Eds.), *The state as parent: International research perspectives on interventions with young persons* (pp. 331–345). Boston: Kluwer.

Petchers, M. K., Biegel, D. E., & Snyder, A. (1991). Barriers to implementation of a cooperative model of respite care. *Journal of Gerontological Social Work, 16,* 17–31.

Pigott, H. E., & Trott, L. T. (1993). Curbing behavioral health costs while enhancing the quality of patient care: The implementation of a crisis intervention, triage and treatment service in the private sector. *American Journal of Medical Quality, 8,* 138–144.

Podvoll, E. (1990). *The seduction of madness.* New York: HarperCollins.

Polak, P. B., Kirby, M. W., & Deitchman, W. S. (1995). Treating acutely psychotic patients in private homes. In R. Warner (Ed.), *Alternatives to the hospital for acute psychiatric treatment* (pp. 213–226). Washington, DC: American Psychiatric Press.

Proehl, K. J., & Berila, R. A. (1997). Psychiatric home care nursing in the United States. In D. Modly, R. Zanotti, P. Poletti, & J. J. Fitzpatrick (Eds.), *Home care nursing services: International lessons* (pp. 157–168). New York: Springer Publishing Co.

Richie, F. & Lusky, K. (1987). Psychiatric home health nursing: A new role in community mental health. *Community Mental Health Journal, 23,* 229–236.

Roberts, R., & Wasik, B. (1990). Home visiting programs for families with children birth to three: Results of a national survey. *Journal of Early Intervention, 14,* 274–284.

Rosenfeld, A., Altman, R., & Kaufman, I. (1997). Foster care. In R. K. Schreter, S. S. Sharfstein, & C. A. Schreter (Eds.), *Managing care, not dollars* (pp. 125–137). Washington, DC: American Psychiatric Press.

Santos, A. B., Henggeler, S. W., Burns, B. J., Arana, G. W., & Meisler, N. (1995). Research on field-based services: Models for reform in the delivery of mental health care to populations with complex clinical problems. *American Journal of Psychiatry, 152,* 1111–1123.

Schreter, R. K., Sharfstein, S. S., & Schreter, C. A. (1997). *Managing care, not dollars: The continuum of mental health services.* Washington DC: American Psychiatric Press.

Singer, G. H. S. (1996). Introduction: Trends affecting home and community care for people with chronic conditions in the United States. In G. H. S. Singer, L. E. Powers, & A. L. Olson (Eds), *Redefining family support: Innovations in public-private partnerships.* Baltimore, MD: Paul H. Brooks.

Spaid, W. M., Lewis, R. E., & Pecora, P. J. (1991). Factors associated with success and failure in family-based and intensive family preservation services. In M. W. Fraser, P. J. Pecora, & D.A. Haapala (Eds.), *Families in crisis: The impact of intensive family preservation services* (pp. 49–58). New York: Aldine De Gruyter.

Stalker, K., & Robinson, C. (1994). Parents' views of different respite care services. *Mental Handicap Research, 7,* 97–117.

Starkey, J., & Sarli, P. (1989). Respite and family support services: Responding to the need. *Child and Adolescent Social Work, 6,* 313–326.

Stone, R. (1986). *Recent developments in respite care services for caregivers of the impaired elderly.* Reported funded by AoA Grant #90-AP003.

Stroul, B. A., & Friedman, R. M. (1986). *A system of care for severely emotionally disturbed children and youth.* Washington, DC: Children and Adolescent Service System Program Technical Assistance Center.

VanDenBerg, J. E., & Grealish, E. M. (1996). Individualized services and supports through the wraparound process: Philosophy and procedures. *Journal of Child and Family Studies, 5,* 7–21.

Watkins, S., Clark, T., Strong, C., & Barringer, D. (1994). The effectiveness of an intervener model of services for young deaf-blind children. *American Annals of the Deaf, 139,* 404–409.

Warner, R. (Ed.). (1995). *Alternatives to the hospital for acute psychiatric treatment.* Washington, DC: American Psychiatric Press.

Wells, K. (1995). Family preservation services in context: Origins, practices, and current issues. In I. M. Schwartz & P. AuClaire (Eds.), *Home-based services for troubled children* (pp. 1–28). Lincoln: University of Nebraska Press.

Woolston, J. L., Berkowitz, S. J., Schaefer, M.C., & Adnopoz, J. A. (1998). Intensive, integrated, in-home psychiatric services. *Child and Adolescent Psychiatric Clinics of North America, 7,* 615–633.

CHAPTER TWO

Issues in In-Home Psychosocial Care

Nancy A. Newton

As clinicians move into the home setting, their theoretical perspectives shift toward a more holistic, functional, and strength-based perspective. Nancy Newton reviews and contrasts the major theoretical approaches used by home-based clinicians. The medical model of treatment contrasts with other systems or ecologically focused models. All shifted when brought into the home. This shift becomes clearer given the new relationship that develops between client and therapist when therapy is on the client's home ground. Moving from theory to pragmatics, Dr. Newton then discusses the funding and staffing issues faced by home-based clinicians.

The physical environment in which mental health treatment occurs has profound implications for the nature of that treatment. Researchers in the 1960s and 1970s observed that much of the pathological behavior of long-institutionalized psychiatric clients reflected adaptation to the particular demands and constraints of living in an environment where there is little privacy, a clearly defined hierarchy, little opportunity for healthy, creative expression, and an emphasis on following set policies and procedures (Goffman, 1961; Goldstein, 1979). Confined to a social world peopled by others struggling with severe disturbance and psychiatric experts who focus on their dysfunction, and managing daily life filled with dehumanizing rituals, pathological behavior can be seen as attempts at adaptive coping. Indeed, research demonstrated that significantly modifying interpersonal and physical aspects of that environment led to remarkable changes in patients' behavior, attitudes, and social skills. As a result, inpatient units developed interventions that maximized the therapeutic benefits of the interpersonal and physical characteristics of their environment. The fact that clients are gathered together, staff control the unit, and certain resources are readily available—all are the basis of interventions such as group therapy, recreation and art therapy, and the roles and responsibilities assigned to various types of mental health staff.

Similarly, clinicians working in their private offices have extensively explored the implications of that setting for psychotherapy. The clearly defined and limited time in which the client and therapist interact, a high degree of privacy, and lack of direct observation of either participant's life—these are all situational variables directly incorporated into current models of outpatient psychotherapy.

Transfer of the practice of mental health professionals into their clients' homes prompts consideration of that environment as a "therapeutic milieu." The home environment presents its own unique challenges. There, both the therapist and client are in the midst of the client's naturally occurring support system (or lack thereof). Inevitably, the client and therapist both know much more about each other through direct observation, and much of that information is of a more informal nature than either obtains in the professional office. Therapists can evaluate client self-reports based on their own observations. They can directly observe their clients' willingness and ability to implement treatment interventions and the real-world obstacles that hamper their effectiveness. Clients observe their therapists' ability to negotiate their world and the land mines within it. It is on their "home turf" that therapists must earn credibility and trust.

Despite these differences from treatment in other settings, home-based programs face the same core issues as do all mental health treatment programs. They require:

- a treatment philosophy that guides understanding of the client, formulation of treatment goals and strategies, and evaluation of treatment effectiveness;
- funding;
- staffing models that provide necessary levels of expertise within inevitable financial constraints.

The home, however, provides a unique setting for addressing these issues. Potential resources to be incorporated into treatment strategies and obstacles that hinder their effectiveness are very different from the clinician's office. Because of the populations they typically serve and the attitudes of mainstream mental health professionals, home-based programs have had to seek funding outside of the private insurance, fee-for-service domain that fund most mental health services. Staffing patterns developed for clinics and hospitals are prohibitively expensive when travel time to and from the client's home is incorporated. Thus, although the issues are familiar, the solutions often require innovation and creativity. Drawing from the literature across the wide spectrum of programs described in chapter 1, this chapter describes the ways in which in-home services address treatment philosophy, funding, and staffing issues.

THEORETICAL MODELS

Theories define the conceptual lenses through which the clinician and client view their work. At their most fundamental level, theoretical models define sanity and insanity; they illuminate strategies for cultivating sanity. Theory provides a way to simplify the complexity of human experience so that it can be understood and worked with in a meaningful way. It draws attention to particular aspects of the client's presentation and experience; it minimizes other aspects. It provides a framework within which observations of the client will be understood and given meaning. Theories provide logic for treatment goals, interventions, and evaluation strategies. Embedded within psychological theories and treatment models are personal and cultural values about mental health and its cultivation, attitudes toward people who are experiencing significant distress, and the role and status of the person providing assistance.

Although the programs described in the preceding chapter varied in many ways, three themes emerged that seem to generally characterize the nature of home-based treatment. First, whatever their original theoretical orientation, the perspectives of staff who work with clients in their homes tend to shift toward a more holistic model. The larger context within which the client's behavior occurs is immediately observable and the importance of that context becomes obvious. Home-based staff cannot help but gain direct information about many aspects of their clients' lives. Inevitably, they seek to incorporate this information in formulating their understanding of their clients' problems and potential solutions. Second, staff tends to shift toward treatment strategies that are based on their clients' strengths. When relating to their natural environment, clients often demonstrate coping strategies and interests they would never spontaneously reveal in the foreign domain of the mental health professional. When observed within the context in which it developed, even problematic behavior can more readily be seen as an effort to cope with often demoralizing circumstances. The drive toward adaptation that fueled it and the strengths inherent within it often become visible. Third, home-based treatment tends to include more pragmatic interventions than does office- or hospital-based therapy. Often staff are addressing the needs of very vulnerable clients with few resources who are negotiating a complex world; meeting concrete needs for housing, employment, food, or transportation is crucial to their emotional well-being. Even when addressing quality-of-life, self-esteem, and other psychological issues, treatment plans often involve practical assistance and attend to daily activities. As a result, home-based treatment draws attention to the ways in which ordinary activities or relationships with ordinary people can be psychologically healing.

It follows that theoretical models that are holistic, address problems by focusing on client strengths, and provide a bridge between the client's psychological issues and actual daily life experiences will be most useful in conceptualizing home-based mental health treatment. This focus, however, generally runs counter to mainstream psychological theory and research over the last number of decades. As immediately evident in the *Diagnostic and Statistical Manual of Mental Disorders* (DSM-IV) (American Psychiatric Association, 1994), clinicians typically focus on delineation of pathology as the crucial determinant for diagnosis and treatment of psychiatric disorders. Whether relying on a medical model that emphasizes the physiological underpinnings of psychiatric disorders or psychodynamic models that focus on analysis of the client's inner world, the practitioner is encouraged to understand clients separate from (rather than embedded within) their social–cultural environment (Woods, 1988). The resulting treatment interventions inevitably focus on bringing about internal changes in clients so that they can deal more effectively with the pragmatic realities of their worlds, rather than directly partnering with the client to address those pragmatic realities.

In the absence of theoretical models developed out of home-based clinical work, mental health professionals who, for a variety of reasons, have been drawn into their clients' homes have applied familiar theories to their work in this new setting. These theories direct the attention of the clinician to a different dimension of the home as a treatment environment. In home health care that is based on the medical model, the focus is on the identified client as the recipient of treatment; interventions are generally directed at the individual client, focusing on the biological or psychological roots of his/her problems (Duffey, Miller, & Parlocha, 1993). In contrast, some home-based treatment programs work primarily with the client and his/her immediate support system, using a family-systems model (Archacki-Stone, 1995; Fraser, 1995; Henggeler & Borduin, 1990; Lindblad-Goldberg, Dore, & Stern, 1998). Others also pay attention to the resources and challenges present within the client's community (Aponte, Zarski, Bixenstine, & Cibik, 1991).

Often, clinicians draw on multiple theories. Interventions in the Yale Intensive Child and Adolescent Psychiatry Services program "are informed by a synthesis of the medical model, developmental psychopathology, systems theory, and wraparound concepts" (Woolston, Berkowitz, Schaefer, & Adnopoz, 1998, p. 619). Family-preservation services draw on four major models: crisis intervention, family systems, social learning, and ecological theories (Barth, 1988; Maluccio, 1988). Family therapists working in the home have often expanded their thinking to include "systems" beyond the immediate family, such as neighbors, schools, and friends (Henggeler et al., 1994). The following sections briefly review the theoretical models most often used to conceptualize in-home psychosocial interventions.

Crisis Intervention Theory

A crisis is a situation in which there is an imbalance between the difficulties the individual faces and the resources he or she has available for coping with it. The result is psychological disequilibrium. In-home services are often initiated as a result of significant crisis, either within an individual or family system. Vulnerable people—whether that vulnerability is the result of age (either very young or old), lack of financial/social resources, or psychological problems—are also more prone to crisis. It is not surprising then that crisis theory has played a significant role in conceptualizing home-based treatment. Nursing models of crisis intervention theory are incorporated in psychiatric home health care assessment and intervention strategies (Duffey et al., 1993). Homebuilders, a prototypical model for intervening with multiproblem families, builds on the assumption that a family in crisis is more amenable to change (Barth, 1988). With the family system in a crisis-related state of instability, family members are assumed to be less likely to deny problems and more willing to confront even long-standing dysfunctional interaction patterns within the family system. Homebuilders' staff takes advantage of this window of opportunity by implementing clinical and practical interventions designed to restabilize the family with more functional patterns and relationships.

Barth (1988) points out the limitations of crisis theory as a model for in-home interventions. By drawing attention to situational factors and precipitating events, crisis theory minimizes the importance of long-standing psychological issues and interpersonal dynamics. Problems in these families are often entrenched even though a particular situation drew attention to them. The assumption that crisis reactions are time-limited and thus interventions also should be time-limited has often proven to be unrealistic. For very vulnerable people and families with long-standing psychological problems, dysfunctional family relationship patterns, and limited external resources, services for an extended period of time may be essential to long-term stabilization. The hypothesis that families are most amenable to intervention when in crisis also may be overly simplistic. Too much stress may overwhelm clients' ability to process and learn from their experience, just as too little stress may fail to motivate change.

FAMILY SYSTEMS

Family systems models extend the focus beyond the individual to the significant people in the client's life. Pathology is understood and addressed within the context of immediate family/interpersonal dynamics. Interventions are directed at changing engrained, dysfunctional family patterns that reflect and contribute to psychological symptoms within individual family members. Woods (1988) identifies a number of reasons why the home can be an ideal setting for family therapy:

1. It makes therapy more accessible and thus likely to be used by families whose economic disadvantages make it difficult to come to the therapist's office.

2. The therapist is more likely to capture all relevant members of the family system—including people such as romantic friends and close neighbors who may spend a lot of time in the home and significantly impact the family system but who would not necessarily be identified or invited to office-based family therapy sessions. Working in the home also makes it more feasible to include young children.

3. Rich and valuable information is spontaneously and immediately available. The physical environment sheds light on family customs, myths, and rituals; discrepancies between client reports and their realities may be immediately evident; family interaction patterns naturally arise in their full force and manifestation. Particularly when the therapist differs from the client in cultural, ethnic, racial, or socioeconomic background, seeing the family in its natural environment can correct therapists' biases and misperceptions and challenge the personal values and attitudes that guide their decisions.

4. The therapist can teach and model more appropriate behaviors and interaction patterns as they naturally arise, increasing the likelihood that interventions will make a difference. Observing therapists develop and modify interventions in "real time" to address the realities of their lives can immediate enhance therapists' salience and credibility.

Intensive family preservation services and in-home services for children and adolescents with severe emotional disturbance frequently include family therapy. These families are often characterized by high rates of conflict, low levels of affection, inconsistent discipline strategies, poor communication patterns, limited problem-solving skills, and ineffectual family structure. It is not surprising then that a variety of models of family therapy have been incorporated into, or are the basis of, these programs. The most frequently used model is Structural Family Therapy (Minuchin, 1974). Fraser (1995) and Archacki-Stone (1995) describe and illustrate the use of in-home structural family therapy for children with severe emotional disturbance. Family therapists are also discovering that working in clients' homes requires modification in their models and treatment strategies. It can be easy to become too personally involved in the family dynamics that one is there to change (Lindblad-Goldberg et al., 1998; Zarski, Sand-Pringle, Greenback, & Cibik, 1991). To address these issues, Zarski et al. (1991) have developed a model for supervising in-home family therapy that incorporates supervisor home visits into the treatment process.

Multisystemic therapy is an approach that has had success with a variety of very difficult to treat adolescent populations, including adolescents with serious antisocial behavior, adolescent sexual offenders, and adolescents in abusive and/or neglecting families (Henggeler & Borduin, 1990; Henggeler et al., 1994; Santos et al., 1995). In multisystemic therapy, family members are viewed as full collaborators, sharing responsibility with the therapist and treatment team for engagement and outcome. In contrast to many other family therapy models, it has a strongly ecological orientation, with focus on enhancing communication and cooperation among families, schools, and community agencies.

BEHAVIOR THEORY

Behavior theory describes basic principles that explain under what conditions behavior increases or decreases in frequency and intensity. Most relevant to home-based interventions is B. F. Skinner's (1974) work on operant conditioning. "Operants" refer to voluntary behaviors that are the target of interventions designed to either increase or decrease their frequency. Operants can be increased in frequency if their occurrence is followed by consequences that the individual finds desirable or reinforcing. The same operants or voluntary behaviors decrease in frequency if followed by removal of desirable consequences or initiation of punishing consequences. Using these principles, behavior therapists design interventions that strive to increase the frequency of desired behavior by following that behavior with consequences that the individual finds reinforcing. For example, behavior management programs are often implemented to help parents change their children's behavior. Working with parents in their homes to develop these programs allows the clinician to be more fully cognizant of the subtle reinforcers that sometimes maintain problematic behavior, to identify the most effective ways of reinforcing the replacement behavior, and to set up realistic regimens for changing behavior. It maximizes the likelihood that clinicians develop a useful and realistic behavior management program and that the parents understand it, are committed to it, and will implement it accurately.

Pinkston and Linsk (1984) exemplify in-home behavior therapy programs. They trained family caregivers of elderly people with dementia, disabling depression, or other psychiatric symptoms to use operant techniques. Caregivers identified specific behaviors in their family members that they wanted to increase or decrease in frequency. Targeted behaviors included urinary incontinence, bizarre verbal behavior, and self-care deficits. Pinkston and Linsk taught the family caregivers to operationally define and quantify the frequency of the targeted behaviors, to choose reinforcements that would be effective with the client, and to implement reward systems designed to increase the frequency of incompatible, adaptive behaviors while ignoring undesirable behaviors. Based on analysis of their data, Pinkston and Linsk found that 78% of the behaviors chosen for intervention improved. Mental status scores improved approximately 15% between pre- and postassessment. Both clients and caregivers reported general improvement, with the greatest impact on increased frequency of home activities and independent abilities.

SOCIAL LEARNING THEORY

Albert Bandura (1977) expanded on Skinner's concepts of how people learn. He suggested that people also learn through observing and then imitating the behavior of others. For this process to be effective, learners must be motivated to change their behavior, observe and accurately perceive the desired behavior as it is performed by a model, remember the behavior, possess the skills to execute it, and observe that the behavior is rewarded. Parent training programs sometimes include in-home interventions to increase the likelihood that what parents have learned will be applied in their real lives. In-home sessions enable staff to individualize the training and model its use in real situations. An example is the primary prevention intervention program designed for families of preschool-aged children at high risk for developing conduct disorder (Miller, 1994). The year-long program includes parent training and support groups, children's play groups in which "incidental teaching" is used to build social skills and discourage disruptive behavior, parent–child interaction training, and a program that encourages reading together between parents and children. A fifth component is twice-monthly home visits designed to individualize the training and facilitate generalization of what the parents have learned.

In programs such as Homebuilders and Program for Assertive Community Treatment (PACT), many interventions are based in behavioral models and social learning theory. Paradigms for teaching stress reduction, parenting, anger management, conflict resolution, and household management skills directly draw from these models (Pecora, 1991). Barth (1988) suggests that social learning theory has made two major contributions to family-preservation programs: it has been the basis for rejecting the belief that changes in thinking and feeling necessarily antecede behavior changes; it provides a model for conceptualizing the ways in which family members learn from each other.

ECOLOGICAL THEORY

Despite their strengths and usefulness, none of these models truly conceptualize the complex interrelationship between individual psychosocial functioning and the context in which that functioning occurs. Typically, when research focuses on the relationship between external events and a person's psychological or behavioral response, it almost exclusively studies specific ways in which people's behavior is shaped by particular aspects of their circumstances. And the vast majority of this work focuses on interpersonal aspects of context. The impact of factors that are less specific or immediate, such as access to economic and other necessary resources for healthy living, is rarely incorporated (Barth, 1988). As a result, these models are limited as a framework for conceptualizing the home and community context as a contributor to dysfunction or an active component of treatment.

To compensate for the limitations of traditional theory in addressing this larger context of behavior, some clinicians have turned to an ecological perspective. Ecological psychology studies "human behavior in an environmental context" (Burnette, 1997, p. 13), focusing on understanding the behavior of normal people within their ordinary world. This model points to a more fluid dynamic orientation to capturing essential aspects of behavior. It draws from ecology, systems theory, anthropology, and organizational theory to provide a broad conceptual lens for analyzing human behavior and social functioning within a natural environment (Maluccio, 1988). Although studies that examine the interrelationship between behavior and environment are few, they support the idea that normal individuals behave differently within different settings.

Often, home-based mental health services describe their programs as working from an ecological perspective (Barth, 1988; Maluccio, 1988). As Barth (1988) notes, this descriptor frequently refers to an attitude rather than an articulated conceptual model. It often means that services include case management to link the client with community resources, coordinate care, or attend to concrete needs. Much work continues to be needed to conceptually bridge the gap between an ecological attitude, these services, and the client's psychological issues.

Ecostructural Model

One attempt to achieve this bridge is the ecostructural model proposed by Aponte et al. (1991). This model conceptualizes the psychological implications of the multiple levels of systems that impact on the client. It combines the insights of structural family therapy and Auerswald's (1968) ecological approach to provide a rationale and structure for conceptualizing cross-family and community-directed interventions that support the interventions within the family.

> The model assumes that the family is not alone in the problems it brings to treatment, but that the problems are part of an ecosystem that includes the individual, the family, and the community. Consequently, the solutions to these problems are both within and among the systems of the social ecosystem. The ecostructural model seeks to repair those systemic structures that are functionally relevant to a family's problems. (p. 404)

Families served by family-preservation programs are often poor, minority, single-parent families residing in communities with limited resources and poor schools. Unable to function successfully on their own, they become dependent on social service agencies. Poor boundaries between families and agencies, lack of control over their own lives, and lack of coordination between families and social service agencies all contribute to, model, and mirror the sense of powerlessness and disorganization that characterizes the family dynamics.

To address these issues, Aponte et al. (1991) suggest a two-tier approach. The first tier is the family-focused family-preservation program. The second tier is a multifamily group organized by the social service agency from among its client families. Aponte suggests that families be encouraged but not required to join these open-ended, geographically organized groups. Holding meetings outside of the agency (i.e., at the library, church, "Y") encourages a community focus. Aponte argues that these groups serve three purposes. They provide sources of mutual support for meeting individual family goals, they help the families enhance their ability to deal with social service agencies, and they act collectively as an advocacy group. A third tier in the ecostructural model is direct community advocacy, in support of changing the community to be more responsive to client needs.

Home

A crucial component of the client's ecology is his/her actual, physical home. Home is a very intimate place. Getting one's own apartment is the most visible sign that one has separated from parents. In late life, moving from one's own home to live with other family or into a group residence is an equally powerful symbol that independent and productive adulthood is past. The degree of choice people have over the location, physical make-up, and appearance of their home is a powerful measure of status in the social hierarchy. The decisions they make among the choices available to them are unavoidably self-expressive. How living space is organized, decorated, and cared for visibly displays important aspects—both conscious and unconscious—of who one is. Home is the space in which one negotiates one's most important relationships and mourns and celebrates one's most powerful experiences. It is a place within which people expect safety and retreat. When those expectations are violated, the personal sense of vulnerability and assault is profound. It is not surprising that their home directly and powerfully reveals peoples' psychological issues. An example from Jacobson (1995):

> The home of a family of four lacked a single interior door, even on the bathroom. The parents verbalized fears about the developing sexuality in their children; they did not want their 14 year old son to masturbate in the bedroom, and believe that bathroom privacy would lead their 12 year old daughter to spend excessive time putting on make-up which would make her look provocative. (p. 312)

Use of space is strongly rooted within cultural traditions. Cultural norms dictate the expected balance between privacy and intimacy and between separated, personal space and shared, communal space. They prescribe the amount of space considered necessary or luxurious for a family unit and who is expected to reside within that family unit. They establish the standards of beauty that serve as criteria within which the family finds its own self-expression. Whereas the absence of doors in the home of the family described by Jacobson has psychological meaning within its cultural context, the same absence of doors would be unremarkable within some cultures. In some cultures, it would be the presence of doors and the expectation of privacy that would shock. Given the intensely personal and deep meaning of home, it is not surprising that the ways in which people in unfamiliar cultures use and organize space often provoke strong reactions. Even small differences from one's own standards can seem highly irregular and unacceptable.

Just as psychological issues influence use of the immediate environment, the environment directly influences one's state of mind. Research on people living in or working in group situations points to the power of architectural structures, layout of space, and even decorative elements such as the color of walls. Organization of space and layout of furniture in nursing homes correlates with the psychological well-being and extent of socialization between residents (Parmelee & Lawton, 1990). Studies of college dorms found that architectural structures such as corridor length and room-sharing configurations influence residents' feelings and behaviors and that this influence generalizes into other arenas (Baum & Valins, 1977).

It follows that one potentially powerful form of in-home psychological intervention is directly working with clients' relationship to their physical environment. Often, services include direct environmental interventions: housekeeping for elderly clients unable to maintain the upkeep of their home or financial assistance with needed home repairs. Conceptualizations of the psychological implications of these concrete interventions are limited, however. In addition, it is rare that clinicians directly work with clients' relationship to their environment in order to facilitate psychological change—whether it is bringing order to a chaotic environment, helping the client to get rid of junk and clutter that fills the space, or helping the client create a home that feels comfortable and safe.

Windhorse Associates (Fortuna, 1995) and Dana Home Care (Newton, chapter 10, this volume) draw from Buddhist psychology to conceptualize the psychological implications of these concrete interventions. Central to this model is the idea that psychological dysfunction is characterized by lack of accurate connection with one's environment and lack of synchronicity between mind and body. Through relating to the client around ordinary activities such as housekeeping, creating a pleasant home environment, daily-life routines and interests such as sports, staff assists clients to cultivate mind–body synchronicity. Clients develop a more accurate appreciation of their environment and relate to that world more effectively. In the process, their thinking becomes clearer. Through these activities, staff's interactions with clients are characterized by attitudes of patience and empathy, labeled "Basic Attendance":

> Basic Attendance is a fundamental skill practiced by Windhorse clinicians in the course of daily activities which is used to focus awareness on the immediate needs of the moment. Basic Attendance has the effect of gently grounding attention in physical reality and strengthening the empathic bond between client and staff. The practice of Basic Attendance cultivates the moments of clarity, humor, and relaxation found in even the most confused state. These "islands of clarity," when recognized and valued, become the seeds of recovery. (Windhorse Associates, 1998, p. 5)

THERAPEUTIC RELATIONSHIP

Theories provide frameworks for conceptualizing the mental health professional's relationship with the client. They identify the interpersonal dimensions considered essential in establishing a "therapeutic" relationship and provide guidelines about the kinds of interactions that maximize the likelihood of positive consequences and minimize the possibility of harm. Three themes emerge in the literature on home-based services that characterize therapeutic relationships in that setting. The first theme is the emphasis on partnership between client and staff. Often in family-preservation and wraparound programs, parents are described as full partners in conceptualizing and making treatment decisions (Henggeler et al., 1994; Maluccio, 1988). One of the goals of these programs is frequently to empower parents to be more effective in advocating for their children and negotiating the maze of community resources (Aponte et al., 1991; Evans et al., 1994). PACT programs for adults with chronic psychiatric problems emphasize the attitude of partnership and empowerment by identifying the people they serve as "consumers" (NAMI, 1999). A second theme is the multiple roles that clinicians often assume when working with clients in their homes. In addition to therapist, staff often function as the client's teacher, educating him or her in new strategies for parenting or managing stress. They may provide mentoring, as they guide clients into more functional roles and life styles; they can serve as models, demonstrating new techniques for relating to family members or disciplining children. Finally, the clinician often functions as the client's advocate, assisting him or her to obtain needed resources or negotiate the maze of social services.

A third theme emerges in the literature on programs such as therapeutic foster care for children and crisis homes for adults (Bennett, 1995; Polak, Kirby, & Deitchman, 1995). In these programs, the majority of client contact is with "ordinary" families with whom the client lives for brief or extended periods of time. The experiences of clinicians involved in this work draw attention to the ways in which relationships with ordinary people can provide their own unique therapeutic impact. These relationships often assume a quality of mutuality that appears helpful. The perspectives of a family who provided a crisis home for 6 years illustrates this interaction (Bennett, 1995):

> Somehow our guests have not stayed strangers for long. With the kaleidoscope of personalities who have come to stay with us, I'm struck by the fact that overwhelmingly we have enjoyed their presence. Yes, there is fragility, awkwardness at times, and wrenching pain that also touches our family in surprising ways. But our guests have been so accepting of us and our fragility. That, far from feeling invaded by people with "problems" it's more as though our family enlarges a little at times.

> Finally, it turns out that, in spite of ourselves, we often are "good for" the person staying with us. As it is for everyone, there are days when a lot happens in our family; we have a lot of chores to tackle, a lot of turmoil to handle in our own lives. There's not always time to consciously channel energy into the role of helper for someone else. Though we acknowledge the emotional challenge facing our guest, it's almost as if circumstances conspire to leave the "disorder" behind for periods in the day; taking such a break seems to fortify the person. It is clear to me that often I have ended up on the *receiving* end of the helping that happens here; this has been the lesson most useful to me about living in a crisis home. (p. 235)

FUNDING FOR SERVICES

There are five general categories of funding for mental health services: public (federal, state, and local) program support, private foundations, Medicaid, Medicare, private health insurance, and managed behavioral health care organizations (MBHCOs). Medicaid, Medicare, private health insurance, and MBHCOs provide mental health benefits for individuals who meet their criteria for coverage. Until very recently, these funding sources rarely covered in-home psychiatric care. In contrast, public social service budgets and private foundations underwrite programs that serve defined populations with specific needs. The vast majority of home-based mental health initiatives were initially funded through public agencies; support of private foundations, such as United Way, has also been key. Often, the incentive was the desire to develop more cost-effective and/or publicly acceptable solutions for problematic social issues. Changes in public values and attitudes, such as toward out-of-home placement of children or institutional care for chronic psychiatric patients, fueled interest in community-based treatment. The three most widely replicated home-based services were all associated with federally legislated changes in public policy: community-based programs for chronic mentally ill adults were encouraged by the federal Mental Retardations and Community Mental Health Centers Construction Act of 1963; family-preservation programs were supported by the 1980 Adoption Assistance and Child Welfare Reform Act, and the 1993 federal Family Preservation and Family Support Initiative; wraparound programs for children with severe emotional disturbance were given impetus by the 1984 federal Child and Adolescent Service System Program (CASSP).

As much as public policy decisions led to the development of these programs however, reliance on government funding has interfered with their growth and dissemination. The impact of inconsistencies in government policies is well illustrated in the history of home-based services for adults with chronic psychiatric disorders (Kiesler, 1982; Torrey, 1990). Between 1960 and 1980, a number of well-designed research studies demonstrated that severely disturbed psychiatric patients could be treated and maintained outside of the hospital if they were provided with sufficient support (Fenton, Tessier, Struening, Smith, & Benoit, 1982; Kiesler, 1982). These studies also demonstrated that community care costs no more and often costs less than inpatient care.

As changes in government policy, however, shifted the care of adult chronic psychiatric clients from large public psychiatric institutions to community mental health centers, financial responsibility for their care also shifted. State mental health budgets that had funded the institutions shrank; sufficient funds were rarely transferred to replacement community programs. Newly developing Medicaid and Medicare programs assumed financial responsibility for the health care of many of these clients. That responsibility, however, was on an individual, client-by-client basis. Medicare and Medicaid contained significant financial incentives favoring hospital care. As a result, decreased rate of hospitalization in state and county mental institutions was more than offset by increased admissions to general hospital psychiatric units, private mental hospitals, and VA hospital psychiatric units (Kiesler, 1982).

The difficulty of influencing public policy decisions even when large scale, well-designed research supports the potential efficacy of programs is a theme in the literature (Olds, O'Brien, Racine, Glazner, & Kitzman, 1998; Santos et al., 1995). In 1990, Torrey observed: "The most remarkable fact about these demonstration projects, however, is how seldom they have been copied and how remarkably little influence they have had on mental health services in general" (p. 526). Lack of implementation results from a variety of factors including funding issues, contradictory policies at the federal, state, and local level, attitudes within the mental health profession, and territorial battles between mental health disciplines and social service agencies. Santos et al. (1995) note that the few states which have widely disseminated community treatment programs for chronic psychiatric adult clients have all had consistency in leadership and policy direction within the state mental health system. Supporters of in-home services have also contributed to the problems. Olds et al. (1998) note that exaggeration of potential benefits, unrealistic expectations that programs will "fix" too many social ills, or difficulty replicating successful programs contributes to disillusionment when programs do not meet high expectations. Often, demonstration projects on which research data is collected are well-funded and carefully implemented. With time, shifts in funding and policies mean that programs are modified in ways that substantially change their effectiveness. In instituting public policy, sufficient attention may not be paid to which elements of a complex program are most crucial to success.

Within the last few years, however, perspectives are shifting. Managed care is increasingly interested in exploring less costly alternatives to hospitalization. Changes in Medicaid and Medicare policies are making more money available for in-home services. Psychiatric clients and their families, through organizations such as the National Alliance for the Mentally Ill (NAMI), are more directly advocating for programs such as PACT. A new generation of innovative programs is emerging in the private sector (McKenzie, Mikkelsen, Stelk, Bereika, & Monack, 1995; Moy & Pigott, 1997; Woolston et al., 1998).

Although these are promising signs, the current confusion and lack of stability in the private-pay market make it difficult to provide continuity in community-based programs over a long period of time. In addition, private insurance is more inclined to fund intensive services for clients in acute crisis rather than less intense but still somewhat costly services for at-risk clients once the crisis has passed. Finally, funding based on individual clients makes it difficult to begin and maintain home-based programs that require full-time staff commitments and continuity. Given these financial realities, it is not surprising that many in-home services seek funding from multiple sources. These include purchase of service contracts with local child welfare agencies and juvenile courts, state mental health budgets, and insurance payments. The complexity of funding sources and differing requirements about who can be served and how adds tremendous complexity to the referral, assessment, and service delivery process (Archacki-Stone, 1995).

Part of the difficulty in funding community-based programs through Medicare, Medicaid, commercial insurance, and managed care is that payment is structured for fee-for-service reimbursement of clearly defined services provided for set periods of time by licensed mental health professionals. Community interventions, particularly with clients and families in crisis, are most effective when the structure and content of services is flexible and individualized; unlicensed paraprofessional staff often plays a key role. Many services that from an ecological perspective are crucial to recovery—linkage to community resources, repairing the clients' homes, and transportation—are hard to justify within the constraints of traditional psychiatric diagnostic categories and treatment plans. Thus, if partnerships are going to develop between these funding sources and innovative in-home psychiatric services, creativity will be required on both sides. The Yale Intensive In-home Child and Adolescent Psychiatry Services (YICAPS) has addressed this issue by bundling levels of service: 5 hours, 8 hours, 12 hours, and 20 hours per week. The bundled levels cover in-home psychiatric services, environmental interventions, and intensive case management.

COST-EFFECTIVENESS

Whether funding is private or public, an inevitable concern for in-home programs is cost. How to provide the optimal breadth and intensity of services within the inevitable reality of limited funds is an ongoing issue. Are community-based mental health services more cost-effective than the alternative? The answer to this question is highly subjective. It depends on: (a) the criteria used to measure treatment success, (b) the "acceptable" alternative, (c) the time frame over which the cost comparisons between different types of services are considered.

Criteria for Measuring Treatment Success

The most universally used measure of success is the extent to which clients remain in their homes during and following treatment. Specific criteria may be avoidance of hospitalization, foster care, or other residential placement and/or decrease in number of hospital days. In general, the research suggests that providing appropriate mental health services in the community results in less frequent or lengthy out-of-home placement compared to similar people without services (Christian-Michaels, 1995; McKenzie et al., 1995; Moy & Pigott, 1997; Pecora, Fraser, & Haapala, 1989). Based on their review of the extensive literature on PACT and family-preservation programs, Santos et al. (1995) argue that these programs are effective and financially feasible. In 1990, Kinney, Haapala, Booth, and Leavitt estimated that costs for Homebuilders services for the clients in their Bronx study averaged about $2,000 less than placement during a 6-month period. PACT currently estimates the costs for their comprehensive community-based service program to be $8,000 to $12,000 a year per client (NAMI, 1999). Cost comparisons between in-home programs and treatment in more restrictive settings imply that the decision to hospitalize or place someone outside the home is objective and a direct measure of the family's functioning or individual's well-being. As the marked fluctuations in hospitalization patterns over the last several decades indicate, this is far from accurate. Placement and hospitalization decisions reflect many other variables not directly related to the identified client's psychological health.

Often the measures cited above are the only objective criteria used to demonstrate program success (Moy & Pigott, 1997). Treatment outcome studies are often based on the implementation of a complex, multidimensional program. What particular components of these programs are most useful and to whom is rarely studied (Kohlert & Pecora, 1991). Rarely have people been asked which they prefer. The emphasis on cost comparisons rather than clinical outcome measures or client satisfaction likely reflects the priorities of the decisionmakers to whom researchers are directing their efforts. Often, the primary concern of these decisionmakers is indeed cost—whether they are public policymakers, state mental health departments, or health insurance or managed-care companies. Client satisfaction and well-being is often a lower priority.

Length of Time

Proponents of community-based services often argue that spending money for preventive services, while more expensive than providing no service, saves money in the long run. Longitudinal studies on home-visiting programs (Government Accounting Office, 1990) give support to this argument. Olds (1997) found that rates of child abuse, out-of-home placement, and involvement in the criminal justice system were significantly lower in families who received home-visiting services when their children were very young than in similar families without services.

What Is the Acceptable Alternative?

Providing a comprehensive community-based program to adult chronic psychiatric patients is less expensive than hospitalization (Warner, 1995), but these programs inevitably cost significantly more than traditional outpatient therapy. That many of these clients are unlikely or unable to follow through with outpatient services on a consistently reliable basis becomes a concern when the priority is providing quality care, but less of a concern when the focus is on cost. From a purely fiscal perspective, when clients don't follow through with outpatient services, they no longer constitute an expense. In-home services obviously cost more than no service, which in too many cases has unfortunately been the real alternative. Thus, although cost would seem to be a crucial issue in determining the worth and value of in-home services, often cultural values, biases within the mental health system, political agendas, and social priorities underlie stated concerns about money.

STAFF

Recruitment, training, and supervision of quality staff is crucial to the success of any home-based program. Although this is obviously true in any psychiatric treatment program, the variety and unpredictability of situations encountered on a daily basis and accompanying demands for flexibility, independent judgment, and responsibility often put more demands on in-home staff than on their hospital-based peers. Clinicians who work in their clients' homes have to be comfortable working in isolation and without easily available peer support. People responsible for staffing and supervising in-home mental health services would agree with Santos et al.'s (1995) description of "ideal" home-based multisystemic therapists: people experienced with a range of human problems, sensitive to cultural and ethnic issues, highly committed to resolving the problems facing their often psychologically and socially vulnerable clients, able to identify and focus on client strengths, highly intelligent and with strong common sense, possessing social and interpersonal flexibility, "streetwise," and self-confident.

Staff who provide in-home and community-based interventions fall into two broad categories:

mental health professionals: social workers, registered nurses, psychiatrists, and psychologists
paraprofessionals: certified nursing assistants, home health aides, foster parents, respite care workers, and B.A. level staff

The term "paraprofessional" is used broadly to include all workers who do not possess formal postgraduate education and credentialing in the mental health field.

MENTAL HEALTH PROFESSIONALS

The full spectrum of mental health professionals—psychiatrists, psychologists, social workers, and nurses—are increasingly involved in home-based services, either as direct care providers or as behind-the-scenes supervisors. Each of these professions has its own education, professional training, and licensing standards. Often, however, this training focuses exclusively on mental health treatment strategies designed for inpatient and outpatient settings. Mental health professionals generally learned models that have limited applicability in conceptualizing in-home interventions. They have often not been exposed to the unique constraints and opportunities of the home as a location for treatment. At worst, their training may be counter to the skills and attitudes that underlie successful in-home assessment and therapy. At best, they are grappling with the uncertainties inherent in trying new strategies in an unfamiliar treatment context.

Nursing and social work each has a long history of community-based care within their discipline. Social work and nursing literature from early in this century discuss the same issues that home-based clinicians encounter today (Whittington, 1987). As psychiatric care shifted, however, into inpatient and outpatient treatment settings during the 1920s to 1990s, psychiatric nurses and social workers followed. Only within the last decade has each of these disciplines aggressively sought out professional roles within the arena of home-based services (Mellon, 1994; Ward-Miller, 1996). Interestingly, each discipline has taken charge of its own domain. Developed within the child welfare system, family-preservation programs and wraparound services for seriously emotionally disturbed children rely heavily on social workers to develop, supervise, and staff these programs. Home health care is the domain of nurses; social workers, along with occupational and physical therapists, are considered adjunct professionals who provide specific, narrowly defined services.

Each discipline brings its own unique perspectives and rationale for a major role in home-based mental health services. Registered nurses argue that their medical training equips them to address the clients' medical needs as well as their psychological issues (Moore, Browne, Forte, & Sherwood, 1996). This is particularly important when clients, such as the elderly, also have significant physical problems or when medication management is a component of the in-home treatment program. Nurses also see educating clients and their families about mental health issues and coordinating care with other medical providers as interventions in which they are particularly skilled (Hellwig, 1993). On the other side, social workers have consistently maintained the most holistic orientation of any mental health discipline and have the most extensive community-based experience working with clients with emotional or psychosocial problems.

PARAPROFESSIONALS

Staff other than highly educated mental health professionals often play a significant role in home-based interventions. Intense family-preservation programs are sometimes staffed by a high proportion of paraprofessionals or workers with baccalaureate degrees (Kohlert & Pecora, 1991). Typical foster-care providers for adult psychiatric patients are middle-aged women with family caretaking experience but little formal education or work experience (Deci & Mattix, 1997). In home health services, it is estimated that 70% to 80% of long-term, medical in-home care is provided by "paraprofessional" home care workers (Eustis, Kane, & Fischer, 1993). As home health care services increasingly care for psychiatric patients, the reliance on paraprofessional workers is likely to follow.

For in-home programs to be a cost-effective strategy for treating clients who require intense intervention, the involvement of paraprofessional workers is crucial. Only with a less costly work force can clients in crisis or at significant risk for crisis receive sufficient monitoring and support. This workforce increases the likelihood that programs can provide particularly vulnerable and fragile clients—whether they be adults with chronic mental illness, children with severe emotional disturbance, or families with multiple problems—with the long-term assistance that diminishes the rate of institutional placement. The challenge, however, is that paraprofessional staff working within clients' homes is inevitably working independently without immediate access to supervisors or peers. Circumstances arise in which even the supervisor who can be paged is an impractical resource. Inevitably, paraprofessional staff often make instant judgment calls and decisions. This is quite different from inpatient and partial hospitalization programs where paraprofessionals provide a high degree of care but have immediate access to professional mental health staff. As a result, identifying appropriate qualifications and training for home-based paraprofessional staff is crucial. Other essential questions are: what specific roles should professionals and paraprofessionals play in home-based treatment and what level of supervision and monitoring is optimal? Gould (chapter 7, this volume) addresses paraprofessional training and supervision. This chapter briefly considers who the paraprofessional caregivers are and what roles they fill.

Paraprofessional Qualifications

Based on their experience with foster families for adult psychiatric patients, Deci and Mattix (1997) suggest that emotional stability, interpersonal warmth, and natural ability to provide a healing environment are more important than credentials, education, age, gender, and marital status in providing such care. Newton and Brauer (1989) identify the same qualities as crucial in selecting home health care workers to work with psychiatric clients. In their study of home visitors in early-intervention programs, Wasik (1993) identified factors such as maturity, flexibility, good judgment, interpersonal skills, and communication skills to be more important than credentials. The National Commission to Prevent Infant Mortality reached similar conclusions (quoted in McCurdy, 1995):

> Experts agree that several personal characteristics of home visitors make them successful across programs. These characteristics include strong skills in observing, organizing, listening, supporting, probing, interpreting, prompting, and gently confronting. Home visitors need to be particularly sensitive to various cultures and to the variety of conditions they face in the homes. It is imperative that they be non-judgmental. Generally, a program should select visitors who have strong 'people' skills and the right mix of medical and social skills appropriate for the needs of the families they serve. Of equal importance are issues of training, supervision, and support. (p. 32)

Recruiting people who have these qualities and are interested in meeting the challenges of this work is not easy. Many programs that rely heavily on the paraprofessional staff have developed extensive recruitment and screening procedures (Eckstein, 1995; Polak et al., 1995). Eckstein (1995) notes that only 1 of the 50 people they recruit as therapeutic foster parents actually completes the screening and training process.

Therapeutic Roles

In therapeutic foster homes, family-preservation programs, PACT programs, wraparound programs, and home visiting programs, paraprofessional staff are often identified as respected members of the treatment team with clearly defined roles and responsibilities. Sometimes the roles of paraprofessional and professional staff are interchangeable. For example, some early-intervention programs for high-risk mothers use nurses as home visitors, and some use paraprofessionals. In her review of research comparing the effectiveness of these staff groups, McCurdy (1995) found conflicting results. Some but not all studies found nurses to be more effective under certain circumstances. McCurdy suggests that other differences between programs using nurses and paraprofessionals, such as program design, intensity, and objectives, may be more important in the findings than the professional qualifications of the home visitors.

Other programs have included paraprofessional workers as part of the treatment team because they believe that their "paraprofessional" status is an asset. A combination of natural "helping" attitudes and skills, direct personal experience with problems or life experiences similar to the clients', and lack of formal mental health training allows them to provide a unique form of psychological assistance. Both Polak et al. (1995) and Bennett (1995) argue that "ordinary" families bring unique qualities to creating respite home environments for acutely disturbed adult clients in crisis. In their wraparound program for children with SED, Evans et al. (1994) use a family support team that includes both a case manager and a parent advocate. Evans et al. note that the parent advocate who has raised a child with SED can play a unique role as the ally of parents who are often at odds with the established mental health system.

Paraprofessional caregivers may be more able to take advantage of treatment opportunities within the client's home environment than their professional colleagues. Many potentially therapeutic activities are pragmatic and time consuming: directly working with clients to bring order to their environment and structure to their day, engaging clients in activities that build self-esteem and competence, and linking them with community resources and programs. Typically, these activities are defined as "nonprofessional." Indeed, skilled paraprofessional staff who are comfortable within the client's world may be more successful in carrying them out (see Newton, chapter 10, this volume). Paraprofessional staff often shares the client's sociodemographic background and has had similar life experiences. This common ground can enable the paraprofessional to become a powerful role model, resource, and confidante to the client.

Home Health Care

Significant differences exist between home health care and community-based programs in the roles and regulation of paraprofessional caregivers. To some extent, these differences reflect the different historical origins of these programs. In contrast to community-based psychosocial programs, home health care resides within the highly regulated arena of medical health care. Despite the extensive regulation and oversight in home health care, however, there is little consistency between job responsibilities and level of training at the paraprofessional level.

Home health care paraprofessionals carry a variety of job titles: home health aides, certified nursing assistants, homemakers, personal care attendants, personal care aides, sitters, and companions. Although some titles (i.e., home health aide and certified nursing assistant) are state regulated with clearly spelled out credentialing processes and criteria, others (companions, sitters, personal care aides) lack clearly defined job responsibilities and training requirements. Despite the differences in titles and training, all of these workers provide similar, "low-tech" services: personal care, housekeeping and meals, companionship and supervision, accompaniment on doctors' visits and outings. Essentially, they provide whatever practical services are required to compensate for clients' limitations and to support their functioning in an independent living setting. Even when there is legal differentiation between job titles, responsibilities and functions, in reality, often overlap. One worker may do the same work under different categories in different agencies or settings. Workers are drawn from the same pool—often lower social economic class, poorly educated, minority, and immigrant women. In contrast to the often brief and focused visits of registered nurses and other professionals, paraprofessionals often spend extended periods of time in the home of the client, and the degree to which that time is structured by specific activities and interventions is quite variable.

Home health aides work in Medicare-certified home health agencies; they are the only paraprofessionals covered by Medicare (Eustis et al., 1993). State laws and accrediting bodies set criteria for home health aides. Generally, these criteria consist of entry-level training requirements—often 75 to 125 hours of training, passing an entry exam, background checks, and tuberculosis vaccinations. Because their work primarily focuses on caring for medical patients with practical needs, little home health aide training focuses on psychiatric patients and the psychosocial meaning of their relationships with these patients. Consistent with Medicare requirements, the specific functions of the home health aide with a particular client are defined in the care plan.

This work force has received a great deal of research attention, consistent with its importance to the home care industry. The paraprofessional workforce is also the bane of the industry. Pay is low and benefits are often nonexistent. Workers often feel disrespected and alienated as they work at the bottom of the medical hierarchy. Rebecca Donovan (1987) described these workers as a "legacy of slavery in the United States" (as quoted in Chichin, 1991, p. 27). Transferring what has been learned about increasing the professionalism, respect, and roles of the paraprofessional work force in community-based programs to the home health care arena may be a helpful starting place.

CONCLUSIONS

In-home mental health services must develop a treatment model that guides their understanding of and interventions with clients; they must hire, train, and supervise staff; they must pay that staff and fund other program costs. In each of these issues, programs are in the midst of a rapid revolution. Conceptual models are increasingly attempting to integrate multiple aspects of the client's experience in their formulations of client's strengths and weaknesses and in their treatment plans. As Medicare, Medicaid, MBHCOs, and private insurance express curiosity about home-based mental health programs, programs are shaping themselves to meet the opportunities and constraints associated with that funding; these issues are often very different than those in program based government or foundation funding. Finally, defining appropriate roles for professional and paraprofessional workers, designing treatment strategies that maximize the effectiveness of each, and creating team models when team members each work so independently present interesting challenges for staffing home-based programs.

REFERENCES

Abaum, A., & Valins, S. (1977). *Architecture and social behavior: Psychological studies of social density.* Hillsdale, NY: Erlbaum.

American Psychiatric Association. (1994). *Diagnostic and statistical manual of mental disorders* (4th ed.). Washington, DC: American Psychiatric Press.

Aponte, H., Zarski, J., Bixenstine, C., & Cibik, P. (1991). Home/community services: A two-tier approach. *American Journal of Orthopsychiatry, 61,* 403–408.

Archacki-Stone, C. (1995). Family-based mental health services. In L. Combrinck-Graham (Ed.), *Children in families at risk: Maintaining the connections* (pp. 107–124). New York: Guilford.

Auerswald, E. H. (1968). Interdisciplinary vs. ecological approach. *Family Process, 7,* 202–215.

Bandura, A. (1977). *Social learning theory.* Englewood Cliffs, NJ: Prentice-Hall.

Barth, R. P. (1988). Theories guiding home-based intensive family preservation services. In J. Whittaker, J. Kinney, E. Tracy, & C. Booth (Eds.), *Improving practice technology for work with high risk families: Lessons from the "Homebuilders" Social Work Education Project* (Monograph No. 6; pp. 89–112). Seattle: University of Washington, Center for Social Welfare Research.

Baum, A., & Valins, S. (1977). *Architecture and social behavior: Psychological studies of social density.* Hillsdale, NJ: Erlbaum.

Bennett, R. (1995). The crisis home program of Dane County. In R. Warner (Ed.), *Alternatives to the hospital for acute psychiatric treatment* (pp. 227–236). Washington, DC: American Psychiatric Press.

Burnette, E. (1997, July). Learning about behavior by studying environment. *APA Monitor,* p. 13.

Chichin, E. R. (1991). The treatment of paraprofessional workers in the home. *Pride Institute Journal of Long Term Health Care, 10,* 26–35.

Christian-Michaels, S. (1995). Psychiatric emergencies and family preservation: Partnerships in an array of community-based services. In L. Combrinck-Graham (Ed.), *Children in families at risk: Maintaining the connections* (pp. 56–82). New York: Guilford.

Deci, P. A., & Mattix, G. N. (1997). Adult foster care: The forgotten alternative. In S. W. Henggeler & A. B. Santos (Eds.), *Innovative approaches to difficult-to-treat populations* (pp. 253–362). Washington, DC: American Psychiatric Press.

Donovan, R. (1987). Homecare work: A legacy of slavery in U.S. health care. *Affilia: Journal of Women and Social Work, 2/3,* 33–44.

Duffey, J., Miller, M. P., & Parlocha, P. (1993). Psychiatric home care: A framework for assessment and intervention. *Home Healthcare Nurse, 11,* 22–28.

Eckstein, M. A. (1995). Foster family clusters: Continuum advocate home network. In L. Combrinck-Graham (Ed.), *Children in families at risk: Maintaining the connections* (pp. 275–298). New York: Guilford.

Eustis, N. N., Kane, R. A., & Fischer, L. R. (1993). Home care quality and the home care worker: Beyond quality assurance as usual. *Gerontologist, 33,* 64–73.

Evans, M. E., Armstrong, M. I., Dollard, N., Kuppinger, A. D., Huz, S., & Wood, V. (1994). Development and evaluation of treatment foster care and family-centered intensive case management in New York. *Journal of Emotional and Behavioral Disorders, 2,* 228–239.

Fenton, F. R., Tessier, L., Struening, E. L., Smith, F. A., & Benoit, C. (1982). *Home and hospital psychiatric treatment.* Pittsburgh, PA: University of Pittsburgh Press.

Fortuna, J. (1995). The Windhorse Program for Recovery. In R. Warner (Ed.), *Alternatives to the hospital for acute psychiatric treatment* (pp. 171–192). Washington, DC: American Psychiatric Press.

Fraser, L. H. (1995). Eastfield Ming Quong: Multiple-impact in-home treatment model. In L. Combrinck-Graham (Ed.), *Children in families at risk: Maintaining the connections* (pp. 83–106). New York: Guilford.

Germain, C. B. (1978, November). Space: An ecological variable in social work practice. *Social Casework,* pp. 515–522.

Goffman, E. (1961). *Essays on the social situation of mental patients and other inmates.* Garden City, NY: Doubleday.

Goldstein, M. S. (1979). The sociology of mental health and illness. *Annual Review of Sociology, 5,* 381–409.

Government Accounting Office. (1990). *Home visiting: A promising early intervention strategy for at-risk families.* GAO/HRD-90-83. Washington, DC: Author.

Hellwig, K. (1993). Psychiatric home care nursing: Managing patients in the community setting. *Journal of Psychosocial Nursing, 31,* 21–24.

Henggeler, S. W., & Borduin, C. M. (1990). *Family therapy and beyond: A multisystemic approach to treating the behavior problems of children and adolescents.* Pacific Grove, CA: Brooks/Cole.

Henggeler, S. W., Schoenwald, S. K., Pickrel, C. S., Brondun, M. J., Borduin, C. M., & Hall, J. A. (1994). *Treatment manual for family preservation using multisystemic therapy.* Columbia, SC: Health and Human Service Finance Commission.

Jacobson, K. D. (1995). Drawing households and other living spaces in the process of assessment and psychotherapy. *Clinical Social Work Journal, 23,* 305–325.

Kiesler, Charles A. (1982). Mental hospitals and alternative care: Noninstitutionalization as potential public policy for mental patients. *American Psychologist, 37,* 349–360.

Kinney, J., Haapala, D., Booth, C., & Leavitt, S. (1990). The Homebuilders model. In J. K. Whittaker, J. Kinney, E. M. Tracy, & C. Booth (Eds.), *Reaching high-risk families: Intensive family preservation in human services* (pp. 31–64). New York: Aldine De Gruyter.

Kohlert, N. M., & Pecora, P. J. (1991). Therapist perceptions of organizational support and job satisfaction. In M. W. Fraser, P. J. Pecora, & D. A. Haapala (Eds.), *Families in crisis: The impact of intensive family preservation services* (pp. 109–129). New York: Aldine De Gruyter.

Lindblad-Goldberg, M., Dore, M., & Stern, L. (1998). *Creating competence from chaos: A comprehensive guide to home-based services.* New York: Norton.

Maluccio, A. N. (1988). Family preservation services and the social work practice sequence. In J. Whittaker, J. Kinney, E. Tracy, & C. Booth (Eds.), *Improving practice technology for work with high risk families: Lessons from the "Homebuilders" Social Work Education Project* (Monograph No. 6, pp. 113–126). Seattle: University of Washington, Center for Social Welfare Research.

McCurdy, K. (1995). *Home visiting* (Working Paper Number 866). Chicago: National Committee to Prevent Child Abuse.

McKenzie, J., Mikkelsen, E. J., Stelk, W., Bereika, G., & Monack, D. (1995). The role of a home-based mentor program in the psychiatric continuum of care for children and adolescents. In L. Combrinck-Graham (Ed.), *Children in families at risk: Maintaining the connections* (pp. 209–227). New York: Guilford.

Mellon, S. K. (1994). Mental health clinical nurse specialist in home care for the 90s. *Issues in Mental Health Nursing, 15,* 229–237.

Miller, L. S. (1994). Primary prevention of conduct disorder. *Psychiatric Quarterly, 65,* 273–285.

Minuchin, S. (1974). *Families and family therapy.* Cambridge, MA: Harvard University Press.

Moore, M. C., Browne, L., Forte, E. M., & Sherwood, D. K. (1996). Mental health home visits for the elderly. *Perspectives in Psychiatric Care, 32,* 5–9.

Moy, S., & Pigott, H. E. (1997). Home-based services. In R. K. Schreter, S. S. Sharfstein, & C. A. Schreter (Eds.), *Managing care, not dollars* (pp. 27–41). Washington, DC: American Psychiatric Press.

National Alliance for the Mentally Ill. (1999). *The PACT advocacy guide* [brochure]. Arlington, VA: Author.

Newton, N. A., & Brauer, W. F. (1989, June). In-home mental health services: A paraprofessional model of care. *Caring,* 16–19.

Olds, D. (1997). The prenatal/early infancy project: Fifteen years later. Issues in children's and families' lives. In G. W. Albee & T. P. Gullota (Eds.), *Primary prevention works.* Thousand Oaks: CA: Sage.

Olds, D., O'Brien, R. A., Racine, D., Glazner, J., & Kitzman, H. (1998). Increasing the policy and program relevance of results from randomized trials of home visitation. *Journal of Community Psychology, 26,* 85–100.

Parmelee, P., & Lawton, M. P. (1990). The design of special environments for the aged. In J. E. Birren & K. W. Schaie (Eds.), *Handbook of the psychology of aging* (3rd ed., pp. 464–487). New York: Academic Press.

Pecora, P. J. (1991). Family-based and intensive family preservation services: A select literature review. In M. W. Fraser, P. J. Pecora, & D. A. Haapala (Eds.), *Families in crisis: The impact of intensive family preservation services* (pp. 17–47). New York: Aldine De Gruyter.

Pecora, P. J., Fraser, M. W., & Haapala, D. A. (1989). Intensive home-based family treatment: Client outcomes and issues for program design. In J. Hudson & B. Galaway (Eds.), *The state as parent: International research perspectives on interventions with young persons* (pp. 331–345). Boston: Kluwer.

Pinkston, E. M., & Linsk, N. L. (1984). *Care of the elderly: A family approach.* New York: Pergamon Press.

Polak, P. B., Kirby, M. W., & Deitchman, W. S. (1995). Treating acutely psychotic patients in private homes. In R. Warner (Ed.), *Alternatives to the hospital for acute psychiatric treatment* (pp. 213–226). Washington, DC: American Psychiatric Press.

Santos, A. B., Henggeler, S. W., Burns, B. J., Arana, G. W., & Meisler, N. (1995). Research on field-based services: Models for reform in the delivery of mental health care to populations with complex clinical problems. *American Journal of Psychiatry, 152,* 1111–1123.

Skinner, B. F. (1974). *About behaviorism.* New York: Knopf.

Torrey, E. F. (1990). Economic barriers to widespread implementation of model programs for the seriously mentally ill. *Hospital and Community Psychiatry, 41,* 526–531.

Ward-Miller, S. (1996). The psychiatric clinical specialist in the home care setting. *Advanced Practice Nursing, 31,* 519–525.

Warner, R. (1995). From patient management to risk management. In R. Warner (Ed.), *Alternatives to the hospital for acute psychiatric treatment* (pp. 237–248). Washington, DC: American Psychiatric Press.

Wasik, B. (1993). Staffing issues for home visiting programs. *Future of Children, 3,* 140–157.

Whittington, R. (1987). The new friendly visitors: A rediscovered role for independent social workers. *Journal of Independent Social Work, 1,* 65–74.

Windhorse Associates. (1998). [Brochure]. Northhampton, MA: Windhorse Associates.

Woolston, J. L., Berkowitz, S. J., Schaefer, M. C., & Adnopoz, J. A. (1998). Intensive, integrated, in-home psychiatric services. *Child and Adolescent Psychiatric Clinics of North America, 7,* 615–633.

Woods, L. J. (1988). Home-based family therapy. *Social Work, 33,* 211–214.

Zarski, J. J., Sand-Pringle, C., Greenback, M., & Cibik, P. (1991). The invisible mirror: In-home family therapy and supervision. *Journal of Marital and Family Therapy, 17,* 133–143.

CHAPTER THREE

Sources of Failure in Home-Based Therapy

Kadi Sprengle

Although home-based treatment can be a rich addition to inpatient and outpatient services, in-home psychiatric treatment for very vulnerable, high-risk clients is an uncertain undertaking. All too often the lack of clearly defined therapist roles and behavior, institutional safeguards, and professional oversight makes home-based treatment seem (and in reality is) dangerous for both clients and the clinicians responsible for their care. In this chapter, Kadi Sprengle draws on her hard-won knowledge of these dangers to remind us of their reality and suggest ways of minimizing the risk.

I started my home health career with no training and many opinions. Having read *One Flew Over the Cuckoo's Nest* by Ken Kesey (1997), I was excited about a job keeping young psychotic adults out of the psychiatric hospital. I had run out of money while working on a master's degree in Black Labor History, and the job offered 36 hours of pay for spending the weekend in an apartment building with eight psychotic young adults. The position would be filled by the vote of the clients. (The social worker running the program was also given one vote.)

Although the other candidates had graduate degrees in psychology, I won the election. After 1 day of orientation by the polite but alarmed social worker, I started out as the only staff on duty for the weekends. The facility was a three-flat building in a run-down neighborhood on the north side of Chicago. On the first floor, one of the bedrooms was considered a staff office, with a foldout couch where I would sleep. I had been instructed to consider myself a guest in the clients' homes. I was given no authority but was expected to use persuasion only. When in public with the clients, I was not to reveal the nature of our relationship. (This was especially tricky when, on a stroll with me, one client shocked the neighbor by French kissing her dog.)

The first night I woke up at 2:00 A.M. to find Roscoe, who lived on the third floor, standing at the foot of my bed staring at me. At least I think he was staring; his dark glasses made it difficult to tell. When I sat up, he chided me for sleeping on the job and proceeded to complain about his roommate. I was too shocked to even protest.

The next night, after I asked him to leave me alone, I was wakened by a strange sound. Roscoe was removing the door to my room. He explained that I had been hired to attend to the needs of the clients and that it was rude of me to isolate myself from the residents who were my employers. I explained that my hiring arrangement had included the right to sleep at night, and he calmly responded by giving me a lecture on the needs of chronic mental patients. He felt that, since he and some of the other residents stayed up at night and slept during the day, I, too, should follow that pattern.

So began my introduction to home-based interventions.

I feel especially well-qualified to write of failure and gross error because failure and error are familiar territory. Working in experimental programs with no training taught me to learn from my mistakes. Later, after I went back to school and completed a doctorate, I discovered, sadly, that an advanced degree did not prevent further error. Trial and error, it turns out, is just another name for the clinical method.

This is hard work, and there is little research to guide us. Failure is common. Over the years, however, I have discovered that certain strategies and principles increase the likelihood of success and recovery. Violating those same principles can lead to failure. The following article outlines principles which seem essential to home-based therapy and then gives examples of blunders caused by disregarding these principles.

PRINCIPLES OF HOME-BASED THERAPY

In reviewing some of the (rather amazing) mistakes that can be made in home-based work, it does not appear that the faults lie with one brand of treatment over another. Good intentions and hard work do not guard against gross error either. Rather, there appear to be principles that lay the basis for solid therapeutic work in the home. When these principles are followed, mistakes can be seen and corrected. When these principles are discarded, errors snowball.

Successful programs and successful individual therapists share certain traits which cut across theoretical divisions:

1. They have a thought-out strategy for determining appropriate boundaries in their work. Clear lines of communication are established between treatment team members and clients. Clear rules of conduct guide the clinician.
2. Home-based clinicians, paraprofessional or professional, are well-trained, have good clinical supervision, and a supportive atmosphere in which to discuss the case.
3. They have a commitment to honesty and the organizational structure to support honesty.
4. Treatment planning is based on the client's needs rather than the program's restrictions. Where the program is time limited, provisions are made for continuity of care.
5. The programs have enough money to provide the services that are needed.

WHY HAVE BOUNDARIES?

In psychodynamic therapy, constructing a "frame" is thought to be an essential part of the treatment. A frame is the structure of limits and boundaries which organize the treatment. For example, working within an office-based "50-minute hour" is often part of the frame. Other common boundaries include a ban against "dual relationships." (For example, the therapist cannot do business with the client or be a friend or relative. Some therapists do not accept gifts from a client.)

The limits on the relationship between the therapist and the client help focus the attention of both. The tension between the strong feelings aroused in therapy and the artificial structure of the limits of the frame serve as a lens to magnify and clarify the client's interpersonal difficulties. The frame helps the client and the therapist see clearly. Suddenly details fall into place, and a pattern is revealed.

Family systems therapists support the need for a frame. They argue that a clinician risks being inducted into the disturbed family system as the clinician attempts to intervene in that system. Attention to boundaries will aid the clinician (and the family) in resisting the pull to participate in the family dynamics.

In the field, it is easy to be caught unawares. For example, a novice case manager who had accompanied an abusive mother to court found himself with his arms around her as she sobbed when the judge ruled against her. Her children watched silently as she thanked him for "being the only one that knows the truth of my innocence." The case manager later decided that the children's report of abuse was not reliable.

Developing and maintaining guidelines regarding boundaries are essential for successful in-home treatment. All lines of communication are part of the boundaries and frame which support (or undermine) the clinical work. Clinicians working in the home need to have an established pattern of communication between team members, clients, and collateral people. Policies on emergency contact, gossip, complaints, and disputes need to be in place before misunderstandings develop.

Common boundary issues that arise in home-based therapy include the following:

- If the TV is on when you arrive for a family therapy appointment, should the therapist ask that it be turned off? What happens when a neighbor drops by or the phone rings? If you planned to see the entire family, how do you handle missing family members? By having a strategy in place to make these decisions, the clinician is freed to focus on the treatment.
- Gifts and favors between clients and treatment team members also need to be thought out. While in the client's home, the therapist will see things that are needed by the client. When, if ever, is it appropriate to privately supply the needed item?
- A therapist in our agency was paged at 2:00 A.M. by a homeless client who had skipped her last two appointments. The client was hungry and cold and needed a place to stay. What response makes sense in that situation?
- A client of mine walked 6 miles each way to her part-time, minimum wage job. I saw a bicycle at a garage sale that would have cut her travel time by two hours. Should I have purchased it? If so, how should it have been given to her?

TRAINING, EXPERIENCE, AND SUFFICIENT SUPERVISION

Home-based psychotherapy is often done by people with little clinical training. Some child welfare agencies regularly assign Bachelor-degreed workers as "therapists"; others use unlicensed master's-level workers. High turnover among home-based clinical staff impedes training efforts. For example, one study found the average length of time clinical staff stay in a family preservation job is just 18 months (Tracy, Bean, Gwatkin, & Hill, 1992).

Studies of novice clinicians found that daily interactions with colleagues are an important part of training (Liddle, 1988), yet clinicians in home-based programs rarely have daily contact with colleagues. Inexperienced clinicians are especially vulnerable to becoming overinvolved with their clients (Zarski, 1991), a problem that is further exacerbated when meeting with clients in their homes.

Given the lack of experience and training, careful supervision is all the more important. When clinicians go into the home independently, with no colleagues or supervisors present, there is no way to ensure professional behavior. Without well-designed systems of supervision, novice therapists can easily run into difficulties.

For example, a new therapist was assigned to the child with Asperger's described in Alice Farrell's chapter (chapter 10, this volume). Unfamiliar with Asperger's, she did not know what she should be doing, so she spent her time (billed as therapy) chatting with the respite worker while the respite worker played with the child. Since she had no regular clinical supervision, this was not corrected although she did not attempt to conceal her lack of knowledge.

Another therapist, with no previous experience working with children, was assigned to do therapy with a mentally ill mother and her son. The mother had lost custody of her son five years before when she became convinced that government agents would kidnap her son if she allowed him to go to school. She was now on medication, and she and her son were court ordered to have therapy to see if reunification would be possible. Mother and son were shy and uneasy with each other; the mother confided that she remembered with shame trying to hide her child and threatening his teacher. She feared her son hated her for her crazy behavior, but she did not know how to talk to him about the devastation her mental illness had brought into their lives.

In the six months of therapy, the therapist never raised the subject of the mother's mental illness. Rather, each week, the therapist engaged the pair in a series of cheerful activities: pizza and cards at home, a trip to a video arcade, shopping in the mall. The therapist explained that he did not want to make them uncomfortable by raising painful topics. In the 6 months of therapy, the therapist received no clinical supervision on the case. At the end of 6 months, the therapist wrote, honestly, in his court report, that the mother and son could only relate on a superficial level; the mother was unable to talk with her son about important issues. The therapist's agency recommended to the court that the mother's parental rights be terminated.

When meeting clients in the community, and when integrating ordinary activities into treatment, it is easy to overlook the lack of genuine communication. In the office, when the client is silent, it is obvious. But at a mall, it is not so obvious when important issues are being avoided.

THE MCDONALD'S SCHOOL OF PSYCHOTHERAPY

The local fast-food chain is often an annex of the child welfare agency. Agencies doing home-based treatment often use the McDonald's as a place to be alone with a child. Some routinely bill for such time as psychotherapy (which is reimbursable at a higher rate than respite care). But time spent with a child at McDonald's is rarely psychotherapy and rarely even a thought-out part of a treatment plan.

There are clinical reasons why a trip to McDonald's might be helpful, but often McDonald's is used because the unskilled clinician does not know what else to do or even the skilled clinician, I might add. This is why we need both the time and support to consider how ordinary activities can be made therapeutic.

PROGRAM RESTRICTIONS ON TREATMENT PLANNING: CONTINUITY OF CARE

Program design is a source of treatment failure in some cases. For example, many home- and community-based programs have been developed to provide intensive interventions on a short-term basis only. When the program is through, the family or individual client is referred to another agency (if one exists), and the case is closed. The treatment needs of the clients often outlast the program. Often, the client decompensates when treatment is removed. If the client completely decompensates, he or she becomes eligible for the program again, and the circle completes itself.

Some public agencies have reorganized to provide treatment to only the most severely emotionally disturbed. (Among children, this has become a catch phrase. The phrase "severely emotionally disturbed," or SED, is treated as if it were a discrete diagnostic category instead of a level of distress.) When the client improves, from severe to moderately disturbed, the client is discharged. For those improved clients without access to private funding, there is no longer a source for inexpensive mental health treatment, therefore, they are often left without treatment. When they decompensate, they again become eligible for treatment. Many programs attend to the crisis without offering the long-term treatment and support needed to maintain the client's improvement.

Until there is sufficient public or private funding to provide affordable mental health treatment to all who require it, problems like these will continue.

ECONOMIC AND POLITICAL PRESSURES ON TREATMENT PLANNING: IS HOSPITAL PREVENTION A VALID TREATMENT GOAL?

Hospital prevention as a program goal in mental health services has the same problems that hospital prevention faces in physical health services: It can be dangerous, and it makes clinical decisions based on program ideology (or finances) rather than a clear assessment of the needs of the patient.

This book, and many others, are filled with articles describing the advantages of innovative use of alternatives to hospitalization and other creative and health-producing interventions. When the program (or clinician), however, takes a position that hospitalization itself is the problem and should be avoided on principle, treatment is no longer based on a clear-eyed assessment of what the client needs at a given moment. By making an a priori decision that inpatient treatment, (or long-term treatment, or expensive treatment) is bad treatment, the clinician or program eliminates a treatment option.

Hospitalization began to be condemned in the 1960s during the movement to deinstitutionalize mental patients. Civil rights and patient rights activists (with help from lawsuits sponsored by the ACLU) advocated increased freedom for mental patients and pointed to programs in other countries where mental illness was successfully treated in the community rather than by isolating mental patients for years in hospitals.

Since the development of antipsychotic medications, people could be free of many of the more disturbing aspects of chronic mental illness, such as delusions and hallucinations, so community-based treatment was possible.

At this time, many clinicians believed that the remaining aspects of schizophrenia, such as extreme apathy and dependency, were being caused not by the disorder but by the hospital itself.

Environmental factors in mental illness were emphasized, and some clinicians became convinced that mental illness was a myth. These clinicians argued that syndromes such as schizophrenia were best understood as bizarre behavior learned in a crazy environment (like a mental hospital).

So, at the height of the movement to "deinstitutionalize" the chronically mentally ill, hospitals were seen as places where people were driven crazy. The goal of deinstitutionalization was not to save money but to free patients by providing them with excellent outpatient care and integrating them into their community.

By increasing the freedom for the mentally ill, these programs increased the dignity and quality of life of many chronically ill. Excellent pilot programs were launched to meet the treatment needs of the newly released mental patients. The idea was to expand these programs as soon as it was clear which ones were the most helpful. But few of the programs ever received permanent funding.

Deinstitutionalization was realized just as the political climate shifted in this country. Tax reductions and dismantling the "welfare state" became the goals of many politicians. Funding for social services was slashed just as the severely mentally ill were turned out of the hospitals. With little community support, chronic mental patients found themselves moved from the back wards of hospitals to flophouses and homeless shelters. Deinstitutionalization finally failed to increase the quality of life overall because it "freed" the mentally ill from treatment at the same time it freed them from confinement.

In fact, in a series of pioneering studies, Dr. Linda Teplin found that the mentally ill were more likely to end up in jail than those without a mental illness. She discovered that jails were, in some cases, the new substitute for mental hospitals (Teplin, 1984; Teplin & Pruett, 1992).

Meanwhile, clinical research on various treatments for mental illness often measured the success of a treatment by whether the treatment reduced the number of days per year spent in the hospital. Length of stay was seen as a solid measure of level of psychopathology. If a patient needed fewer days in the hospital, he or she must be more sane.

Insurance companies began to fund studies on length of stay in psychiatric and medical hospitals. Concerns over cost gave birth to managed care companies whose mission was to reduce health care costs and reduce the hospital length of stay. Eventually, length of stay, once seen as a marker of recovery from mental illness, became a goal in itself.

Renewed interest in home-based treatment was spurred both by the brief flowering of altruistic interest in alternatives to hospitalization and by the search for cheaper mental health services. Advocates of home-based mental health services found a new hearing only after slashes in public funding and private insurance led to increased experiments in alternatives to hospitalizations.

Faced with major budget cuts, agencies hired those people who strongly believed that home-based care was the best form of care. Clinicians who felt that hospitalization was detrimental found they had an edge in the hiring line.

For economic reasons, advocates for home-based services were offered funding for their programs. We saw a merging of ideology and economics. Since the people hired to run the programs often firmly believed that they were rescuing patients from poor treatment in hospitals, the cost-saving benefits of these programs were seen as only the frosting on the cake. The leaders of these programs did not see the mandate to decrease hospitalization or long-term therapy as a conflict of interest. For a while, there was yet another flowering of these programs, and some excellent innovative work was done, but now, as cuts continue, even these programs are in financial difficulty.

Today we see alternatives to hospitalization reduced to the absurd. Partial hospitalization programs were originally developed to replace long-term hospitalization so that the chronic mental patient would be able to remain in the community for the many months or years of intensive treatment they needed. Now, long-term hospitalization does not exist as a treatment option for the vast majority of severely disturbed patients. Long-term partial programs are also being wiped out and being replaced by short-term crisis stabilization programs. Often, the stay is marked in days, not months or even weeks.

Hospital prevention and treatment reduction are now seen as valid treatment goals. Entire programs have been developed whose funding depends on their ability to reduce hospitalization (as opposed to reducing symptoms).

One of the best of such programs was described by Christian-Michaels (1995). In Illinois, all requests for admission to a state-funded bed in a psychiatric hospital are screened in person by a state "SASS" agent. The agent is authorized to put into place emergency crisis stabilization programs if the family will accept a decision to attempt to maintain the child outside the hospital. The SASS program guarantees a face-to-face intake interview on site within two hours of the request. The program runs 24 hours daily.

As Christian-Michaels' article points out, the program has succeeded in reducing the number of psychiatric hospitalizations. In fact, the only state psychiatric hospital for children has been closed.

The SASS program is based on the belief that community-based treatment is superior to hospitalization in almost all cases and that deflection from hospitalization is to be applauded. Some of the work done by SASS programs is outstanding. However, at times biases against hospitalization lead to mistakes and misjudgments. Here are some examples of difficulties:

• An emergency worker was called by the DuPage County Youth Home (the jail for adolescents) to assess an adolescent for hospitalization. The young man was paranoid and delusional, seemed terrified, and was scaring the other residents (a difficult thing to do). The SASS worker who called to make arrangements to hospitalize the young man was told she was being unnecessarily restrictive. Her SASS supervisor suggested they put wraparound services in the youth home to stabilize the young man "and avoid the trauma of hospitalization."

• A family who insisted that their daughter needed to be hospitalized rather than have home-based treatment was advised that, if she was hospitalized, she ran the risk of being raped in the hospital. This advice was offered by the director of the assessment team and was never corrected.

• On a Friday, the crisis hot line received a call from the worried parents of a delusional adult son. He was threatening to set fire to their home. A crisis worker went to their home and determined that he was not in need of hospitalization. On Monday, the man set fire to his home. This is the sort of incident that crisis workers have nightmares about.

When pressured to manage even the most harrowing cases without seeing hospitalization as a legitimate alternative, the nightmares can too easily become reality. When mistakes do occur, honest discussion allows clinicians to develop an informed knowledge base. However, that discussion can only occur when staff have the resources and support to act on the knowledge they accumulate.

IS THERE AN APPROPRIATE USE OF HOSPITALIZATION?

Pressure to keep children out of the hospital can disrupt already tenuous family systems. Parents can find a psychotic or suicidal child frightening. To demand that they also be in charge of supervising that child while he or she is hallucinating or trying to cut himself or herself is to demand more than most parents can handle. Parents need to know that the safety of their child and themselves is important. They are not betraying the child if they want him or her hospitalized. When a child shows up with a rope burn around his neck, or is found to be concealing knives, or is threatening to kill his brother, physical safety must be the priority. Increased respite care is no substitute for 24-hour containment.

When foster parents are not allowed the option of hospitalization, they are more likely to request the removal of psychotic children from their home. The child then loses the placement and the foster family. A child ejected from a foster home due to psychotic behavior will likely "bounce." Bouncing is a local term for what happens to children too disturbed to be able to stabilize in foster care. They bounce around the system, never spending more than 6 months to a year in one foster placement. Their treatment team often changes with every move: new home, new parents, new therapist, new family, new school. No one supports these "bounces," even those who fear the hospital. But there is often no alternative in agency budgets.

By the criteria of the "less is more" advocates, keeping a child out of the hospital or a residential program is saving the child. And because funding for long-term, restrictive programs has all but disappeared, the few programs left usually have serious problems. There is not a clear way to evaluate the few options for long-term care. Case workers ask around, send out packets of information, and hope for the best.

RECORDS

Clients referred for home-based services often have a long history of psychiatric interventions. Thick records scattered through multiple agencies document these treatment attempts. Few people have the time to gather, let alone read them. And no one wants to read about record-keeping, so I offer a truly hair-raising cautionary tale to keep your interest.

Our agency was offered a fascinating case for outpatient treatment. Luckily, the case manager honestly filled us in about the case. Due to a policy change, all children in out-of-state placements were to be returned to the state then, as quickly as possible, returned to a community-based placement. This young man, now a teenager, had sampled several programs without success. He had been returned to his mother's care for 9 months, but had been in and out of the youth home for a variety of acts of disobedience, threats, and fights. He was now in the youth home and about to be returned home once again.

His case had been assigned to a team specializing in placement stabilization who took pride in their ability to offer community-based services to children thought to be only treatable in a residential setting. This team had convinced a wary judge that wraparound services could help and that the wishes of the boy and his mother for reunion should be honored.

The boy's mother was adamant in her demands that her son be returned. She had written the press and several politicians asking for their help in ensuring a quick return for her child.

The case worker doubted the safety of the reunification plan and had asked for a therapist, in addition to the wrap services, to help with an ongoing assessment of the safety of home-based services.

Somehow she managed the near-impossible feat of wrangling permission to use therapy money to pay me and a social worker to read the entire chart.

We spent 20 hours reading the massive chart, comparing notes, and reading to each other aloud from what we had uncovered. No one had ever had the time to read the entire chart, and the case had been changed from agency to agency so many times that no one now involved with the case knew the family when the case was opened.

We found that, over the life of this child, time after time his mother had called the police for emergency help with her son, then denied problems whenever the case came to court. For example, she claimed that he had attempted to murder his crippled sister by setting up wire traps to trip her at the top of stairs, but in court she stated that the police had misunderstood her. Her son had done nothing wrong.

She shared her bed with her teen-age son and had been observed by several workers to kiss him on the lips. A home-based case worker had reported feeling uncomfortable with the kisses, but felt that they must be innocent because they were being done in his presence.

Buried deep in a blurry copy of records from the mother's own treatment, we found that she had confessed to her therapist that, 10 years ago, she had helped bury the body of a women shot by her lover. There was no record that the therapist ever followed up on this report. The lover was still in prison for murder.

Also in the notes, however, were reports by the treatment team complaining about the mother's regular threats to shoot her son and bury him. Current staff, not having read about the murder, had assessed her threats as bad tempered, but did not take them seriously.

We decided not to take the case and recommended that the young man be returned to residential treatment. Nevertheless, he was returned home until his crippled sister was injured in a fall down the stairs. The boy had pushed her.

Anyone who has worked in this field can give you (usually less spine-tingling) stories of their own. The Munchausen's case described by Julia Klco in chapter 7 would have never been uncovered if not for reading records.

Past records are cumbersome and, even collecting them can be a daunting task. Few home-based workers are reimbursed for time spent reading records. Many do not even have ready access to the records.

Policies need to be changed to allow for a thorough record review on every case considered for home-based treatment. Until then, read the records anyway, obtain releases, and send for records, and read them when they arrive.

SUMMARY

Home-based therapy has many pitfalls. It is easier to fail at home-based therapy, and mistakes in the client's home can snowball into disasters. Nevertheless, when appropriately applied, home-based assessment and treatment can lead to remarkable recovery. Adherence to principles, however, is essential. Providers of home-based treatment need to be well-trained and well-supervised at both the professional and paraprofessional level.

Accurate assessment and plain honesty is so important in this work that any agency doing home-based assessment needs to develop organizational methods of increasing and rewarding honesty.

Within a larger organization, clinical reviews of work should be based on the client's needs rather than the program's needs.

Records for these cases need to be carefully reviewed, whether or not funding is available to pay for the time spent in record review. Staff who take time to gather data before developing a treatment plan need to be rewarded.

Treatment plans need to be developed based on the needs of the client. If the client needs services that are not available, document that need.

Funding continues to be slashed for mental health services. While most experienced home-based clinicians will agree with many of the principles listed here, many have come to believe that it is impossible to carry these principles out due to funding restrictions. At least in the child welfare world, agencies are left with budgets too small to cover the clinical needs of the people on their case load. These agencies are left with difficult dilemmas.

The pressure to rationalize insufficient treatment is great. Today, mental health workers face triage decisions that echo *Sophie's Choice.*

Each professional in this field will need to make difficult ethical decisions about how they will participate in a mental health delivery system which denies complete treatment to the majority of Americans. Some home care agencies are closing. Individual clinicians are leaving the field. Some (like our agency) are limiting our home-based child welfare cases to about 25% of their caseloads. Other agencies and individuals are drifting into incompetent work as they struggle with impossible case loads. Work in our field has never been more challenging.

Clinicians entering the homes of their clients must accept that mistakes are inevitable and clear answers are rare, but with solid organizational support and a commitment to principles, we can maintain decent standards as we work in the home.

REFERENCES

Christian-Michaels, S. (1995). Psychiatric emergencies and family preservation: Partnerships in an array of community based services. In L. Comrinick-Graham (Ed.), *Children in families at risk*. New York: Guilford.

Kesey, K. (1977). *One flew over the cuckoo's nest*. New York: Penguin.

Liddle, H. A. (1988). Systemic supervision: Conceptual overlays and pragmatic guidelines. In H. A. Liddle, D. C. Breulin, & R. C. Schwartz (Eds.), *Handbook of family therapy training and supervision* (pp. 153–171). New York: Guilford.

Teplin, L. A. (1984). Criminalizing mental disorder: The comparative arrest rate of the mentally ill. *American Psychologist, 39*, 794–803.

Teplin, L. A., & Pruett, N. (1992). Police as street corner psychiatrist: Managing the mentally ill. *International Journal of Law and Psychiatry, 15*, 139–156.

Tracy, E. M., Bean, N., Gwatkin, S., & Hill, B. (1992). Family preservation workers: Sources of job satisfaction and job stress. *Research on Social Work Practice, 2*, 465–479.

Zarski, J. J., Sand-Pringle, C., Greenback, M., & Cibik, P. (1991). The invisible mirror: In-home family therapy and supervision. *Journal of Marital and Family Therapy, 17*, 133–143.

CHAPTER FOUR

In-Home Managed Behavioral Health Care: Usage, Credentialing, and Quality Issues

Diane Stephenson

Funding issues continue to impede the development of home-based ser-vices. Medicare will only fund such services for acute, rather than chronic conditions. Private insurance has been slow to alter their coverage to include home mental health services.

Clinicians and program managers seeking reimbursement from private insurance will find the following chapter helpful. Diane Stephenson is well placed to provide us with a guided tour of managed care in the men-tal health field. She has extensive experience developing and implement-ing mental health care delivery systems in both the private and public sector. She serves as a consultant to the federal government and to pri-vate managed care companies. Dr. Stephenson is also a clinical psychol-ogist in private practice.

I n-home behavioral health care is a mode and site of treatment that is used by managed behavioral health care organizations, though not always to maximum potential or to optimal benefit for the patient. This chapter discusses the pluses, minuses, and potential problems with in-home behavioral health care from the perspective of the managed behavioral health care organization (MBHO).

Many Americans receive their medical insurance for psychotherapy, inpatient psychiatric treatment, drug and alcohol counseling, and other behavioral health care under MBHOs through their employers or through their parents' or spouses' employers. Large and small corporations; businesses; and governmental units such as counties, states, or other large organizations such as churches contract with a large local or nationwide behavioral health care organization to manage behavioral health care for that contracted company's or organization's beneficiaries (employees and dependents).

MANAGING BEHAVIORAL HEALTH CARE

MBHOs hire *care managers* to manage the care of persons seeking services. Care managers (sometimes called *case managers* or *clinical care managers*) are generally master's level clinicians. They are licensed in their professions, such as social work, clinical counseling, or nursing, and have a number of years of direct clinical experience. By referencing the MBHO's written clinical criteria, the care manager assists the provider of care (e.g., psychologist, psychiatrist, hospital) to determine the appropriate level of care for the patient (e.g., inpatient, partial hospitalization, outpatient psychotherapy), as well as the appropriate length of stay of treatment or number of sessions, given the clinical situation. A corporation, organization, or other employer would not have the resources available within its organization to evaluate the behavioral health care its employees were receiving, nor should a company have detailed knowledge about the behavioral health care treatment of its employees. Just as insurance companies review and authorize certain medical procedures and treatments based on medical necessity, so will MBHOs review and authorize the clinical appropriateness of behavioral health care.

Ideally, one of the benefits of the care-management system is that the care manager would have the knowledge and authority to creatively meet the patient's needs in the most cost-effective manner. The innovative use of home health services is a means of reaching this worthwhile objective of care management. The care management system as it operates today, however, would benefit from some changes in order to make the process operate optimally, as will be discussed later.

MEDICAL NECESSITY CRITERIA

The main goal of the MBHO is to determine the most clinically appropriate type of behavioral health treatment at the most appropriate level of care (e.g., inpatient stay, partial hospitalization, outpatient therapy, home health, etc.) to result in clinical improvement and ongoing stabilization of the patient. The cost side of the equation follows from this. The "medical necessity" criteria developed by the MBHO spell out criteria appropriate for a level of care for a patient at that specific time. Medical necessity criteria are based on patient symptomatology, his or her functioning at work and home, risk factors such as suicidality or homicidality, support systems, past behavioral health history, medical issues, and other clinical and practical indicators that indicate what a level of care and type of treatment will be the most effective and least restrictive for treating the patient. If the most appropriate level of care and modality of treatment is at a lesser degree of restrictiveness, then costs of total care are generally less, for example, using a partial hospitalization program rather than an inpatient program. If in-home psychiatric services stabilize or maintain the psychiatric stability of a patient, averting decompensation of the patient and avoiding inpatient hospitalization, then in-home care is not only of clinical benefit to the patient, but also likely to be cost-effective. MBHOs have both clinical and financial rationale to support home health care.

MEDICAL NECESSITY CRITERIA FOR IN-HOME CARE

Most MBHOs have level-of-care descriptive criteria for in-home behavioral health care. What are the indicators for in-home psychiatric care? Under what circumstances is it the "best" care, given the patient's problems and needs? Level of care criteria take into account the patient's symptoms and intensity of those symptoms, functioning level, family and community supports, and risk for harm to self or others as would the assessment for any determination of level of care. In-home criteria, however, also needs to spell out the rationale for using the in-home site of treatment rather than a provider's office. This may include:

- patient is not ambulatory;
- patient shows an extensive history of noncompliance with office visits resulting in extreme destabilization and need for higher levels of care;
- other persons in the home need to be included in the assessment and/or intervention, such as, other family members, parents or children;
- other home-based factors need to be assessed to determine their influence on the patient's destabilization or inability to show improvement, such as nutrition and safety.

BENEFITS OF IN-HOME PSYCHIATRIC CARE

The benefits of in-home behavioral health care can best be exemplified through real life examples that take into consideration both medical necessity factors as well as the unique aspects of in-home care.

MEDICAL PSYCHIATRIC CARE AND MOBILITY CONCERNS

Example 1

An elderly widowed woman, Mrs. T, has had depressive symptomatology intermittently for years. She is on a limited income, has vision problems, and is diabetic. She is on antidepressants. Mrs. T has no immediate family members in the area, lives in her own home, and does not drive. She appears to be forgetful but, to date, medical tests have not diagnosed a medical cause for the forgetfulness.

Medical Necessity. Mrs. T meets medical necessity criteria for ongoing medication management for her antidepressants. She is stable on the antidepressants but needs to be monitored regularly for compliance based on her forgetfulness and for dosage side effects given her age and issues regarding the interface with any other over-the-counter or prescribed medications she may be taking.

Mobility. Mrs. T would have great difficulty making it to an outpatient psychiatrist's office on her own.

Compliance and Health Concerns. A home health nurse was assigned to make regular visits to Mrs. T's home between infrequent visits to the psychiatrist's office. The nurse evaluated Mrs. T's psychiatric symptoms and her psychiatric stability at each visit. The nurse arranged a weekly system for Mrs. T to take her antidepressants and checked to see if they were taken. The nurse reviewed the medication diary and all medications left in the designated medication area in Mrs. T's kitchen. The nurse also determined what type of food was in the house, ascertained if Mrs. T was continuing to get meals delivered once a day, and how much she ate of those meals. In addition to assuring that Mrs. T was getting necessary nutrition, changes in diet could affect the potency of the medication and could indicate a revised dosage level. The nurse checked to see if there were other medications that Mrs. T had begun taking to evaluate interactions between medications. Mrs. T looked forward to and appreciated the home visits. She remained stable psychiatrically.

Example 2

A late-night fight between an adolescent and her parents presents another opportunity for clinically and cost-effective use of in-home care. Where such a fight includes physical violence and/or threats of harm to the adolescent, parents, or others, an in-home crisis team dispatched immediately from a treatment center or program can often defuse the situation. The team conducted an in-home evaluation, determined if any psychiatric issues indicated placement in a psychiatric facility or program, and assessed whether options other than psychiatric placement would be workable. The adolescent did not need psychiatric placement but needed to be out of the home for a few days to defuse the home situation and to allow the parents and child to have some outpatient sessions addressing key issues prior to the adolescent's returning to the home. In the past, circumstances like a fight between an adolescent and her parent often resulted in the adolescent's admission to an inpatient unit. In this instance, an immediate in-home assessment, crisis intervention, and a sound outpatient treatment plan avoided a facility placement.

Example 3

A single woman recently adopted twin, four-year-old girls from an orphanage in an Eastern European country. The twins were exhibiting persistent, destructive acting-out behaviors, suggestive of reacting to the trauma of the changes and continuing attachment issues. The adoptive mother had a chronic but not progressive physical condition that caused her to tire readily. The adoption was headed on a collision course, despite the good intentions of the adoptive mother, her involvement in an adoption support group, a psychological assessment, and some play therapy being offered to the girls. An assessment indicated that creative wraparound, in-home services to support the mother, to give her concrete parental guidance, and to demonstrate useful behavioral techniques in the home setting were clinically necessary for the mother and daughters and would help stabilize the adoptive family and save the adoption. A psychiatrically trained master's level child guidance specialist came to the home several times a week over several months and intermittently thereafter to model for the mother and work with her on structured behavioral techniques to reinforce positive behaviors and provide clear structure and expectations for the children. It had the secondary benefit of providing much needed support for the mother. She then had someone who clearly observed and was empathic to the stress she was under but was able to provide care and a different perspective, as she observed and learned.

These three examples exemplify several of the uses and concrete benefits of in-home care: enhancing treatment compliance, averting escalation of a problem requiring placement in a higher level of care, incorporation of therapeutic lessons learned in a day-to-day home setting, and support and evaluation of factors in the home that would never have been known had the patient been seen only in an office setting—diet, safety, cleanliness, availability of toys and appropriate creative play activities for children, and capability of handling the activities of daily living (ADLs) on a day-to-day basis. Secondary benefits include: greater likelihood for the patient to remain stable at an outpatient treatment level of care and reduction in total costs since maintaining the patient's stability through in-home treatment reduces the likelihood of decompensation and the subsequent need for a higher level of care, such as inpatient hospitalization.

STRUCTURE OF THE MANAGED BEHAVIORAL HEALTH CARE ORGANIZATION

To better understand the framework and constraints the managed behavioral health care organization's (MBHO) care managers face, the financial structure, intent, and focus of the MBHO should be clarified.

CAPITATION

The MBHO may contract to provide all care for all the covered beneficiaries for a set amount of money, often set up as a PEPY (per employee per year) or PEPM (per employee per month) arrangement. This is referred to as capitation (of which there are a number of different forms). In general, the MBHO is paid the same amount of money every month or every year for a member (each covered beneficiary) regardless of how many or how few services are used by the member or the costs of the services used. The total dollar amount paid to the MBHO will often include: the cost of care managers to manage, review, and determine medical necessity for the care; all administrative costs of the MBHO for administering that contract (e.g., account management liaison, clerical and administrative services, quality management staff); the costs of all patient care (e.g., all costs for inpatient psychiatric stay, costs of psychotherapy, costs of all other approved care); and any profit margin the MBHO builds in. If the MBHO miscalculated its costs, however, or if the claims costs for patient care were particularly high for a period of time, costing the MBHO more than the PEPY originally assessed, the MBHO may need to absorb those unplanned extra financial amounts and operate without a profit or at a loss for that particular contracted organization.

For other companies, however, the MBHO charges for administrative services only (ASO). This includes the costs of care managers to review prospective and concurrent care for medical necessity and all associated administrative costs to keep the MBHO functioning, growing, and profiting. It does not include the actual direct costs of patient care—inpatient treatment, psychiatrists' fees, psychotherapy, and all other claims costs. These fees are paid from the company's or organization's own insurance funding, that is, the company may be self-insured and only contract for the MBHO to manage the behavioral health care since the MBHO employs clinical staff who would have an understanding of medically necessary psychiatric care. There are a number of other financial and operational structures for the management and provision of behavioral health services. There are also variations on the two major models of funding structures for the MBHO services, but those provided are two of the more common, basic models.

REIMBURSEMENT TO PROVIDERS OF BEHAVIORAL HEALTH SERVICES

The MBHO, which manages the provision of behavioral health care for members, establishes arrangements for payment reimbursement to the providers (e.g., hospitals, psychiatrists, psychologists) who actually provide the clinical treatment. The MBHO may have a capitation agreement with a provider group. The provider group, which may provide services at a single level of care, such as outpatient therapy, or services at a number of levels of care, such as inpatient and partial hospitalization and intensive outpatient care, could have a capitation agreement with the MBHO where the group receives a set amount of money per year to provide services to an agreed-upon member population. Or, the MBHO may have a fee-for-service arrangement with providers, that is, the MBHO contracts with individual and facility (hospital) providers of care to pay the provider a set amount of money for *each* service provided to each patient.

BENEFIT PLAN AND CREDENTIALING

Research and clinical studies support the use of psychiatric home health programs (Amundson, 1989; Pigott & Trott, 1993; Thobaben & Kozlak, 1990). The clinical, practical, and financial benefits of in-home care are evident from the previous examples. For MBHOs that serve private sector client organizations (e.g., corporations), however, a matrix of quality and systems factors must come together before in-home care can be used on an individual basis for a particular patient with a particular set of circumstances. These factors include the following:

- The benefit plan coverage must include provisions to cover the costs of in-home care as well as various types and forms of in-home care.
- Providers of the in-home care and the in-home programs need to meet certain credentialing, licensing, and quality standards.
- The in-home programs need to be easily located in any given community throughout the country to enable the MBHO's clinical care managers to know of the programs, to refer patients to them, and to approve/certify the care and payment for the home health care services.

BENEFIT PLAN COVERAGE

The health benefit plans for most employers cover certain standard levels of care and treatment modalities for psychiatric/mental health conditions. These are spelled out in the plan's SPD (summary plan description). The SPD is a document most employer companies and employer organizations develop that includes, in greater or lesser detail, the services that are covered by and the services that are excluded from coverage in the employee health benefit plan. The SPD describes the medical diagnoses and treatments that are covered by the benefit plan as well as the behavioral health diagnoses and treatments that are covered by the plan, or those that will be paid for in part or in whole through the plan coverage. Regarding behavioral health coverage, the benefit plans usually speak to covering the basic levels of behavioral health care: inpatient hospitalization, partial hospitalization, intensive outpatient programs, outpatient psychotherapy, and outpatient medication management. The benefit plans of many corporations and organizations, however, do not include in-home care. Plans often do not state specifically that in-home care for behavioral health diagnoses is a covered benefit that would be paid for through the health insurance coverage.

This is unlike plans and services that are available to public sector patients, those entitled to Medicaid or Medicare benefits. The benefits managers who established the benefit plan coverage for private sector corporations and organizations did not perceive that their employee and covered dependent population would need in-home psychiatric services. Because the covered population consisted of employed persons and their dependents, the employee's family unit was considered to be high functioning and to have resources, so the family's access to support persons and services precluded the need for in-home services. Also, when the SPDs for many corporations and organizations were originally developed, in-home *psychiatric* care services were not fully developed in many communities so they were not thought of as a readily available, sound, or usable treatment modality for psychiatric care and, hence, were not even spoken to in the SPDs.

BENEFIT PLAN "FLEXES"

Because most benefit plans for private sector corporations and organizations do not address psychiatric in-home care services, the care manager or other MBHO clinician involved in managing the patient's care often needs to "flex" services to approve, arrange, and refer someone to in-home services. "Flexing" services means counting in-home services against a standard level of care already approved under the benefit plan. For instance, if a psychiatric RN makes weekly visits to a homebound schizophrenic patient for monitoring and medication management, this may be counted against the standard outpatient services on a one-for-one basis. Often, benefit flexes need to be approved by the company's benefit administrator. This is a cumbersome process requiring final approval by persons without behavioral health clinical backgrounds.

CREDENTIALING CRITERIA

MBHOs have established processes in place to add individual providers, groups, and program treatment services to their network of providers and treatment programs. This is called *credentialing.* The MBHO sets criteria for individual behavioral health practitioners and for behavioral health treatment programs. Credentialing criteria for individual psychotherapists might include: Master's degree or higher in a mental health field; license to practice independently at the highest clinical level granted by the state; at least five years of direct clinical psychotherapy experience; and malpractice insurance.

MBHOs will generally credential in-home psychiatric care services by specific service or treatment program rather than credentialing en masse all types of in-home programs offered by a particular organization or hospital. That means that an MBHO's provider credentialing department will need to review each and every type of in-home service offered by the organization to assure that each service meets the MBHO's standards. Once an MBHO credentials an individual practitioner or treatment program, that entity becomes a part of the MBHO's provider network. The clinicians (care managers) employed by the MBHO to evaluate and manage the patient's behavioral health care will reference, via computer search, the MBHO's provider network of credentialed practitioners and programs as treatment sources for patients.

The following subsections indicate typical criteria required by MBHOs to credential different forms of in-home behavioral health programs.

24-Hour Crisis Services

- Meet state licensing criteria and applicable state, local, and federal laws
- Offer telephonic and face-to-face mobilization availability 24 hours a day, 7 days a week
- Offer essential program components such as comprehensive crisis evaluation services both telephonically and face-to-face
- Program staff must include: MD/DOs or RNs, licensed mental health professionals, other trained staff.

The roles of these "program staff" and how they are used in the provision of crisis services is of concern to the MBHO. In general, the MBHO expects that program oversight and responsibility are held by the MD or other higher-level, licensed and degreed mental health professional. Clinical mental health and chemical dependency assessments of both the patient and the family must be conducted by licensed, master's level, mental health professionals. These assessments may be supplemented by non-clinical assessments conducted by experienced paraprofessional staff. Those assessments may include:

- Evaluation of the patient's living necessities—how he/she is getting food, shelter, medical care, medications, employment.
- How the patient is getting to and from medical and behavioral health appointments.
- Whether the patient needs referrals to job placement or job training programs, shelters, community services.
- If there are other support services in use or that could be pulled in.

Assertive Community Treatment Programs

These programs provide and arrange for the provision of services for clients with chronic mental illness so they can live, work, and socialize in the community environment. The programs assist the client in the development of daily living skills, social skills, and vocational skills.

Credentialing criteria may include:

- Meet state licensing criteria and applicable state, local, and federal laws
- Formal, written agreement with a provider of inpatient services in case of need for both emergency medical and emergency psychiatric care
- Telephonic and mobilization availability 24 hours a day, 7 days a week
- Qualitative program components including: capability and expertise in making assessments and referrals to services offering assistance with basic needs such as housing and food; knowledge, use and coordination of support systems such as community services, religious organizations, self-help groups; and coordination of services for vocational, job-training goals, and skill development
- Offer monitoring of treatment and medication management
- Conduct crisis intervention
- Conduct complete mental health/substance abuse assessments as well as assessments of daily living needs
- Program staff must include: MD/DOs or RNs, licensed mental health professionals, other trained staff.

Psychiatric/Mental Health Home Care

These services include the more traditional home health services, comparable to medical home health services that have been in existence for many years. Services may entail a psychiatric nurse going to the home of a homebound patient at regular intervals to assure that psychotropic medications are being taken as prescribed or to administer injections of antipsychotic medications. The nurse or another staff person may, at the same time, conduct an "eyeball" survey of the home to assure that there is adequate nutritional food and that there are no evident home health hazards. Because the use of home health for medical services is well established, there are more structured local and nation-wide credentialing criteria for these traditional services in existence than for the other behavioral health home services. Adding psychiatric services to these established programs has merit. The credentialing for psychiatric services has piggy-backed on the credentialing for medical home health services. For example, the Joint Commission on Accreditation of Healthcare Organizations (JCAHO) accredits home health agencies; states have licensing criteria for home health agencies.

Credentialing criteria for these psychiatric home health services include:

- State licensing as a home health care service
- Licensed staff and a program director who is a licensed, master's level or above, mental health professional
- JCAHO accreditation
- Formal, written agreement with a JCAHO-accredited provider of medical and psychiatric inpatient services in case of need for either emergency medical or emergency psychiatric care
- Structured program components must include the capability for providing certain services such as: 24-hour crisis services and crisis evaluation; referral arrangement capabilities; a staff or consulting psychiatrist; capacity for psychiatric, medical, and psychological evaluations; family and individual assessments, evaluations, and therapies; and medication monitoring.

These are sample credentialing criteria for a number of in-home psychiatric services. For every form of in-home service, MBHOs have separate and distinct credentialing criteria, enabling the in-home program to be a part of the MBHO's provider network. Once part of the MBHO's provider network, the program will receive direct patient referrals from the MBHO's care managers.

PROVIDER AND NETWORK DEVELOPMENT ISSUES

In addition to the specialized credentialing criteria specified above, there are many other aspects to home health programs that are of concern and interest to MBHOs. Those include: scope and services offered through the home health organization; continuity of care for the patient; clinical background of staff; and training and supervision provided to staff. In addition to these quality issues, the MBHOs must consider a practical issue of primary importance; that is, given the time it takes to review and credential each program, how can many in-home services and programs be added to the MBHO's provider network so they are readily accessible to the care managers who must access them and refer patients to them?

IN-HOME SERVICES OFFERED THROUGH HEALTH CARE ORGANIZATIONS

Many different mental health services may involve some in-home services. In *traditional psychiatric home care,* modeled after medical home care services, a nurse may go to the home to assess the patient on a regular basis, monitor the patient's condition, administer medication injections, or manage medications. *Crisis programs* involve a crisis team making an emergency visit to the home in the case of an escalated home/family situation. *Multisystemic therapies,* effective with adolescent offenders, are family- and community-based treatment systems. Professional clinicians (PhD, MSW, RN) as well as BA level paraprofessionals conduct counseling with the family in the home or community setting and establish intervention and coordination plans with schools, youth groups, churches, and other community programs and sites. *Assertive community treatment programs* provide for services necessary to enable persons with a chronic mental illness to live, work, and socialize in the community environment. *Wraparound programs* are generally used for family situations where a combination of parental support, child guidance, and other family support activities reduce the psychiatric symptomatology of one or more family members. Other variations of these major clinical interventions involving in-home services or a combination of in-home and community services exist in many forms.

Given the vast array of types of in-home behavioral health programs and the creative new pilot programs that community mental health centers and private and public agencies frequently establish to address the needs in their communities, the MBHO with nationwide accounts can find it an enormous administrative and clinical task to evaluate the quality, consistency, and effectiveness of each program and to bring each program into the MBHO's nationwide network of provider organizations.

In addition, the many forms of in-home behavioral health services are often provided by different types of organizations. The traditional in-home RN psychiatric services may be offered by home health agencies that specialize in medical home health care. These agencies are often not staffed or equipped to handle crisis services. The adolescent crisis services may be offered by psychiatric hospitals or community mental health or health departments. An MBHO, therefore, may need to locate and review the programs of, and contract with, many different organizations, each of which may offer one form of in-home care.

CERTIFYING CARE

MBHOs are familiar with and have historically contracted with licensed psychologists, social workers, and psychiatrists for outpatient clinical services. They contract with hospitals and community agencies for inpatient, partial hospitalization, and intensive outpatient services.

The array of available in-home services, however, do not often fit into the neat packages of the standard treatment modalities cited previously. If a homebound person needs therapy once a week and a clinical psychologist goes to the home to conduct the therapy, this form of in-home treatment equates nicely with one session of outpatient therapy and may so be justified under a company's benefit plan. If a child guidance specialist, however, visits a home on a regular basis to model behavioral techniques for the parent(s) in the child's home environment, this activity does not offer such a neat package for approval of services under the mental health plan. The service is generally not offered by a licensed mental health professional but by a BA or MA level professional trained in child guidance but not clinical treatment. Most companies' benefit plans state that mental health services must be performed by licensed mental health professionals. Also, the service provided is not, strictly speaking, a clinical psychiatric service even though behavioral child guidance may be the best service to treat the problem situation. So, the wraparound treatment service may not be allowable under a company's benefit plan. Likewise, the use of a certified nursing assistant (CNA) to work a full shift in a patient's home to monitor a patient with a serious history of self-abuse and suicide attempts is not a covered benefit under the behavioral health sections of most benefit plans.

MEDICAL VERSUS PSYCHIATRIC COVERAGE

Other types of in-home services provided to patients with behavioral health problems by paraprofessionals may fall under the medical portion of the benefit plan (as opposed to the behavioral health portion), such as personal care services for a patient with dementia or brain damage. When patient care and treatment overlap the medical and the psychiatric domains, bureaucratic nightmares can result. Care managers of the company managing the medical care and the company managing the behavioral health care can agree that the care is appropriate and necessary, however, representatives from both companies may assert that the service does not fall under their portion of the benefit plan and that they would have no contractual basis on which to pay the claims. Although the "who pays?" dilemma can result any time there is interface between behavioral health and medical care, it is more likely to occur in the provision of home health care since a higher proportion of patients will have joint medical/behavioral problems. Many telephone calls, e-mails, and conversations may be needed to clarify who the claims payor should be, an activity that many home health patients may not be capable of handling on their own.

CONTINUITY OF CARE

Continuity of a patient's care throughout all of his or her treatment in a behavioral health care system is of concern related to both in-home services and health care in general. *Continuity of care* refers to the coordination of services as the patient moves from one service provider or organization to another. For instance, if a patient moves from a psychiatric inpatient hospitalization to a partial hospitalization program at the same hospital while continuing to have the same primary psychiatrist and therapist, this would be an indicator of strong continuity of care. If the patient moves to a partial hospitalization program at a different facility and with different primary clinicians, the continuity of care may not be strong or effective unless the two program clinicians involved have excellent communication and share all pertinent information about the patient. Even then, the patient may have difficulty adjusting to changing venues and clinicians.

How does the continuity of care issue relate to in-home behavioral health care? Again, the importance of coordination and communication between the providers of care cannot be over-emphasized. If the in-home services are provided by the hospital that provided inpatient care or by the organization that provided outpatient services, the in-home providers would have access to records and would be able to pick up where the previous program and treatment left off. Often, however, less than comprehensive information is provided to new providers. Sometimes critical information is missing in the handover of the case, such as all the medications prescribed, complete past history, support persons who have been involved in treatment, and all aspects of the treatment plan. Even if the same umbrella organization provides both outpatient office treatment and in-home treatment, the home health team is often comprised of entirely different members than the in-office treatment team, resulting in gaps in communication, disruption to the patient, and inconsistencies in treatment.

CLINICAL BACKGROUND OF STAFF

The two aspects to this issue are: (a) what credentials the MBHO will pay for, and (b) what credentials are clinically appropriate for the specific clinical services being provided. The two are not always in agreement.

The typical credentialing criteria of MBHOs cited previously require that home health programs be directed by licensed master's level (or higher) degreed staff. The MBHO may require that the initial in-home assessment must be conducted by a master's level, licensed, experienced clinician. Although a paraprofessional may accompany the clinician for the initial assessment to conduct the health and safety survey of the patient's living situation, the MBHO may determine that the services of two staff members are not necessary except in a family crisis situation. So, the MBHO is likely to pay only for the services of the licensed clinician whether a paraprofessional provided some services or not. Under the MBHO's standards and policies, specific services can only be reimbursed if they are provided by persons with specific credentials.

The issue of who (with what credentials) should be providing the in-home service is open to considerable debate. Although the credentials needed by the service provider are clear cut in some instances (e.g., an RN to provide medication monitoring, or an MSW or PhD psychologist to provide traditional psychotherapy), in other instances it may be argued that a BA or a non-degreed person may be able to provide the service. The initial in-home assessment is critical in identifying the full range of clinical, diagnostic, and situational issues the patient is confronting, so it should be conducted by a master's-level, licensed clinician. A routine check-in might be provided by a well-trained paraprofessional with a clear checklist and guidelines on what to look for and whom to call if anything out-of-the-ordinary is expected. The MBHO, however, is not likely to pay for that person's services since, if it did not require a clinical professional, it may not be considered a medically necessary service.

MBHO contracts providing behavioral health services to public sector clients/patients are an exception. Supportive services *are* often considered medically necessary for public sector clients since, if the support service were not available, the client may not be able to maintain behavioral health stability or to access or make maximum use of the clinical services. Government contracts often require that supportive services be built into the contract; contracts with private companies or organizations seldom, if ever, include extensive supportive services, which means that those services would not be paid for under the medical benefit plan. This is unfortunate since, in reality, many persons need a full scope of support services whether they are covered under private or public sector funding.

TRAINING AND SUPERVISION OF IN-HOME STAFF

In-home care sets up a different dynamic for the providers of the services than office-based care, whether those providing care are licensed clinicians or paraprofessionals. In the office, the therapist is on his or her own territory, generally has access to other clinicians, and has a greater sense of structure and control than when providing services at another site. Roles and boundaries are less clearly defined. The clinician may be at the home of a bed-ridden, depressed patient for the purpose of conducting psychotherapy when the patient requests assistance getting to the bathroom and using the toilet. This brings both a service role and a degree of intimacy that is otherwise far outside the boundaries of the traditional therapist-patient relationship. In the provision of in-home services such as wraparound or adolescent/parent therapy, the therapist or other professional becomes more a participant of the family constellation than in office-based treatment. Though licensed and experienced clinicians may be more conscious of what the issues are in these situations than paraprofessionals, both groups are likely to need and to benefit from intensive training and ongoing supervision and/or consultation. The therapist or paraprofessional is likely to encounter a broader range of unanticipated situations than he or she has encountered in office-based treatment settings. In working with complicated family situations, with patients with unstable personality disorders, or with highly dependent patients, an unhealthy or maladaptive dynamic could result with the home health staff member being drawn into the situation.

This situation could impact the progress and health of the patient or family in treatment, but could also severely stress and destabilize the home health care giver who may not have the resources to restructure the maladaptive situation. Eustis, Kane, and Fischer (1993) present a thoughtful analysis of the burnout, stress, and boundary issues confronting the home care worker. They present a strong case for thorough training and ongoing supervisory support, structure, and consultation for the home care worker. Although JCAHO requires training and supervision of staff in order to receive JCAHO accreditation, not all in-home behavioral health programs are subject to the purview of JCAHO. Supervision and training of staff is critical in all behavioral health care settings, and many inpatient and day hospital settings heavily employ paraprofessional staff. In facility settings, however, the staff operate as part of a treatment team, observe each other's behavior, have staff meetings and patient staffings, and, in general, have greater opportunity to provide ongoing support and feedback to each other. This opportunity is lacking in the home care setting.

One implication of these issues for the MBHO is that the in-home services become harder to monitor without site visits or extensive paperwork submission on the part of the in-home service and subsequent extensive and costly review time by the MBHO staff. There is also the likelihood for problems to occur that put the MBHO at legal risk.

NETWORK DEVELOPMENT OF IN-HOME SERVICES

When the MBHO's care managers determine that a particular level of care at a particular type of treatment site is appropriate for a specific patient, the care manager references the MBHO's computer-based directory of network providers of those services. These are providers that have applied to be in the MBHO's provider network and completed the extensive applications required—essentially, those that have met the MBHO's credentialing standards. At this time in the development of the MBHO industry, most have an extensive network of individual providers (social workers, psychologists, psychiatrists) as well as facility-based programs (inpatient, partial hospitalization). Most MBHOs, however, do not have a nationwide network of providers of home-based, psychiatric-related care. Although some community agencies offer creative programs than may meet the needs for in-home services at reasonable costs, programs differ greatly from agency to agency in type of services offered, requiring that the MBHO review each program individually. Some nationwide home health care companies are now in the process of expanding their home-based psychiatric treatment programs and are becoming part of the nationwide MBHO networks. Each local program of a nationwide home health care company would not need to be reviewed separately if they all conformed to the same structure, standards, and services, but the most interesting, promising, community- and home-based programs for severe psychiatric patients tend to be grass-roots, local, and small. Yet, MBHOs tend to cater to the traditional home health care models that have nationwide programs in order to maintain efficient and cost-effective nationwide network credentialing and monitoring activities. It will take a long time for the full range of home-based services to be readily available in all the locations nationwide serviced by the MBHOs and for the MBHO's care managers to seek out home-based services. Without availability and use proceeding hand-in-hand, without programs being up, running, and having an established track record, and without care managers and other professionals simultaneously seeking out home-based behavioral health program, availability and demand may never meet in the same place. If this is the case, home-based psychiatric programs may never be able to meet the true need.

ACCREDITATION AND LEGAL ISSUES

Home health services may be the recipients of legal action, as may any treatment provider or program. Liability for inadequate care, breach of confidentiality, patient harm to self or others, and other issues related to the care given psychiatric patients is generally ascribed to the provider of care and the hospital or other organization that is providing the direct care to the patient. The managed care organization, the MBHO, may also be the recipient of legal action if it did not provide appropriate oversight of the care. This again gives the MBHO cause for concern about the supervision, training, support, and safety precautions that the home health program is providing its staff.

The National Committee for Quality Assurance (NCQA) has established standards for accreditation of MBHOs. This accreditation process can be compared with the JCAHO accreditation for hospitals and other facility-based programs. In order to achieve NCQA accreditation, the MBHO must meet NCQA-established standards in such content areas as accessibility, availability, and referral; credentialing and recredentialing; preventive behavioral health services; quality management; members' rights; and utilization management. NCQA representatives inspect how the MBHO conducts its business in these areas. Certainly, the MBHO seeks to have the best quality providers of care for its members, with or without consideration of NCQA accreditation. It is to the advantage of the MBHO, however, to receive NCQA accreditation. NCQA accreditation can put the MBHO in a more competitive position when seeking new business since prospective client companies and client organizations will know that the MBHO has been scrutinized by NCQA and has been found to meet certain standards in prescribed areas. Also, some client organizations such as governmental entities and health plans like HMOs require that the MBHO managing the care of its members have NCQA accreditation.

What does NCQA accreditation of MBHOs have to do with home health care and home health care providers? Although the NCQA standards speak primarily to the systems, policies, procedures, and practices of the MBHO, a number of the standards also directly or indirectly address the MBHO's providers, which would include the home health provider and program. Because NCQA states that the MBHO has "a responsibility to safeguard the public," it is of the utmost importance to the MBHO that the home health provider and program have staff with appropriate credentials, especially considering the potential patient care problems that are unique to in-home services. If the in-home care program does not have systems in place to adequately train, monitor, supervise, and support staff, harm could befall the patient and/or the in-home provider. This would indicate to NCQA that the MBHO, through its lack of oversight of the in-home provider or program, failed to "safeguard the public." Failing an NCQA accreditation process shakes the confidence client companies and client organizations have in the MBHO and would likely have significant financial implications as well.

WHAT CAN BEHAVIORAL-CARE IN-HOME PROVIDERS DO TO WORK WELL WITH MBHOS?

In-home behavioral health care providers and in-home behavioral health care programs and organizations can take several steps to work more efficiently and productively with MBHOs, both at the organizational and individual levels.

MBHO CREDENTIALING STANDARDS

At the organizational level, the agency providing in-home behavioral health services should obtain credentialing information from the major MBHOs so the agency can work toward meeting the MBHO's credentialing standards, including gaining JCAHO or Commission for Accreditation of Rehabilitation Facilities accreditation, employing staff with the appropriate credentials, and offering baseline services. It would certainly be to the advantage of the home health agency to become credentialed by the MBHO and to become a part of the MBHO's provider network. This would help to assure referrals to its in-home services. In-home services that are part of a larger system of services and levels of care would be likely to obtain more patient referrals than stand-alone programs. For instance, if a hospital offers inpatient psychiatric hospitalization *and* in-home RN follow-up and medication administration, the MBHO might be more likely to approve or certify the in-home care since it would offer the opportunity for strong continuity of care for the patient. Or, if a community mental health center offers family and individual counseling as well as in-home crisis services, the MBHO may be more likely to refer an adolescent for treatment to that center, with the expectation that crisis services could be mobilized if a family situation escalated. Continuity of care between the crisis services and the outpatient family counseling services would be maintained.

PROVIDE STRONG RATIONALE

An individual providing in-home psychiatric services or a representative of a home health service seeking to gain approval or certification from an MBHO for in-home services for a particular patient should be able to provide certain information to the MBHO's care manager. In addition to offering standard clinical assessment information, the in-home representative should be specific in identifying why this particular patient or situation needs to be treated in the home versus an office setting. Is the patient bedridden or not ambulatory? Is the patient very disorganized and does he/she have a significant history of missing office appointments with subsequent decompensation? Does the whole family or domicile unit need to be involved in the treatment, such as in adolescent/family crisis situations? Is the home situation a necessary part of the treatment process, as in the wraparound services described previously? The in-home representative may suggest that the in-home care be "flexed" if such care is not offered by the member's health benefit plan. If the in-home care overlaps between the medical and psychiatric health benefits, such as depression medication administration by an RN for a depressed patient with Alzheimer's disease, the in-home representative may suggest that different services be covered under the medical and the psychiatric benefit plans.

SUGGEST THE BENEFITS OF HOME-HEALTH CARE

Unfortunately, over the past few years care managers for the commercial insurance programs (the non-public sector programs) have been acclimated to think only of the traditional level of care options—inpatient, partial hospitalization, outpatient psychotherapy—and not of the innovative programs that may actually provide the best care for the patient's needs. The in-home provider may be in the position to suggest certain innovative programs to the MBHO care manager.

The provider of in-home services may seek creative solutions and partnerships with the MBHO through the care manager. For instance, the Alzheimer's patient may need in-home monitoring by a psychiatric RN, but may also require a paraprofessional to assess the safety and nutritional conditions and possibly a CNA to perform some day-to-day daily living activities. For some conditions, whereas the MBHO arranges for the RN's visits with payment through the benefit plan of the company the patient retired from, community services and public funding through Medicare or Medicaid programs may be drawn in to provide the full scope of services the patient needs. In addition, MBHOs often do not provide full case management services, that is, the MBHO is unlikely to identify the full scope of services the patient needs in such areas as meals-on-wheels, home cleaning, or nursing assistance and then to arrange for such services to be provided. This type of traditional case management is beyond the scope of the psychiatric and chemical dependency benefit plan description, so the MBHO would not receive funding from the private sector to pay for these services. Community mental health centers and similar agencies are more likely to provide these forms of case management services. Creative partnerships can be arranged, utilizing both private sector (the health benefits received through an employer or previous employer) and public sector funding (Medicare, Medicaid, special state-funded programs). For instance, *medically necessary* clinical services such as psychotherapy or medication monitoring may be provided through the employer's health benefit plan while the environmental assessments and check-ins conducted by paraprofessionals may be provided through public sector funding. This may require coordination between the MBHO care manager and the community-based mental health center's case manager. The time and effort involved are deterrents to this optimal, effective, and thorough coordination of care.

Although a mental health professional may feel strongly that the MBHO *should* provide the full scope of in-home services a psychiatric patient needs, the current claims payment and contractual agreements between the MBHO and the client company or organization may not allow for the payment of such services through the psychiatric section of the company's benefit plan (commonly called "mental/nervous" in the insurance industry). If some of the services (e.g., a patient nutritional analysis) are not direct psychiatric services, they are generally not covered for payment under the psychiatric portion of the benefit plan. It is unfortunate that in this country many of the services an individual needs are provided and funded separately by different organizations (e.g., medical care, psychiatric care, nutritional and safety services), so the holistic approach to full patient/person care is missing. Care is provided through separate "silos." Although many states are now in the process of establishing linkages and coordination of services for their Medicaid populations, that service linkage is missing for most employed persons, though some of the more forward-thinking, creative, employee assistance programs (EAPs) perform some linkages in services for their company's employees.

SUMMARY OF MBHO CONCERNS WITH PSYCHIATRIC HOME HEALTH CARE

In-home behavioral health services are a newer treatment modality. Their acceptance and use is hampered by a number of issues. One of the mandates of the MBHO is the protection of the consumer (the individual client/patient) and the protection of the client organization (the company or organization contracting with the MBHO to provide care management). The lack of control over care provided in the home inevitably makes monitoring more difficult and the risk higher. Extending coverage into a more comprehensive domain than the traditional levels of care may be beyond the funding capabilities of MBHOs, or at least of MBHOs in their present form. Therefore, it is safer, easier, and, in the short run, more economical to use the levels of care currently in the MBHO networks and not to add additional levels. The smaller, local MBHOs and local HMOs may be able to make greater strides in the creative use of psychiatric home health services than the nationwide MBHOs.

Psychiatric home health care and behavioral health programs that involve in-home treatment have been shown to be clinically sound, to result in positive outcomes, and to help maintain the patient in the home environment. They are often cost-effective forms of psychiatric treatment. Before MBHOs offering services for private sector patients can fully embrace these programs, however, a number of factors need to be considered and operationalized. The benefit plan through which the employee and his/her dependents receives the behavioral health benefit ("mental/nervous") must allow payment for such services. The agency or program providing the home health services must be easy to identify and locate by the MBHO's clinical care managers. Home health programs need to meet certain credentialing standards established by the MBHO. The home health program or service must have training, monitoring, supervision, support, and guidance systems in place to provide its professional and paraprofessional home health staff the skills to handle professionally the specific issues that arise in the provision of home health care. Since many MBHOs manage behavioral health services for patients nationwide throughout the United States, there must be consistency in in-home program services. The MBHOs, the in-home programs, and the behavioral health industry in general need to work together in partnerships to develop new programs and new ways of authorizing, delivering, and funding behavioral health care that will assure the availability and provision of the best comprehensive behavioral health care for each person's needs.

REFERENCES

Amundson, M. J. (1989). Family crisis care. *Issues in Mental Health Nursing, 10,* 285–296.

Eustis, N. N., Kane, R. A., & Fischer, L. R. (1993). Home care quality and the home care worker: Beyond quality assurance as usual. *Gerontologist, 33,* 64–73.

Pigott, H. E., & Trott, L. (1993). Translating research into practice: The implementation of an in-home crisis intervention triage and treatment service in the private sector. *American Journal of Medical Quality, 8,* 138–144.

Thobaben, M., & Kozlak, J. (1990). Home health care's unique role in serving the elderly mentally ill. *Home Healthcare Nurse, 8,* 37–39.

Legal Minefields of Psychiatric Home Care

Mark Epstein

Mark Epstein, JD, concentrates in mental health law and has litigated some of the leading mental health law cases in Illinois.

His law firm, Epstein and Epstein, is a general and litigation firm concentrating in the areas of mental health law, elder law, probate law, and related matters. He is also an adjunct Professor of Law at Northwestern Law School, currently teaching Law and Psychiatry.

The following chapter reviews legal issues relevant to anyone attempting to provide mental health services in the home of a client.

THE LAW PROTECTS AMERICANS IN THEIR HOMES

The law protects Americans in their homes. It has since at least 1607 when the law of England became the law of the American colonies. Lord Coke in his *Commentaries* said "A man's house is his castle—for where shall a man be safe if it be not in his house?" And, long before Coke, another English commentator said, "One's home is the safest refuge for every one" (see *People v. Eatman*, 1950).

In addition to place, the law protects the person. Justice Benjamin Cardozo wrote:

> Every human being of adult years and sound mind has a right to determine what shall be done with his own body; and a surgeon who performs an operation without his patient's consent commits an assault, for which he is liable in damages. (*Schloendorff v. Society of New York Hospital*, 1914)

So, "A man's home is his castle"; a woman's hers. And a health professional who enters the home to intervene in a person's life—notwithstanding presumably good motives—enters a legally sanctified zone.

OBTAINING CONSENT

The first question as you approach the door should be: "Who has given you consent?" Generally speaking, if you are entering the home of the person you are seeking to treat, and that person has given you consent to enter and to treat, you will be on solid legal ground unless and until that person revokes her consent. This applies even if the person suffers from a mental disability; for, initially, all adults are presumed legally competent to direct their legal affairs (e.g., see *In re Phyllis P.,* 1998).

OBTAINING INFORMED CONSENT

Nevertheless, be cautious of accepting consent too readily. In 1990 the United States Supreme Court decided that a Florida state mental hospital may have deprived a Mr. Burch of his rights by improperly accepting his "voluntary" admission. Justice Harry Blackmun, speaking for the majority, said:

> The very risks created by the application of the informed-consent requirement to the special context of mental health care are borne out by the facts alleged in this case. It appears from the exhibits accompanying Burch's complaint that he was simply given admission forms to sign by clerical workers, and, after he signed, was considered a voluntary patient. Burch alleges that [the state health care authorities] knew or should have known that he was incapable of informed consent. This allegation is supported . . . by the psychiatrist's admission notes. (*Zinermon v. Burch,* 1990)

So, accepting the treatment consent of a mentally disabled person can be problematic.

THE CONSTITUTIONAL LIBERTY INTEREST TO BE FREE FROM UNWANTED PSYCHIATRIC TREATMENT

If accepting the treatment consent of a mentally disabled person can be problematic, treating a mentally disabled person with psychotropic medications—however therapeutic—maybe even more so. In 1990, the United States Supreme Court ruled, for the first time, that a person has a constitutionally protected liberty interest to be free from unwanted psychotropic medications. Justice Stevens explained, in fiery terms, his concerns:

> [U]nder the Fourteenth Amendment "respondent possesses a significant liberty interest in avoiding the unwanted administration of antipsychotic drugs." [There are] several dimensions of that liberty. They are both physical and intellectual. Every violation of a person's bodily integrity is an invasion of his or her liberty. The invasion is particularly intrusive if it creates a substantial risk of permanent injury and premature death. Moreover, any such action is degrading if it overrides a competent person's choice to reject a specific form of medical treatment. And when the purpose or effect of forced drugging is to alter the will and the mind of the subject, it constitutes a deprivation of liberty in the most literal and fundamental sense.
>
> "The makers of our Constitution undertook to secure conditions favorable to the pursuit of happiness. They recognized the significance of man's spiritual nature, of his feelings and of his intellect. They knew that only a part of the pain, pleasure and satisfactions of life are to be found in material things. They sought to protect Americans in their beliefs, their thoughts, their emotions and their sensations. They conferred, as against the Government, the right to be let alone—the most comprehensive of rights and the right most valued by civilized men (*Olmstead v. United States,* 1928) (Brandeis, J., dissenting)."
>
> The liberty of citizens to resist the administration of mind-altering drugs arises from our Nation's most basic values. (*Washington v. Harper,* 1990; Justice Stevens was writing for himself and Justices Blackmun and Marshall).

CONSENT AS A PROCESS, NOT A FORM

When entering a person's home, then, and proceeding to treat that person, you must take care that you have obtained his or her consent. Many people think of consent as a form, a document that a person "signs off" on. That is a mistake. Consent is a process, not a form. It is the dialogue between the patient and the provider of services in which both parties exchange information and questions culminating in the patient's agreeing to a specific intervention. On the one hand, the patient needs certain basic details in order to decide whether to accept the treatment. On the other, the service provider also needs information from the patient in order to tailor the disclosure of risks and benefits to her. This process, if it is to be effective, requires active give-and-take from both parties (Rozovsky, 1990).

GUIDELINES FOR DETERMINING CAPACITY
TO GIVE INFORMED CONSENT

How can you tell whether the person has the capacity to consent or refuse treatment? Several courts have formulated guidelines. For example: (a) Does the person know he or she has a choice to make? (b) Does the person have the ability to understand the available options, their advantages and disadvantages? (c) Is the person under some form of involuntary legal commitment or guardianship? (d) Has the person previously received the type of medication or treatment at issue? (e) If so, can the person describe what happened as a result and how the effects were beneficial or harmful? (f) Are there any interfering pathological perceptions or beliefs or interfering emotional states that might prevent an understanding of legitimate risks and benefits (see *In re Israel,* 1996).

OBTAINING SUBSTITUTED INFORMED CONSENT

If the person does not have the capacity to give informed consent, is there someone else authorized to give "substituted" informed consent? For example, has the person signed an "advance directive" giving an *agent* authority to make health care decisions when he or she is unable? Or, has the person been adjudicated legally disabled and had a *guardian* appointed by the court to make health care decisions for him or her? If the person has neither an agent nor a guardian is there a *statutory surrogate* available? A statutory surrogate is a person—usually a close relative or friend—who, without necessity of a court hearing, is authorized by state statute to make health care decisions for a patient who has been certified by his or her doctor as being mentally incapacitated. Depending upon the laws of the particular state, if you are unable to obtain informed consent from your patient/client, you may be able to obtain "substituted" informed consent from an agent, a guardian, or a statutory surrogate.

THE STANDARD FOR SUBSTITUTED INFORMED CONSENT:
"SUBSTITUTED JUDGMENT" VERSUS "BEST INTERESTS"

It is generally thought that someone making substitute decisions for an incapacitated person—a guardian, a health care agent, or a statutory surrogate—makes a decision based on the "best interests" of the person he or she is making the decision for, but current thinking is moving in a somewhat different direction. Applying "best interests" alone is seen as being overly paternalistic. It is seen as too much the product of the substitute decision-maker's own viewpoints. The more current preference is for the substitute decision-maker to set aside her own biases and, instead, "step into the shoes" of the incapacitated person to see what he or she would decide if he or she were capable of making his/her own decisions. Thus, for example, say that Doug is at the end of his life. Catherine is Doug's closest relative and has become Doug's statutory surrogate. Doug has always believed that people should not be left to suffer when their chances for quality of life is gone, even when extraordinary measures could keep a person alive for a long time. Catherine, on the other hand, believes that a miracle is always possible or that it's not for one person to cut short the life-span of another. Normally, Catherine, using her perception of Doug's "best interests" would require sustained extraordinary measures to keep Doug alive. The more current thinking, however, is that Catherine should apply the "substituted judgment" approach and, notwithstanding her own predilections, make the decision for Doug that Doug would make for himself.

Similarly, if the shoe were on the other foot and it was Catherine on life supports, Doug, notwithstanding his own philosophy, would make the decision for Catherine that Catherine would make for herself.

Substitute decisionmaking is not limited to end-of-life decisions. It applies whenever an incapacitated person needs another to make a decision for him or her. In the case of guardians making decisions for their wards, one state has formulated the approach this way:

> Decisions made by a guardian on behalf of a ward shall be made in accordance with the following standards for decision making. Decisions made by a guardian on behalf of a ward may be made by conforming as closely as possible to what the ward, if competent, would have done or intended under the circumstances, taking into account evidence that includes, but is not limited to, the ward's personal, philosophical, religious and moral beliefs, and ethical values relative to the decision to be made by the guardian. Where possible, the guardian shall determine how the ward would have made a decision based on the ward's previously expressed preferences, and make decisions in accordance with the preferences of the ward. If the ward's wishes are unknown and remain unknown after reasonable efforts to discern them, the decision shall be made on the basis of the ward's best interests as determined by the guardian. In determining the ward's best interests, the guardian shall weigh the reason for and nature of the proposed action, the benefit or necessity of the action, the possible risks and other consequences of the

proposed action, and any available alternatives and their risks, consequences and benefits, and shall take into account any other information, including the views of family and friends, that the guardian believes the ward would have considered if able to act for herself or himself [755 ILCS 5/11a-17(e).

This approach recognizes the autonomy and dignity of the individual. Although you will not be in a position to make substitute decisions for your patients, those close to your patient may often look to you for support and guidance. Keeping these principles in mind may help you help them. "It's what Mom would have wanted."

WHAT TO DO IF YOU ARE UNABLE TO OBTAIN CONSENT

What if you are unable to obtain consent from your patient/client and there is no agent, guardian, or statutory surrogate to give substituted informed consent? Then you may not proceed. What if, for example, your patient/client objects to your presence in his or her home and objects to your treating him or her; yet, the person's daughter wants you to intervene and wants you to treat and will let you into the house? If the daughter is not authorized—she does not have an advance directive, she has not been appointed legal guardian, and she is not authorized under the state surrogacy laws—you may not proceed. Certainly, double-check with your lawyer, but do not proceed unless and until you have received informed consent from an appropriate source. You may be violating statutory and common law rights of privacy and constitutional rights to be free from unwanted treatment. If the family insists that something must be done, then they should be advised to pursue legal remedies such as guardianship in order to properly assert their viewpoint.

Finally, let's say that you have obtained informed consent—either from the patient/client or from a legally authorized substitute—and you have begun to treat. What are your obligations regarding confidentiality? What are your obligations regarding mandatory reporting?

WHAT TO DO, OR NOT DO, WITH CONFIDENTIAL MENTAL HEALTH INFORMATION

The professional working in a hospital or nursing home is inured to the routine of protocols and paperwork that surrounds, protects, even alienates the professional from the client. The professional working in the home may feel free of those strictures. Yet, while the aura of legal flim-flam may be less present in the home, the law protects the individual there nonetheless, and the professional should be watchful, wherever, for legal strictures impinging client care.

Watch for confidentiality. Who must keep confidences? What confidences must be kept? Watch, also, for mandated reporting. If I see something wrong, must I tell someone? Or, can I just leave well enough alone (*People v. Eatmon,* 1950)?

We live in an information age. We then must navigate between the Scylla of too much information ("Loose lips sink ships") and the Charybdis of too little ("I don't want to get involved").

WHO MUST KEEP CONFIDENCES?

Mental health information is usually considered to be the equivalent of "top secret, for your eyes only." The reason is clear. Mental health information may include one's most personal and sacred thoughts and secrets, and mental health treatment remains widely stigmatized. Revelation of mental health treatment has literally brought down a vice-presidential candidate.

Who is required to keep mental health information confidential? The scope of confidential mental health information is usually defined by the nature of the relationship with the patient/client. The confidential relationship is often referred to as the "therapist–patient" relationship, but "therapist" is often given a broad definition. Thus, in one state "therapist" is defined as a

> psychiatrist, physician, psychologist, social worker, or nurse providing mental health or developmental disabilities services or any other person not prohibited by law from providing such services or from holding himself out as a therapist if the recipient reasonably believes that such person is permitted to do so (740 ILCS 110/2).

Pursuant to this definition it was determined that although a "pharmacist" who disclosed information about a customer's psychotropic medications was not bound by the confidentiality strictures of the "therapist–patient" relationship, a marriage counselor was.

WHAT CONFIDENCES MUST BE KEPT?

What kind of mental health information is considered confidential? Virtually all information between a therapist and a client relating to the therapeutic services are considered confidential. For example, one state law defines "confidential communication" as "any communication made by a recipient or other person to a therapist or to or in the presence of other persons during or in connection with providing mental health or developmental disability services to a recipient" (740 ILCS 110/2).

In turn, "mental health or developmental services" are typically defined as including but not limited to "examination, diagnosis, evaluation, treatment, training, pharmaceuticals, aftercare, habilitation or rehabilitation" (740 ILCS 110/2). Pretty broad. But the law goes even further: "[Confidential communication] includes information which indicates that a person is a recipient." So, virtually all communications and information involved in a therapist-client relationship is considered confidential—including the *name and identity* of the client.

Rare exceptions are made. One exception may pertain to the needed flow of information between the therapist and the therapist's employer as well as other members of the current treatment team. Also, the therapist can usually discuss the details with his or her lawyer where necessary to determine the therapist's rights and obligations vis-à-vis the client.

Also, the therapist may be required to disclose information in court proceedings. For example, the therapist's records and communications may be subpoenaed in, say, a divorce/custody proceeding. A subpoena, however, can also lay a trap for a therapist. Usually subpoenas come in the form of a command from the Clerk of the Court to disclose information. The subpoena has a very official-looking seal from the Clerk of the Court and says that if you refuse to deliver the information you will most certainly and grievously be held in contempt of court! Yet, another law may direct the therapist to disregard any subpoena that asks for confidential mental health information unless the subpoena is accompanied by a specific court order authorizing it. What is a therapist to do? The bare subpoena gives no clue that it should be disregarded if the information demanded is confidential mental health information! As a matter of good practice, this author advises his therapist clients not to disclose mental health information pursuant to subpoena unless each disclosure has been reviewed by the therapist's own attorney. Even then, good practice often dictates that the information be sealed and delivered to the presiding judge to determine if the information is properly disclosable. If the therapist believes that disclosure of any of the information may be harmful to the client or to others, or that disclosure is unnecessary because it will not further the proceedings, the therapist often can request the judge to sift through the information, in chambers, and decide bit by bit which information must be disclosed and which may remain confidential.

WHEN IS A MENTAL HEALTH PROFESSIONAL PERMITTED OR REQUIRED TO INITIATE DISCLOSURE OF CONFIDENTIAL MENTAL HEALTH INFORMATION?

Although your patient's private mental health information is carefully guarded, at times you may be required to step forward and initiate disclosure even without being asked to. For example, state and/or federal law may require you to report suspected child abuse or neglect. Also, the well-known California case, *Tarasoff v. Regents of the University of California* (1976), adopted in various forms by many other states, may require you to warn authorities or a potential victim if your patient expresses to you a serious credible threat to an identifiable victim.

Perhaps the most likely problem for home health care workers will be suspicion of elder abuse. This may be most difficult for you because the suspected abuser may also be the one paying your bill or may be the only person—short of institutionalization—available to care for the patient.

It is important to double-check your duties with a local attorney. *Do you have an affirmative duty to report? Or are you merely "permitted" to report if you wish to? If your reporting is based upon a "suspicion" how strong must your "suspicion" be?*

CONCLUSIONS

The law protects Americans in their homes. The law may even protect Americans in their homes *against you!* But properly rendered home care may be the blessing that keeps a person safe and independent enough to remain in his or her own home—in that place of "safest refuge"—in every man and woman's own "castle."

REFERENCES

In re Israel, 278 Ill. App.3d 24, 664 N.E. 2d 1032 (1996).
In re Phyllis P., 182 Ill.2d 400, 695 N.E. 2d 851 (Ill. 1998).
Olmstead v. United States, 277 U.S. 438, 478 (1928).
People v. Eatman, 91 N.E. 2d 387, 390 (Ill. 1950).

Rozovsky, (1990). *Consent to treatment: A practical guide* (2nd ed.). Boston: Little, Brown.

Schloendorff v. Society of New York Hospital, 211 N.Y. 125, 129–130, 105 N.E. 92, 93 (1914).

Tarasoff v. Regents of the University of California, 17 Cal.3d 425, 131 Cal. Rptr. 14, 551 P 2d 334 (1976).

Washington v. Harper, 494 U.S. 210, 239 (1990).

Zinermon v. Burch, 494 U.S. 113 (1990).

PART TWO

Assessment in the Home

Assessment, Attention, and Intervention

Kadi Sprengle

Moving assessments from the office into the home has reawakened interest in the fundamental issues of assessment. Is objectivity possible? What is the relationship between the observer and the observed? And does any of this have anything to do with truth?

In the following chapter, Kadi Sprengle reviews how clinicians have grappled with these questions.

To see what is directly under your nose requires a constant struggle.
—George Orwell

How do we pay attention? What should be the focus of our observations? What is the best method of observation? Do different methods of observation affect our final understanding of phenomenon? Clinicians discover over time how the way they pay attention helps determine what they see and what they conclude.

The move to home-based assessment has led researchers and clinicians from diverse fields to similar changes in perspective. The site of the assessment affects the nature of the assessment and the perspective of the assessor.

We will briefly review the assessment methods used by clinicians and researchers in four fields: human attachment research, early-childhood intervention programs, family systems therapy in family reunification programs, and psychosocial rehabilitation programs for the chronically mentally ill.

In each of these areas, there has been a shift toward a new model of assessment where the focus is on the interaction between the individual and the environment. Assessment and treatment are no longer discrete but form a dynamic exchange in which assessment can be treatment and treatment can be assessment. The individual being observed is seen as inherently interdependent rather than independent.

RESEARCH ON ATTACHMENT AND DEVELOPMENT

Some of the most thoughtful home-based assessment techniques were developed by investigators looking at the interactions between parents and small children from an ethological perspective. Ethology is an approach toward behavioral observation done in natural settings rather than in the laboratory (Lorenz, 1970–71).

Investigators such as the psychiatrist John Bowlby (1969, 1973, 1980) attempted to understand attachment between mothers and their children. To do so he used controlled observations in the homes and institutions where children lived to better understand attachment between parents and children. He observed separations and reunions of parents and children when the children were at different stages of development and in different settings.

Mary Ainsworth, a student of Bowlby's, developed a method of assessing the quality of the attachment bond between children and their parents. She called this technique the "Strange Situation" (Ainsworth, 1979).

The Strange Situation is a series of controlled observations of young children alone, with a parent, and with a stranger. This strategy revealed that young children from a variety of cultures respond similarly to separation from their parents and to meeting strangers. Ainsworth and others suggested that the Strange Situation illustrates the nature and strength of the bond that exists between a child and a parent (Ainsworth, 1977; Lester, Kotelchuk, Spelke, Sellers, & Klein, 1974). These patterns of attachment can predict later social adjustment or problem-solving abilities for the growing child (Sroufe, 1979).

Some of the observation techniques developed as research instruments became part of clinical assessment tools. For example, Marianne Marschak (1960, 1980) developed a set of structured observations of parent-child interaction which is now widely used in clinical work in the home and in the office (Jernberg, Booth, Koller, & Allert, 1991). Marschak, like Ainsworth, pioneered the use of structured methods of observation of adult-child interaction in home settings.

These research methods have strongly influenced the development of home-based assessment techniques.

EARLY CHILDHOOD INTERVENTION ASSESSMENTS

"Beginning as a downward extension of conventional, standardized testing, early childhood assessment has gradually moved out of the tester's office and into more familiar settings (e.g., homes, child care locations, early intervention programs) and has begun to use teams of assessors and many more innovative and contextually relevant techniques than ever before" (Meisels & Fenichel, 1996, p. 32).

Clinical staff and researchers in early childhood intervention programs, working with the 0 to 3 population of infants and toddlers, are in the forefront of developing new approaches to assessment which focus on the interaction between the child and the child's family, home, and environment. This orientation comes naturally when trying to study the development of toddlers.

Early-childhood intervention programs were developed to provide services to children whose development was considered to be at risk, often due to suspected disabilities. Assessment was needed to better understand the clinical needs of these children. Yet assessment also served a gate-keeping function. Scores on tests and assessment measures could determine a child's access to treatment and money. With limited space in programs, the methods of assessment came under close critical review of both parents and clinicians.

Initially, assessment was geared toward testing the individual child, separated from his or her parents. Early attempts at assessment were guided by the example of IQ tests and other standardized measures. These measures had been designed to isolate certain traits or abilities and quantify them. Researchers attempted to adapt these measures to disabled toddlers, with mixed results.

The goals of this strategy design were to construct tests that were value- and culture-free. A test was "good" if it isolated a given quality or trait away from the influence of environment. For example, in constructing IQ tests, psychologists strove to design a test that could measure native intelligence and filter out the effects of education or class background. These tests were based on the idea that intelligence existed independently of education or environment. In this view, it was possible to isolate intelligence within an individual and, in doing so, it was assumed we could learn something valuable about that person.

Because the results of these assessments often determined which children would receive special treatments and education, parents and clinicians engaged in a critical debate over the assessment process. Several issues were highlighted:

1. Should the assessment focus on the child as an individual or on the interaction between the child, the family, and the environment?

Should the assessment strive to evaluate the child independent of the environment or as a part of the environment?

2. Does assessment in a controlled setting, such as a clinic, give more accurate results than an assessment in a naturalistic setting, such as the home or a day care center?

3. Should the assessment focus on measuring disabilities or on measuring areas of competence?

4. What is the relationship between assessment and intervention? Is the relationship linear, with assessment leading to intervention leading to reassessment? Is the relationship bidirectional, with assessment and intervention each influencing the other? Is the relationship a dynamic interaction?

These discussions challenged the value and even legitimacy of context-free assessment. Yet, as clinicians and parents debated assessment, many became convinced that independent assessment of independent abilities was neither desirable nor possible with small children. Rather, the goal of assessment was to understand the disabled child in the context of his or her family and to try to determine his or her highest possible level of functioning under optimal circumstances.

Some of those advocating this radical view of inherent interdependence had watched or participated in the national debate over intelligence and IQ testing. A review of that debate may help clarify the assessment issues that continue to concern those interested in home-based assessment.

THE DEBATE OVER INTELLIGENCE AND RACE

The national debate during the 1970s over intelligence testing brought these issues into sharper focus. African Americans as a group scored lower on IQ tests than Caucasians as a group. What did this mean? A few academics proposed that African Americans were, as a group, less intelligent and that their inferior intelligence was the cause of their less fortunate economic and social standing (Jensen, 1979). Others maintained that racism and oppression caused the social inequality between Blacks and Whites, and that IQ tests themselves were biased and racist (Block & Dworkin, 1976). Controversy among academics spilled over into the larger community; on college campuses, well-attended public debates were held in the raucous atmosphere of sporting events, complete with jeering, applause, and a few fist fights.

Did the tests really measure intelligence or something else? Did the oppression and poverty that accompanies racism result in lower test scores? Did economic class have an influence on IQ scores?

Part of the conflict centered on basic issues of assessment. Is there such a thing as true intelligence, which is innate, and, like height or eye color, can be measured? Is it possible to separate out contextual influences on intelligence, such as nutrition, social economic standing, or education? Could we determine the weight of each influence? If we could separate out each influence, then we would be able to distill true intelligence out of its context.

Test developers intensified the search for a culture-free test of innate intelligence, and later versions of major IQ tests reflected these concerns.

But a gap remained between the mean IQ scores of various economic and racial groups. Those who saw IQ scores as a sign of an independent quality called intelligence continued to offer the conclusion that different racial or ethnic groups varied in their native intelligence (not just in their scores).

Some researchers disagreed. Their findings challenged the idea of context-free assessments and of context-free abilities. They argued that the search for a culture-free quality called "intelligence" was futile. Rather, they offered a view of people as inherently interdependent with, and in constant interaction with, their environment.

For example, in New York state, Sameroff studied families over a 10-year period for the presence of protective and risk factors thought to be essential to the functioning of 4-year-old children (Sameroff, Siefer, Barocas, Zax, & Greenspan, 1987). Sameroff's team of investigators found that the majority of variance in 4-year-old's verbal IQ could be explained by environmental factors. If a child had four or more risk factors in his or her environment, she or he was 20% more likely to have marginal cognitive functioning. In other words, this research found that environment played a major role in IQ.

Other research added to the growing picture of intelligence, not as an independent quality but simply as a level of functioning created by the dynamic relationship between the individual and family, environment, culture, and community (Garbarino, 1990).

Clinicians working with the disabled had established a tradition of administering evaluations in such a way to encourage the best possible performance from their disabled clients. This technique, called testing the limits, was used to get the most accurate picture of the potential functioning of a child. This strategy contrasted with academic testing which was for the purpose of comparing students with each other.

Academic tests (and most IQ tests) used a standardized administration of tests to bring fairness to the competition between students. The focus of academic testing was to uncover differences among students. Assessment of the disabled focused on differences in performance within one person. When the goal of the assessment is to discover ways to enhance performance, the distinction between assessment and intervention disappears.

The Zero to Three Work Group on Developmental Assessment formed to address these issues. Early on, members of the group agreed that assessment was for the purpose of "discovering the capacities and resources in the child and in the caregiving environment that can sustain and enhance developmental momentum" (Meisels & Fenichel, 1996, p. 6).

That simple description contains within it positions on the debates we just reviewed. Assessment should focus on the daily life of the child, including the interactions between the child, the family, and the larger environment. Assessment is not separate from interventions, and the assessment process is not a linear one. "Although areas of development can be addressed separately, they are not necessarily independent. Rather, they are interdependent" (Greenspan & Meisels, 1996, p. 13).

FAMILY SYSTEMS THERAPY

At the same time that home-based assessment measures were being developed in the field of early childhood intervention, family systems therapists were working on ways to sharpen their ongoing assessment of families being treated in the home. In many ways, a family systems perspective is especially compatible to home-based services. Like clinicians in early childhood assessment, family systems therapists saw the individual client as part of a dynamic, interactive system. Effective treatment required treatment of the system rather than the individual.

The family systems theory itself pointed to ways of adjusting therapy to best take place in the home. For example, the theory suggests that the family will induct the therapist into the family system at the same time that the therapist is trying to change that system. In the home, the pressure toward induction will be even greater (Zarski, Sand-Pringle, Greenbank, & Cibik, 1991).

Writing about their home-based family therapy program, Lindblad-Goldberg, Dore, and Stern (1998) describe the challenge: ". . . being effective on someone else's turf involves the clinical skill of working in proximity while guarding against induction into the family's dysfunctional patterns" (p. 133).

To help the therapist or assessor keep balanced, family systems theorists advocate that the therapist have the support of good, regular clinical supervision, peer support, and a sufficient discussion of the case to counterbalance the pull from the family. In this view, accurate assessment requires the development of a social support system around the assessor.

Some of the traditional assessment tactics of family therapy are enriched in the home setting. For example, the genogram (or family tree) can be drawn by the family on large sheets of paper spread over the dining room table. As this is going on, the family is participating in both assessment and treatment, as they recreate family history (Lindblad-Goldberg et al., 1998).

Although some home-based family therapy programs still bring the family into the office for a supervision session, Zarski and others (1991) bring the supervisor into the home for a special session. This session, with the supervisor acting as a consultant to the family and the therapist, fuses supervision, assessment, and treatment.

COMMUNITY-BASED ASSESSMENT WITH THE CHRONICALLY MENTALLY ILL: THE PACT MODEL OF CONTINUOUS ASSESSMENT AND TREATMENT PLANNING

The object of PACT's client-centered approach is rather simple: to help persons with severe mental illness live as autonomously as possible.
—D. Allness & W. Knoedler

Developing independently from the fields described previously, new assessment strategies grew out of the innovative work with chronically mentally ill adults lead by the PACT teams in Wisconsin.

PACT is described as a hospital without walls (Allness & Knoedler, 1998). Well-trained staff provide comprehensive treatment for their caseload of severely disturbed adults. The program is long term, as their clientele have ongoing needs for services.

Although PACT has offices, the staff spends 75% of its time in the community with clients. PACT provides most of the services needed by a client, including case management, psychiatric care, psychotherapy, help with housing and employment, and so on. Each client is served by a team of providers who meet daily to discuss their cases.

PACT's approach to assessment is thoughtful and comprehensive. For example, the admissions interview is often done wherever the client is staying. If a new client is still in the hospital, PACT staff will begin the assessment there. Once the client has agreed to services, PACT next drives the client to the PACT offices to meet staff.

Assessment and treatment planning, like the treatment itself, are done as a team. The team approach is central to assessment; the team is an assessment tool. Communications within the team, and between the team and the clients, are considered an essential part of the assessment methodology. Daily case reviews ensure that all staff are familiar with each client. Treatment planning meetings are open to all staff as well. The daily staff meeting is considered a part of the assessment and treatment planning process.

This approach is reminiscent of milieu therapy done on long-term psychiatric hospital units (when they still existed). The patients and staff were considered to have formed a community which had its own atmosphere that could either promote or obstruct healing. Interactions and communications within this community were assessed daily as an essential part of the treatment.

The beginning assessment done on new clients is a month-long process starting with intake interviews and moving on to comprehensive assessments of all spheres of functioning. In addition to over 130 pages of assessment questionnaires and guidelines, the staff relies on collecting a complete set of medical, legal, mental health, and school records. The assessments are also based on interviews with the client and the family and friends of the client.

One of the most interesting assessment tools used by the team is the Psychiatric/Social Functioning History Time Line. The time line is built by the members of the treatment team, using a chart set up for each client. As a team member reads a part of the past treatment record, she or he records the information on the time line. As the time line is constructed, patterns of decompensation and possible precipitant are revealed. Conflicting histories and blank spots also show up. Treatment failures can be seen.

> Completing the time line is labor intensive for the team staff. The older the client and more extensive the treatment records is, the longer it takes to review the record and put together the time line. However, there is no better training for the staff than learning about the problems clients with severe and persistent mental illnesses experience because of the lack of continuity of services in their care. The time line invariably turns staff into advocates for their clients and service delivery. (Allness & Knoedler, 1998, p. 47)

The time line also fulfills another important team-building and training function. Records are often neglected in home-based work. As the staff fill out the time line, they are demonstrating to each other the importance of reading and understanding the records. They are also making certain they actually do the record review.

The PACT model organizes the treatment team to become an assessment team. The team approach is central to the success of their assessments.

SUCCESSFUL STRATEGIES FOR HOME-BASED ASSESSMENTS

As assessment moves into the home, assessors from different fields are discovering similar challenges and are developing successful strategies.

Accurate assessment in the home requires extra support for the assessor. Since assessors are their own main assessment tool, we have to develop compensatory strategies to achieve clarity.

Seeing a client in the office can increase the clarity of the clinician. The same room, the same time, and the same length of time helps the therapist focus. These frames are not constructed because the therapist is special. They are constructed because the therapist is ordinary.

The office and clearly defined roles frame the behavior of the client and the therapist so that it is easier to observe subtle changes in the client. In a home setting, the clinician needs to be acutely aware of the way in which he or she comes to decisions. Objectivity is difficult to maintain as the clinician becomes part of the family system.

The shift in home-based assessments has highlighted that fact. Home-based assessment and treatment is changing to find ways of moderating the influence of the family and home on the clinician while helping the clinician stay open to and respectful of the family and the client.

Clinicians and researchers working with distinct populations are coming to similar conclusions about the assessment techniques best suited to helping the assessor see clearly. Successful programs usually contain the following strategies:

STANDARD ASSESSMENT PROTOCOLS

By approaching each new case using the same structure whether it be a list of questions, checklist of areas to cover, structured procedures or interviews, a standard approach gives the assessor increased clarity.

TEAMWORK

A team approach to assessment has proven successful. Some programs regularly schedule two therapists or assessors to meet with the family together, or bring other clinicians into the home to aid with the assessment (Lindblad-Goldberg et al., 1998; Rathbun, Lord, Koop, & McArthur, 1995; Zarski et al., 1991).

In the PACT model described earlier, all assessment and treatment is done by a team working to provide continuous assessment and treatment planning.

Other programs offer intensive case management, which, if done correctly, can become an assessment process in its own right. By introducing school, medical, and mental health professionals to each other and by collecting the records, opinions, and insights of all, the case manager can create an assessment team out of previously isolated professionals and the client (Christian-Michaels, 1995; Santos, Henggeler, Burns, Arana, & Meisler, 1995).

SUPERVISION AND CASE PRESENTATIONS ARE PART OF THE ASSESSMENT PROCESS

When the treatment team cannot come into the home to support the individual assessor, many programs have thoughtful ways of bringing the home to the treatment team.

Some teams use videotapes (Lindblad-Goldberg et al., 1998). Some assessment measures, such as the Marschak Interaction Method, are regularly videotaped so that other clinicians and the family can view and comment on the tape (Jernberg, 1985). Videotapes give the assessor a valuable second chance to notice what might have been missed on site.

Regular case presentations can also be extremely valuable (Fraser, 1995), and supervision and training are all essential to increase the accuracy of each assessment (Allness & Knoedler, 1998; Gould, chapter 7, this volume; Kinney & Dittmar, 1995; Santos et al., 1995). Unfortunately, good training and regular clinical supervision are often neglected in response to cost-cutting measures. But when the assessment moves to the home, clinical supervision is essential.

GUIDELINES FOR ENHANCING OBJECTIVITY

In home-based assessments, keeping an objective stance is more difficult. The assessor no longer has easy access to peers to discuss the case or confide strong feelings.

Successful programs have developed strategies to aid the assessor in being as objective as possible. These guidelines help the assessor maintain balance and increase clarity.

1. Talk to others about the case. Staff the case on a regular basis, either with a peer, a supervisor, or at agency-wide case conferences or rounds. If possible, use a team rather than an individual assessor.

2. If you are confused, arrange to have another person go into the home and compare notes.

3. Work to be aware of your feelings about the case, and discuss those feelings with a colleague. If you do not have a good program of supervision available to you, arrange for regular peer supervision.

4. Be clear on the limits of what you can conclude and of the weak points in your conclusions. Be aware of other conclusions or diagnoses that might fit the evidence. State in your assessment report the limits of your conclusions and possible steps to improve the accuracy of your assessment.

5. Develop a protocol for home-based assessments and follow it. By using the same approach in every house, the clinician will develop a framework for understanding families or clients in their homes.

6. Watch for parallel process, or what family systems theorists call induction into the family system. Pay special attention to any members of the treatment team who disagree with you. In some cases, staff disputes reflect important conflicts within the client or client's family. Is the client presenting one side to one provider and another side to another?

CONCLUSIONS

As the site of assessment is shifted to the home, the nature of assessment is changing as well (Meisels & Fenichel, 1996; Lindblad-Goldberg et al., 1998). Assessment is now being driven more often by an ethological, ecological, expanded family system or multisystems model of client functioning. The context is now key.

Even when a specific theoretical framework does not guide the work, as clinicians bring the treatment into the home, the home changes the treatment. Clinicians working in the home follow up new leads and develop new treatment strategies.

For example, family systems work expands to include other systems of community, culture, class, and social network. Developmental assessment of small children becomes assessment of the interplay between the child, the family, the home environment, and the treatment team. Assessment of a chronically mentally ill client leads to the development of a long-term social network woven to support the individual client within the community.

Assessment and treatment are no longer distinct. Supervision and ongoing treatment fold into assessment. Team treatment and the relationships between the treatment team, the client, and the family of the client also become part of the assessment.

As clinicians from different fields working with different populations and different theoretical orientations move their work into the home or neighborhood of the client, the clinicians themselves begin to change in a similar direction. Most find themselves drawn toward a focus on the interplay of interconnections that hold the client and the symptoms of the client in a vibrant, dynamic network where change and influence come from all directions.

REFERENCES

Allness, D., & Knoedler, W. (1998). *The PACT model of community-based treatment for persons with severe and persistent mental illness: A manual for PACT startup.* Arlington, VA: Programs of Assertive Community Treatment, Inc.

Ainsworth, M. (1977). Attachment theory and its utility in cross cultural research. In P. H. Liederman, S. R. Tulkin, & A. Rosenfeld (Eds.), *Culture and infancy: Variations in the human experience.* New York: Academic Press.

Ainsworth, M. (1979). Infant–mother attachment. *American Psychologist, 34,* 932–937.

Block, N., & Dworkin, G. (Eds.). (1976). *The IQ controversy.* New York: Pantheon.

Bowlby, J. (1969). *Attachment and loss* (Volume I, Attachment). New York: Basic Books.

Bowlby, J. (1973). *Attachment and loss* (Volume II: Separation, Anxiety, and Anger). London: Hogarth.

Bowlby, J. (1980). *Attachment and loss* (Volume III: Loss, Sadness and Depression). New York: Basic Books.

Christian-Michaels, S. (1995). Psychiatric emergencies and family preservation: Partnerships in an array of community based services. In L. Combrinick-Graham (Ed.), *Children in families at risk: Maintaining the connections* (pp. 56–80). New York: Guilford Press.

Fraser, L. (1995). Eastfield Ming Quong: Multiple-impact in-home treatment model. In L. Combrinck-Graham (Ed.), *Children in families at risk: Maintaining the connections* (pp. 83–106). New York: Guilford.

Garbarino, J. (1990). The human ecology of early risk. In S. J. Meisels & J. P. Shonkoff (Eds.), *Handbook of early childhood intervention* (pp. 78–96). New York: Cambridge University Press.

Greenspan, S. I., & Meisels, S. J. (1996). Toward a new vision for the developmental assessment of infants and young children. In S. J. Meisels & E. Fenichel (Eds.), *New visions for the developmental assessment of infants and young children* (pp 11–26). Washington, DC: Zero to Three: National Center for Infants, Toddlers, and Families.

Jensen, A. (1979). *Bias in mental testing.* Riverside: Free Press.

Jernberg, A. (1985) Assessing parent–child interactions with the Marschak Interaction Method (MIM). In C. Schaefer, K. Gitlin, & A. Sandgrund (Eds.), *Play diagnosis and assessment.* New York: Wiley.

Jernberg, A., Booth, P., Koller, T., & Allert, A. (1991). *Manual for the administration and the clinical interpretation of the Marschak interaction method (MIM): Preschool and school age.* Chicago: Theraplay Institute.

Kinney, J., & Dittmar, K. (1995). Homebuilders: Helping families help themselves. In I. M. Schwartz & P. AuClaire (Eds.), *Home-based services for troubled children* (pp. 29–54). Lincoln: University of Nebraska Press.

Lester, B. M., Kotelchuck, M., Spelke, E., Sellers, M. J., & Klein, R. E. (1974). Separation protest in Guatemalan infants: Cross-cultural and cognitive findings. *Developmental Psychology, 10,* 79–85.

Lindblad-Goldberg, M., Dore, M. M., & Stern, L. (1998). *Creating competence from chaos: A comprehensive guide to home-based services.* New York: Norton.

Lorenz, K. (1970–71). *Studies in animal and human behavior/Konrad Lorenz* (R. Martin, Trans.). Cambridge, MA: Harvard University Press.

Marschak, M. (1960). A Method for evaluating child-parent interaction under controlled conditions. *Journal of Genetic Psychology, 97,* 3–22.

Marschak, M. (1980). *Parent child interaction and youth rebellion.* New York: Gardner Press.

Meisels, S. J. (1996). Charting the continuum of assessment and intervention. In S. J. Meisels & E. Fenichel (Eds.), *New visions for the developmental assessment of infants and young children* (pp. 27–52). Washington, DC: Zero to Three.

Meisels, S. J., & Fenichel, E. (Eds.). (1996). *New visions for the developmental assessment of infants and young children.* Washington, DC: Zero to Three.

Rathbturn, S. W., Lord, D. R., Koop, F. A., & McArthur, V. B. (1995). Families in their own evaluations. In L. Combrinck-Graham (Ed.), *Children in families at risk: Maintaining the connections* (pp. 3–31). New York: Guilford.

Sameroff, A. J., Seifer, R., Barocas, R., Zax, M., & Greenspan, S. (1987). IQ scores of 4 year old children: Social environmental risk factors. *Pediatrics, 79,* 349–350.

Santos, A. B., Henggler, S. W., Burns, B. J., Arana, G. W., & Meisler, N. (1995). Research on field-based services: Models for reform in the delivery of mental health care to populations with complex clinical problems. *American Journal of Psychiatry, 152,* 1111–1123.

Sroufe, L. A. (1979). The coherence of individual development: Early care, attachment, and subsequent development issues. *American Psychologist, 34,* 834–841.

Zarski, J., Sand-Pringle, C., Greenbank, M., & Cibik, P. (1991). The invisible mirror: In-home family therapy and supervision. *Journal of Marital and Family Therapy, 17,* 133–143.

Munchausen Syndrome by Proxy

Julia M. Klco

Therapists are often the last to know about ongoing criminal activity by their clients. By working to be open and understanding, many of us disable our suspicions. By taking the assessment into the home, the assessor can gain direct information that may contradict a client's self-report.

Julia Klco uncovered a case of Munchausen Syndrome while working as a graduate student. Her account of how she came to her conclusions offers insight into the process clinicians go through when they begin to suspect their client is intentionally misleading them.

Being in the home provides the assessor with information that may reveal dishonesty or manipulation on the part of the client. On the other hand, working in the home also can lead clinicians to become so overly engaged with the client that they fail to take full advantage of the wealth of information available to them. In the home, assessors are more likely to be pulled from the role of objective observer to involved participant. Finding balance requires special attention.

Home-based assessment can be particularly illuminating when one is faced with unusual or confusing data. Having access to the family home allows the assessor to evaluate the individual in the context of the environment in which he or she lives. Sociocultural factors may be either minimized or emphasized in the home.

The additional information gained during this type of assessment can help clarify unanswered and often difficult clinical questions. The home-based assessor who is tuned to the surroundings gains information not available in a structured office interview. Sometimes what you see contradicts what you have heard; at other times, visual cues help to confirm hypotheses. For example, in one case I had been told that a child was terrified of fire, yet when I entered the family home, there was a fire in the fireplace and candles everywhere.

In the case that follows, home-based assessment was only the beginning of a lengthy and difficult search for the truth. Observations during my first home visit later helped to pull the entire case together. Names, circumstances, and identifying information have been changed to protect the children's identities and to ensure confidentiality.

The clinic where I was working received a referral from a private child welfare agency. After many years of therapy, Brian, a gangly, 11-year-old adopted child, was not getting better. Two younger siblings, Corey, age 8, and Amber, age 5, who were also adopted, were described as having behavior problems that were also resistant to intervention. The agency wanted psychological evaluations on these three children to help clarify Brian's diagnosis and to identify treatment needs for Corey and Amber. A fourth child (biological) born with cerebral palsy was still too young to be formally assessed. The caseworker reported that the children's mother, Ms. Smith, had recently been diagnosed with breast cancer and may not have long to live.

We were told that the single mother, Ms. Smith, was overwhelmed with four special-needs children. Despite intensive intervention and home-based services, the family continued to have significant difficulties. Many different agencies had worked with the family, yet there had been no progress. In fact, the children's symptoms worsened. There were recent concerns by Ms. Smith, a respite worker, and a caseworker, that Brian and Amber were engaging in inappropriate sexual behavior.

Although the case had been in the child welfare system for over 10 years, the children's behavior problems were escalating rather than remediating. We spoke with many caseworkers and therapists who had worked on this case. All were sympathetic to Ms. Smith and to the problems she encountered with her children. Despite this, the many good interventions that were attempted by therapists and welfare agency workers were without apparent benefit.

Psychological testing is almost always done in the office. There are exceptions, however, particularly when working with underserved populations. Ms. Smith's car had recently broken down and there was no money for repairs. In an attempt to accommodate the family, the caseworker hoped that psychological testing could be conducted in the home. Ms. Smith arranged for her other children to be with a respite worker while I worked with each individually.

On my first visit to the home, I met a young man outside who I assumed to be the oldest of the children I was to evaluate. I asked if his mother was inside and he responded 'Yeah, but she's not my mother." It was later learned that this was a child of a man that Ms. Smith had invited into her home because he had nowhere else to stay.

Ms. Smith's boyfriend had recently been jailed for domestic battery and was awaiting trial. Thus, we expected the family unit to consist of the four children and their mother. It was later learned that Ms. Smith's new boyfriend and his three children were also living in the home (I had first suspected this when I observed a man's shoes lined up under the mother's bed).

Prior to my first visit, Ms. Smith reported during a phone conversation that her son Brian wanted to hurt animals and would attempt it at every opportunity. She also reported that on at least one occasion he had acted on this impulse and choked a rabbit to death. Surprisingly, the house was full of pets. There were dogs, rabbits, fish, guinea pigs, and ferrets.

On entering the home, I was surprised not only by the multitude of animals but also by how clean and neat the home was, given that four "out-of-control" children lived there. One of the children led me to a hallway closet that contained games and toys. They were neatly stacked with all the pieces intact!

Ms. Smith was still in her pajamas, chain smoking, and busily working on a computer. She barely acknowledged my presence, treating me like an intruder, rather than someone who had come to her home to evaluate her children. She continued to work on her computer, virtually ignoring me until Corey became quite disruptive.

During my first visit to the home I had planned to begin a psychological evaluation of Corey, who was reportedly physically violent with his mother. Corey was initially hostile and, on meeting me, threw his hat across the room and ran into his bedroom, slamming the door. At that point in time I still didn't know that I wouldn't be evaluating any of the children that day.

After Corey went into his room and refused to come out, Ms. Smith spontaneously brought me copies of medical, psychological, and school records, and she spent over 4 hours filling me in on the case. She told me that she had been "everywhere" trying to get help for her children. She offered me copies of the records to document her extraordinary efforts. I was quite impressed with Ms. Smith's ability to advocate for her children.

Ms. Smith showed me pictures of grave markers for her children who had died either at birth or shortly thereafter. She also showed me a picture of a gravestone for Corey's twin whom she was also going to adopt, but who died shortly after birth. During this time, I was also shown file after file of records on her adopted children, Brian in particular. She pointed out all the pictures on the wall of family members, including an ex-husband's younger sister, a child who had died in a car accident at the age of 6. This little girl looked eerily like Brian's 5-year-old sister Amber. As she showed me this photograph, Ms. Smith told me that Amber had been sexually abused by a babysitter, but that the child welfare investigators never found enough evidence to prove the abuse.

On this first visit to the home, Brian was the least disruptive of the three children. A respite worker who returned with the children noted that they had been "well behaved" on their outing. Brian remained aloof while his siblings argued. He entertained himself without demanding attention. Ms. Smith ignored bad behavior, such as hitting and spitting, by the other children.

As Corey and Amber fought with each other, I noticed four poster-size sheets of paper taped to the dining room wall. The posters were behavior charts with numbers 1 to 20 written on the bottom. There was one poster for each child and each poster had house rules written on it. This list of rules included such things as no hitting, no screaming, no kicking, etc. Although I did not observe any of the rules to be enforced (although they were broken numerous times), Ms. Smith frequently threatened the children that if they continued to break the rules they would be taken to the hospital.

Over the many hours it took for Ms. Smith to tell me the story of her children and of her many losses, the children actively vied for her attention. Amber and Brian frequently went to her and hugged her. Ms. Smith's response was surprisingly stiff and cold. Her focus remained on telling me her story.

Throughout this first visit Ms. Smith continued to tell me about all the traumas the family had suffered. She related how her first husband and several consecutive boyfriends had beaten her in front of the children. These beatings resulted in multiple calls to the police and trips to the hospital. She reported having had her ribs broken at least twice, her jaw shattered, and too many black eyes and bruises to count. She told me that two of her adopted children were born prematurely as the result of horrible car accidents. She also told me that Corey's (Corey was also reported to be premature and born by emergency C-section) twin had died in the ambulance on the way to the hospital. At the time of evaluation, Corey reported suicidal ideation and a wish to join his twin in death. Ms. Smith often visited the grave of Corey's twin with him and the other children. When asked how she had obtained the details of her adopted children's births, she reported that all of her children were the result of open adoptions and that she had tracked down their histories in an effort to understand their current problems.

Ms. Smith told me that Brian had once broken Amber's arm in a rage. She reported that Brian pinned Amber on the floor and repeatedly jumped on her arm until it broke. She reported how Brian once had trouble opening the door to come inside so, instead of asking for help, he put his fist through the window, breaking the glass. Once, when a glass fell out of the cupboard and hit him in the head, he proceeded to throw all the dishes and glasses out of the cupboard onto the floor.

Ms. Smith complained that Corey beat her up almost daily and that her daughter Amber was provocative, hit, kicked, and bit her, and refused to listen. Even the baby caused her grief as he cried incessantly and had chronic urinary tract infections.

After telling me all about her children, Ms. Smith filled me in on her own traumatic history. She told me how she had been diagnosed with breast cancer over the past year and might not survive. I had earlier been informed of this by Ms. Smith's caseworker who was very concerned and wasn't even sure how long Ms. Smith would live. Ms. Smith told me how she had also been adopted, but that she was taken from her biological mother at the age of 3 and then adopted by a family she had never met.

Ms. Smith reported that as a toddler, she was hospitalized at least 20 times for asthma and had many other medical problems while growing up. She finished her story by telling me that in her early teens she had been brutally raped by a family member and that for many years she blocked out most memory of it. She also stated that the man who raped her had later died after a tragic fall at a construction site. She happened to be in the area and was present when he died.

Ms. Smith had recently found her biological mother and learned that one of her relatives suffered from paranoid schizophrenia and another from bipolar disorder. She also reported that her biological mother had cerebral palsy and was mentally retarded. Ms. Smith believed that most members of her biological family were alcoholics and/or drug users.

I left this first interview feeling quite overwhelmed and wondering how one family could survive so much trauma. It was hard to think of a bad experience that they hadn't had. I found this mother to be zealous in her efforts to get the proper care for her children, and I applauded her efforts and her struggles. That evening I sat down with the records.

A review of records provided by Ms. Smith revealed a long history of psychiatric hospitalizations and medical tests on the oldest child, Brian. In one report Ms. Smith told a social worker that his father had sexually abused Brian when the boy was a toddler. On further record review, however, it was found that these accusations were never reported to the child welfare system.

As soon as Brian was adopted, Ms. Smith sought numerous medical tests on him, including chromosome screenings, allergy tests, PKU testing, a CT scan, MRI, EEGs, and so on. She reported behavior that was out of control almost from infancy, citing inconsolable crying and aggression. When Brian was between 2 and 3 years of age, a counselor from the local health department confirmed some of Ms. Smith's reports, describing tantrums, biting, screaming, and kicking in a summary report. During this same time Ms. Smith reported that Brian refused to eat. He was diagnosed with failure to thrive, but the possibility of neglect was never considered.

Brian's first psychiatric hospitalization occurred when he was 3½. The hospital notes spoke in glowing terms of Brian. At that time he was noted to have good coping skills, was bright, and capable of dealing with others as well as expressing his feelings (notations in hospital case file). This was in considerable contrast to Ms. Smith's reports. Although children often behave better in the structure of a hospital away from their family, the contradictions were fairly dramatic. I was suddenly alarmed and concerned by the discrepancies.

By the time Brian was 9 years of age he had been through many doctors and had a chain of diagnoses: posttraumatic stress disorder, attention deficit hyperactivity disorder, bipolar disorder, separation anxiety, depression NOS, over anxious disorder, major depression, impulse disorder, explosive disorder and psychosis, asthma, and possible scoliosis.

Ms. Smith also had detailed information about Corey's history. She reported that Corey was a premature baby (32 weeks' gestation), born early as the result of a car accident and that his biological mother had required an emergency C-section. She stated that Corey weighed only 1 lb. 8 oz. She also reported that Corey had a twin, Robin, who died on the way to the hospital in the ambulance.

Ms. Smith then reported that she had a biological daughter who had also died at birth. No record of any of this has ever been found, although Ms. Smith showed me pictures of grave markers for Robin and for her biological daughter who died at birth.

As I pored over the records, I learned that in addition to Brian, Corey, Amber, and the baby were all reported to have asthma. It was also reported that Amber had had pneumonia several times and had been very sickly. I remembered that Ms. Smith was smoking heavily on my first visit to the home. It is unlikely that in a home where four children suffered from respiratory disorders that smoke and the number of animals would be tolerable for them without serious consequences.

I was beginning to question some of the information given to me by Ms. Smith. My second visit to the home brought up even more concerns. On this visit Ms. Smith provided me with a home videotape as evidence of Brian's out of control behavior. Brian, however, was again well behaved during my visit.

Amber took me by the hand on a tour of the house during which I noted all of the children's rooms to be neat and orderly. Again, a man's belongings were noted in Ms. Smith's bedroom. Amber told me that she slept on the floor in the same room with her brother Brian because another child was staying in her room. When Ms. Smith heard this she corrected Amber and said, "But that was a long time ago, you have your own room now." Amber looked down and said nothing.

Later that day, I again returned to stacks of records. Some troubling and pervasive questions emerged. There had been many failed interventions as well as reports of children who were well behaved with other caretakers and in school. Even notations during Brian's psychiatric hospitalizations painted a picture of a child very different from the one Ms. Smith had described.

An interview with Ms. Smith's jailed boyfriend cast suspicion on the existence of Corey's twin. He felt that there had never been a twin and that other biological children who the mother reported had died had never really existed. I called the cemetery where the children's headstones were and found that no one was ever buried there.

The boyfriend also reported that he and Ms. Smith had appeared on a syndicated talk show with Brian and Corey. The show was titled "My Ten-Year-Old Will Be a Serial Killer." During this show, Ms. Smith claimed that Brian had attempted to murder his brother Corey. The boyfriend further reported that Ms. Smith's motivation for wanting to do the show was to try to get more help for her children.

Ms. Smith's boyfriend told me that he was suddenly learning things about his girlfriend that he never knew. When he began to compare stories with her relatives, he realized that she had lied about many things. He told me that he had met Ms. Smith on the Internet. He suspected she had a new boyfriend whom she had acquired in the same manner. He also reported that another man she had met through the Internet had raped Ms. Smith earlier in the year at a shopping mall.

These reports by Ms. Smith's boyfriend led to a more thorough and detailed search of medical records and more collateral interviews, such as with Ms. Smith's adoptive mother. The child welfare agency assisted with subpoenas for many of the records. The information we gathered from these searches was quite startling.

It was confirmed that Corey never had a twin, that he was a full-term baby, that his mother had requested a C-section, and that it had not been an emergency. We also learned that one of Ms. Smith's boyfriends, not Brian, had broken Amber's arm. None of the children had any documented medical history of asthma or pneumonia nor were they born prematurely. Most startling was the fact that Ms. Smith had no medical history of asthma or cancer, and she never had any children who died at birth.

Instead of convincing me that her child was a monster, a critical review and evaluation of the home videotape helped to show me how Ms. Smith was provoking her child into misbehavior. For example, Ms. Smith taped Brian as he tantrumed uncontrollably and screamed incomprehensibly about something that had to do with his favorite stuffed toy. On another part of the videotape it looked like Brian was "hanging" this stuffed toy from the top of his bed. During interviews with Brian and with Ms. Smith's adoptive mother, it was learned that prior to taping Brian, Ms. Smith had put Brian's stuffed toy in the oven and then let the dog chew on it. Brian was tying the stuffed animal to the top of his bed to keep it away from the dog. Ms. Smith was so convincing in her reports to professionals involved in her case that no one ever questioned or challenged what she said or what was seen on the video. Instead, she gained everyone's sympathy and support.

Fortunately, in addition to the subpoenaed records, Ms. Smith had signed numerous releases to obtain information. Some of the agencies involved in the case either did not respond to our record requests or put roadblocks in our way. Early on in this case, many treatment professionals took sides supporting or opposing Ms. Smith, and were unable to take an objective look at the data.

Consultation with other child psychologists and a thorough literature review led me to suspect Munchausen Syndrome by Proxy. Munchausen Syndrome is a well-recognized disorder first characterized by Asher (1951), although the subject after whom it was named, Karl Friedrich Hieronymus, Baron von Munchausen, did not suffer from the condition (Goodwin, 1998; Smith & Killam, 1994). The baron was essentially an enthusiastic storyteller who embellished tales about his travels, entertaining many and gaining a reputation for not being truthful.

Munchausen Syndrome by Proxy was identified in 1977 by Meadow (Parnell & Day, 1998; Schreier & Libow, 1993). It is a disorder in a seemingly caring parent, most frequently the mother. The parent causes symptoms of an illness in an otherwise healthy or only mildly ill child. The symptoms are usually physical, but case reports of psychological illness are emerging as well. The mother's aim is to maintain ongoing contact with hospitals and physicians as well as other professionals such as psychologists and social workers. In doing this, the parent receives attention and sympathy and, in a circumspect way, has her own needs met. In cases of Munchausen Syndrome by Proxy, the child's acute physical and/or psychological symptoms often disappear when the mother's access to him or her is restricted. In fact, that is one way of confirming the diagnosis (particularly in medical cases).

There are those who believe that "the concept of factitious disorder (equivalent to Munchausen Syndrome), for the most part, remains empirically unsubstantiated" (Rogers, Bagby, & Rector, 1989, p. 1312) and therefore should not be diagnosed. However, an investigation can proceed by simply documenting the facts of the case as one would with any form of child abuse.

One of the warning signs of Munchausen Syndrome by Proxy is prolonged illness that is unexpected, extraordinary, and resistant to intervention. Appropriate treatment is often ineffective or poorly tolerated.

The mother often provides an elaborate medical history to the doctors and appears to cooperate with the medical team. Ms. Smith provided me with Brian's extensive medical and psychiatric history, along with the records to document it. Additionally, both Brian and Corey had been on numerous trials of medication with negative results. The entire family had received intervention from numerous agencies with no measurable improvement.

Another indicator of Munchausen Syndrome by Proxy is that signs and symptoms are inappropriate and incongruous and are typically observed only by the mother (Parnell & Day, 1998). School staff, respite workers, and the maternal grandmother did not report the same severe symptoms reported by Ms. Smith. Despite this, most staff never questioned her stories. While in the family home I didn't observe any of the severe symptoms reported by Ms. Smith.

Ms. Smith initiated all of Brian's psychiatric hospitalizations. She reported that Brian, Corey, and Amber had asthma, however, no one else had observed or documented this in the children.

Often in Munchausen Syndrome by Proxy, multiple medical evaluations from several physicians consistently have negative diagnostic findings. Numerous diagnostic tests such as x-ray, MRI, and chromosome screen, were negative during Brian's early hospitalizations. Physicians' (psychiatric) reports also often conflicted with reports by Brian's mother.

According to Miller (1996), in cases of Munchausen Syndrome by Proxy, the investigator often finds a history of serious illness and unusual deaths in the mother's family. Ms. Smith visits "Robin's" grave with the children and Corey stated he wanted to die to be with his sister. Ms. Smith also reported that between the time she adopted Corey and Amber she gave birth to another baby who was stillborn. Ms. Smith's adoptive mother reported that Ms. Smith had a very early miscarriage but not a stillborn baby. Ms. Smith had shown pictures of "her children's" gravestones to family counselors, school personnel, and me in an apparent effort to gain sympathy.

The more we uncovered, the more alarmed I felt. Were the children safe? Ms. Smith appeared not just concerned but obsessed with her children's psychiatric illnesses. She had sought numerous psychiatric evaluations for Brian and more recently Corey. The children's latest psychiatrist (who was also Ms. Smith's psychiatrist) reported that he had recently evaluated Amber as well. Brian was apparently seen as so fragile by Ms. Smith, that she was able to obtain a generous care grant for him, and she received funding for 18 hours of respite care per week.

Through further investigation and multiple interviews with Ms. Smith's adoptive mother, it was found that Ms. Smith had her own psychiatric history dating back to adolescence. Ms. Smith had already admitted to the examiner that she suffered from depression and panic attacks. She refused any counseling, however. Without complete medical records and a complete psychiatric and psychological evaluation of Ms. Smith, I could only speculate as to the extent of her own illness.

I searched for more information about Munchausen Syndrome by Proxy. What little information was available indicated that Munchausen Syndrome by Proxy was rare. One study in 1990 found that of 1,288 medical inpatients referred for psychiatric consultation, only 0.8% warranted the diagnosis of factitious disorder and only one qualified for factitious disorder with psychological symptoms (Miller, 1996). I found that a few researchers had published reviews of many of the papers published. A literature search in 1993 yielded 178 articles on Munchausen Syndrome by Proxy. Of these, 143 were found in medical journals and only 19 in the psychiatric and psychological literature (Schreier & Libow, 1993). By 1994, only two additional cases were found in the literature (Miller, 1996). To date, there is only one documented report of Munchausen Syndrome by Proxy with psychiatric illness in the literature (Fisher, Mitchell, & Murdoch, 1993). I was discovering that I was entering into an area of which little is known. There may actually be much larger numbers of Munchausen Syndrome by Proxy, and many of them are not being diagnosed (Miller, 1996; Schreier & Libow, 1993).

In my search for information, I also found that, in 25% to 33% of Munchausen Syndrome by Proxy cases, there is more than one child in a family involved (Parnell & Day, 1998; Schreier & Lebow, 1993). I also discovered that in about 20% to 33% of cases of Munchausen Syndrome by Proxy, there is evidence of Munchausen Syndrome in the mother (Parnell & Day, 1998; Miller, 1990). This again made me think about Ms. Smith's own history. Medical records indicated that Ms. Smith had a cyst and a twisted fallopian tube but no breast cancer. Her adoptive mother said she had never been hospitalized for asthma.

Once documentation was received regarding conflicting information and concerns grew regarding the children's safety, a report of possible child abuse, Munchausen Syndrome by Proxy, was made to the Child Welfare Department. If a diagnosis of Munchausen Syndrome by Proxy has been firmly established, it is necessary to make a hotline report to the Child Welfare Department. Munchausen Syndrome by Proxy qualifies as abuse under the Child Abuse Prevention and Treatment Act of 1974, which sets the standard for state reporting laws. The act defines abuse and neglect as follows:

> The physical or mental injury, sexual abuse, negligent treatment, or maltreatment of a child under the age of 18 by a person who is responsible for the child's welfare under circumstances which indicate the child's health or welfare is harmed or threatened thereby as determined in accordance with regulations prescribed. (Parnell & Day, 1998, p. 97)

My report in this case led to the children's being placed in protective custody. A shelter care hearing, which is usually a fairly brief court procedure (half day at most), lasted 3 days.

During the shelter care hearing, Ms. Smith appeared in court wearing white pancake make-up (which gave her the appearance of being very pale) and had dark circles under her eyes. In an apparent attempt to complete her presentation as a grieving mother and victim, she wore a little girl's bow in her hair and a frilly dress. During court recesses she sobbed about the loss of her children. Members of various agencies were seen to put their arms around her and comfort her. When she thought no one was around, her crying would mysteriously stop. Despite Ms. Smith's valiant efforts to prove otherwise, cause was found for the children to have been placed in protective custody.

One of the very basic and core problems of Munchausen Syndrome by Proxy is that you can't diagnose it unless you think of it, and even to many knowledgeable professionals it is unthinkable. Were it not for the contrasts I first observed in the home, I may not have been alert to the many contradictions and conflicting presentations of the mother. The mothers are so good at their deceit that it requires a very critical eye to look at these cases in an objective light. Both child maltreatment and Munchausen Syndrome by Proxy need to be part of the differential diagnosis when the clinical picture is atypical.

Once Munchausen Syndrome by Proxy is considered, the entire case and the medical record must be reviewed. All medical symptoms and diagnoses the mother reports should be substantiated by lab or test results and by clinic/medical records and family history when available. Records from any and all involved physicians and hospitals should be obtained and reviewed very carefully by someone who is skilled in this area. Nothing can be taken at face value.

When Munchausen Syndrome by Proxy is suspected, it will most likely be necessary to have the court order release of past medical histories as there is often a lack of cooperation from the mother (Miller, 1996). This may be particularly important in cases such as this in which psychological symptoms predominate. Keep in mind that as you try to gather the records most workers will be unfamiliar with the diagnosis of Munchausen Syndrome by Proxy and you will most likely need to be prepared to offer written materials and summaries about the syndrome. Reactions of skepticism and disbelief can and should be anticipated, as should sympathy for these mothers. These reactions are likely to be encountered among service providers as well as within the courts.

One study yielded information that an average length of time to diagnose Munchausen Syndrome by Proxy was more than a year in 19% of cases and more than 6 months in 33% of cases with a mean of 14.9 months. The range was from a few days to 240 months (20 years!) (Schreier & Libow, 1993). This case had been in the system for over 10 years.

Psychiatrists often find no evidence of pathology and often do not support the diagnosis (Miller, 1996). In this particular case, Ms. Smith's psychiatrist commented to a child welfare worker that I was simply on a witch-hunt. Although it is appropriate to obtain a psychiatric consultation, again, psychiatric evaluations are often noncontributory and overreliance on them is to be avoided.

One of the reasons psychiatrists have not been helpful is that Munchausen Syndrome by Proxy is diagnosed not by the presence of symptoms in the client but by documentation of their behavior outside the office. Diagnosis requires an appreciation of a pattern and careful examination of the history, accompanied by reports and documentation. Home-based assessment may be particularly illuminating in such cases. Longitudinal data is crucial to the diagnosis of Munchausen Syndrome by Proxy, as is the observed response to treatment.

Bemused by Ms. Smith's contradictions and presentation in court as well as the reactions of the various treatment team members, I continued to pursue the topic even after the case had been reported to the Child Welfare Department. I found that approximately 10% of the Munchausen Syndrome by Proxy cases are fatal. Of those killed, 20% of the children had been removed from the home and then returned (Miller, 1996). McGuire and Feldman (1989) reported that in their experience "it is difficult to convince courts of the diagnosis and dangers of ongoing risk." I recently learned that in this particular case the children have, in fact, been returned home.

Several theories have been postulated about the perpetrator's motivation in Munchausen Syndrome by Proxy (Folks, 1995; Goodwin, 1988; Libow & Schreier, 1986; McGuire & Feldman, 1989; Parnell & Day, 1998; Smith & Killam, 1994; Trask & Sigman, 1997). Some clinicians maintain that the mother may need attention, possibly because of early childhood deprivation or abuse (sexual abuse figures prominently). The mother in this case fit into this category as she reported having been removed from her parents at the age of 3 and placed in state custody. She was later adopted. She reported that as a teenager an uncle raped her.

No single psychological test profile yet emerges of the "classic" Munchausen Syndrome by Proxy mother. Consistency in patterns of these mothers' profiles, however, is beginning to emerge. Many of these mothers are very rigid and have a denying, defensive style. This can mask an underlying rebelliousness, emotional immaturity and instability, self-centeredness, a lack of social conformity, and intense passive resentment and anger. These mothers also present themselves as victims (Libow & Schreier, 1985).

As was Ms. Smith, these mothers are masters at eliciting sympathy. In a fairly dramatic way, one of their strengths is to fabricate believable stories. Given the history, Ms. Smith was quite successful in this area. From the moment I entered her home she dramatized her plight.

Ms. Smith had also sought out professional after professional for treatment of her children. This is a common characteristic in Munchausen Syndrome by Proxy. There had been at least five psychiatrists involved in Brian's case. He had had three psychiatric hospitalizations and numerous therapists. It is also interesting to note that Munchausen Syndrome by Proxy often co-occurs with reports of sexual abuse (Meadow, 1993). Both Brian and Amber had reportedly been victims of sexual abuse, although these reports were unfounded. Additionally, there had been reports of sexual play between the two. Despite these concerns, Amber showed me the room she claimed to share with Brian. Although Ms. Smith found this highly disturbing, she was not concerned enough to have Amber and Brian sleep in separate rooms.

Most reports estimate that 25% to 35% (however, there is a much wider range in the literature) of children victimized by Munchausen Syndrome by Proxy had siblings who were also victims of Munchausen Syndrome by Proxy (Parnell & Day, 1998; Schreier & Libow, 1993). It appears that Corey and Amber may be following in Brian's footsteps.

In evaluating these cases it should be noted that a real, confirmed, medical or psychiatric illness does not rule out the diagnosis of Munchausen Syndrome by Proxy. Combinations of real, exaggerated, and invented symptoms can co-occur. This obviously complicates the presentation and makes correct diagnosis difficult.

It is important that nonmedical information provided by the mother also be checked and confirmed. As was the case here, it is useful to also inquire about the mother's health. She may have a history of fabricating or inducing symptoms in herself. Caution in these investigations is indicated, however, because, if the mother is alerted to your suspicions, she may flee the area with the child, only to reappear elsewhere to a different care provider.

If Munchausen Syndrome by Proxy is suspected, ongoing case conferences are needed to bring together the child's primary physician, specialists involved in the evaluation process, nursing, and social work. If the health care team feels it is getting close to establishing the diagnosis of Munchausen Syndrome by Proxy, the hospital or clinic's attorney or administrator should be notified. Patients with factitious disorders are not likely to be cooperative with attempts to trace past medical histories. As stated previously, it may be necessary to have the court order release of those records.

Assessment of Munchausen Syndrome by Proxy is always difficult. Starting in the home as was done in this case helped set the stage for the remainder of the investigation. It was conflicting data found in the home environment that first alerted me to contradictions in the mother's reports.

Although the majority of cases in the literature involve physical symptoms, it is believed that those cases involving psychiatric diagnosis are more common than we would expect and are just beginning to be recognized. These cases are probably much more difficult to detect and even harder to prove. Further efforts in education and awareness, particularly for those who work in the child welfare system, are necessary to uncover and diagnose these cases and to protect the child victims.

REFERENCES

Asher, R. (1951) Munchausen syndrome. *Lancet, 1,* 339–341.

Fisher, G. C., Mitchell, I., & Murdoch, D. (1993). Munchausen's syndrome by proxy: The question of psychiatric illness in a child. *British Journal of Psychiatry, 162,* 701–703.

Folks, D. G. (1995). Munchausen's syndrome and other factitious disorders— Special Issue: Malingering and conversion reactions. *Neurologic Clinics, 13,* 267–282.

Goodwin, J. (1988). Munchausen's syndrome as a dissociative disorder. *Dissociation, 1* (1), 54–60.

Libow, J. A., & Schreier, J. A. (1985). Three forms of factitious illness in children: When is it Munchausen Syndrome by Proxy? *American Journal of Orthopsychiatry, 56,* 602–611.

Meadow, R. (1993). False allegations of abuse and Munchausen syndrome by proxy. *Archives of Disease in Childhood, 68,* 444–447.

Miller, A. (1996). Forensic aspects of factitious disorder. In L. B. Schlesinger (Ed.), *Explorations in criminal psychopathology* (pp. 50–73). Springfield, IL: Charles C Thomas.

McGuire, T. L., & Feldman, K. W. (1989). Psychologic morbidity of children subjected to Munchausen syndrome by proxy. *Pediatrics, 83,* 289–292.

Parnell, T. F., & Day, D. O. (Eds.). (1998). *Munchausen by proxy syndrome: Misunderstood child abuse.* Thousand Oaks, CA: Sage.

Rogers, R., Bagby, M., & Rector, N. (1989). Diagnostic legitimacy of factitious disorder with psychological symptoms. *American Journal of Psychiatry, 146,* 1312–1314.

Schreier, H. A., & Libow, J. A. (1993). Munchausen syndrome by proxy: Diagnosis and prevalence. *American Journal of Orthopsychiatry, 63,* 318–321.

Smith, K., & Killam, P. (1994, July–August). Munchausen syndrome. *Maternal Child Nursing, 19,* 214–221.

Trask, P. C., & Saigmon, S. T. (1997). Munchausen syndrome: A review and new conceptualization. *Clinical Psychology Science and Practice, 4,* 346–358.

PART THREE

Paraprofessional Interventions in the Home

CHAPTER EIGHT

Training Home Visitors

Diane L. Gould

In clinic-based day programs and in hospitals, paraprofessionals have always played a major role in treatment. Recognized as part of the treatment team, they are well integrated into the group of clinicians staffing a unit or program.

When treatment moves into the client's home, paraprofessionals no longer have daily collaboration with other staff or daily direct contact with clinical supervisors. They spend most of their working day isolated from colleagues. They are likely to be called on to make clinical decisions on their own. Therefore, programs employing paraprofessionals need to develop strategies for integrating them into the treatment team and providing them with sufficient training and clinical supervision.

In the first chapter of this section, Diane Gould discusses training volunteers, paraprofessionals, and professionals as home visitors. She then introduced us to a variety of training strategies.

Ms. Gould is a licensed clinical social worker whose experiences with residential treatment convinced her of the power of home based interventions. When she began working in community agencies and schools, she advocated for the necessity of adding home visits to complement traditional services. At the Jewish Childrens Bureau of Metropolitan Chicago, she administered a home visiting prevention program for high-risk new mothers.

In the vast majority of professions from plumber to surgeon, the protégé in training is observed and coached while being observed doing the actual work he or she will one day be doing on his or her own. This hands-on training has always been the accepted way to ensure proficiency. When on the operating table having an appendix removed, one would not be pleased to learn that this is the resident's first appendectomy. It would be even more horrifying if an experienced surgeon was not standing next to him or her, directly supervising every move. Only in the field of home-based mental health services are people trained in a classroom setting and then sent out alone into a client's living room to use their skills unwitnessed. To complicate this further, due to the nature of the professions involved and the characteristics of client populations served, if the client rejects the home visitor or the intended service, the home visitor may blame this failure on the client. In turn, colleagues or a supervisor may believe that the service was unsuccessful due to denial on the part of the client or that the client does not have the emotional or mental capacity to make use of the service offered. The privacy inherent in this type of work makes the issue of training even more important than in other therapeutic modalities. How can we successfully train volunteers, paraprofessionals, and professionals alike to become competent home visitors who can both perform the tasks and evaluate accurately the interaction? The purpose of this chapter is to:

1. discuss the challenges involved in training home visitors,
2. review characteristics of existing training programs,
3. outline critical components of effective training programs.

CHALLENGES INVOLVED IN TRAINING HOME VISITORS

There are many challenges involved in training home visitors. Some are the result of the different educational levels of home visitors. Home visiting is unique because there cannot be an assumption that highly educated home visitors are more skilled than a volunteer. In some instances there may be an inverse relationship between level of education and the ease with which one becomes a successful home visitor. It can be more difficult to teach how to do a skill differently than to teach a new skill. That balance between what can be taught and what is intuitive is a constant. Meeting with a client in his or her own home shifts the balance of power, rattling the traditional roles with which mental health professionals are comfortable.

The home environment introduces many things to the experience for both the client and the worker. While engaging in a conversation concerning infant care, the client may be distracted, worrying about how worn her furniture is and if the worker had noticed. The worker may be also distracted, worrying if there are roaches under the chair she is sitting in or if it would be all right to use the bathroom. A good home visitor needs to use his or her observation skills to assess the situation. It may be relevant whether or not there are family pictures in the home, how many beds there are in the house, and whether there are toys for the children. An inadequate home visitor will note these things in a way that appears nosy or intrusive. It is difficult to teach home visitors how to stay in control of the interaction while allowing the client control of the environment. So much of the ability to provide therapeutic help to others is instinctual. Klass (1996) classifies home visitors as artisans. As artisans, home visitors learn much on the job. It is an evolving practice. Home visiting calls for a sharp set of innate skills to achieve the careful dance between worker and client. The worker cannot use the safe confines of an office to protect himself or herself from emotions, either those expressed by the client or stirred within the worker. It is far more difficult to act like a professional in an informal setting, yet not appear cold and judgmental. Inexperienced workers may not know how to act professionally while displaying empathy and compassion. These issues may be somewhat different with volunteer home visitors who may not understand their role and the concept of therapeutic boundaries. The notion of a one-way relationship may be strange and unsettling for someone who becomes a volunteer out of a desire to give of themselves to others. If a client is experiencing stress due to having limited access to transportation, a volunteer may have to fight the desire to lend her own car. A paraprofessional who is insecure of his or her skills may come on too strong to a client in order to position himself or herself as the expert. This may be intensified in programs when the home visitor is from the same community or shares other similarities with the client.

All of these issues have relevance for training. Most of these issues cannot be taught in a curriculum format but must be addressed as part of the training program. Any good training program must provide the opportunity for participants to discuss their feelings about boundaries, comfort levels in client's homes, the intimacy of the relationship, and other difficult emotional issues. As with most things in this field, becoming a skilled home visitor is a process. Most home visitors' approaches to the work change over time. This calls for not only initial training for home visitors but also ongoing training as well. Home visitors also need intense supervision due to isolation. Because of the nature of the work, home visitors are often in the office less than most other workers. Without support from supervisors and co-workers, it can become difficult to maintain the necessary boundaries with clients when they are the primary source of interaction. To put it simply, if no one is asking the worker how he or she is and the client asks him or her, he or she may have difficulty holding back an emotional response if the day is very stressful. Training programs must lay the ground-work for supporting the home visitor while teaching the skills necessary to get the job done.

It is common to minimize the impact of home visits on the client and on the therapeutic process as a whole. If home visits are viewed as temporary and are done as a way to get the client "ready" to come to an office for psychotherapy, the full benefits of home-based approaches will not be achieved. The decision to see clients in their own homes rather than another setting is as important as whether someone should be seen in individual or group therapy. The goals of treatment need to be clear. For example, one of the programs I administer is a parenting program for mothers who have cognitive disabilities. The clients' lack of ability for generalization due to their disability requires that some of the parenting skills must be taught in the home. These clients would not be able to listen to a lecture on child-proofing in a center and be able to apply the lesson to their own homes.

Home visitors need to feel secure on the rationale behind the home visiting approach in order to benefit from training and supervision. Wasik, Bryant, and Lyons (1990) also note that it is useful to present information about the program's philosophy and goals to clarify expectations of the home visitors. They also point out that the role home visitors play should be included in that philosophy. The worker must be very certain of the specific requirements of the position. This will also include tasks such as record keeping, agency policies, and procedures.

It is important to keep in mind that a home visiting component can be used as an adjunct modality to other programs. One year, as a school social worker for a special education program for children with behavior and emotional disorders, I visited each child's home in September. The visits differed due to the nature of the families who dictated the length and type of visit. In many cases I was invited for a family meal. In one case, I ended up playing a game of darts with a resistant, alcoholic father. In all cases, that one home visit influenced my work with those children and their parents throughout the school year. I made more headway with that father during the course of the year than any of the past social workers. One nine-year-old boy referred to that home visit constantly in our therapy sessions. Even if the statement was an innocuous as "I played baseball with my lucky blue bat . . . you remember it don't you . . . it's the one that leans against my closet door." The home visit created a bridge between home and school for him that was so powerful he clung onto it all year. This argues the point that all practitioners would benefit from some training in home visiting even if that is not their primary job responsibility.

CHARACTERISTICS OF EXISTING PROGRAMS

There are many types of training programs used for home-based services. They originate from primarily the nursing, education, or social work disciplines. The home visitors themselves range from volunteers to paraprofessionals to professionally trained individuals. Most of the literature involves training paraprofessionals, but even that is limited. Gordon and Arbuthnot (1988) state that the difficulty with studies reporting on the use of paraprofessionals is the lack of detail in training procedures. Wasik et al. (1990) define professionals as those who have earned credentials in a recognized field such as education, nursing, or social work. Some of the literature uses lay visitor interchangeably with the term paraprofessional. For the purposes of this chapter, lay visitor will be used as a term referring to volunteer. Paraprofessional will be the term for a paid home visitor with less experience or education than necessary to earn credentials. Training needs obviously differ between the three groups. There is a need for more research comparing the training needs of the three groups. Most agencies or institutions that offer home visiting programs utilize one type of home visitor. This may be the result of philosophy, certification, agency structure, or budgetary concerns.

When the literature includes highly educated home visitors, the goal of the visits may be to train the professional. Kates, Webb, and LePage (1991) discuss using home visits to train psychiatry residents. They acknowledge that seeing patients in their own homes requires additional skills on the part of the therapists. Zarski et al. (1991) advocate for an in-home supervision model for master's level therapists. Even at these higher educational levels, training most often is necessary by the employing organization. Weissbound (1987) states that in-service training is necessary because few educational institutions provide this training. It is clear that in-service training is necessary regardless of the educational level of the home visitor. Norris and Baker (1998) make the distinction between initial training and ongoing training. Most experts agree that training can not be an isolated event in the career of home visitors. Unfortunately it is sometimes assumed by some professionals that home visiting is fine for those in training or inexperienced therapists, but when a certain level of expertise is mastered, one would "move beyond" this type of work. As home visiting can be viewed as work "in the trenches," some may feel rewarded when they are promoted to the confines of office psychotherapy. Training for professionals should include a discussion that home visiting is not a lesser form of therapy but instead viewed as a different but equally important modality. It has been my experience that novice professionals and senior clinicians are the most successful home visitors. It is those in the middle who struggle most. Highly trained, experienced clinicians who are comfortable with their own skills do not need an office with their diplomas displayed on the walls to feel secure that they are truly a therapist. A beginning therapist may accept new challenges as necessary learning experiences and be more available to do the hard work of home visiting. I maintain that I did the best therapy in my 20-year career standing shoulder to shoulder washing dishes in a client's home during my first year in the field. The lack of forced eye contact and the intimacy of the interaction allowed an unrestricted sharing of feelings on behalf of the client that has been unparalleled in my fancy corner office with the customary potted plants and Kleenex box.

It is important to keep in mind that the training for home visitors must include two tracks. Home visitors must be taught both the "how to's" of being a home visitor and the skills that are related to the specific program. In some instances a third track of teaching skills to others is added (Danish et al., 1978). The first track is sometimes described as "basic helping skills." Successful training programs have a strong emphasis in these skills. They include: communicating effectively, giving feedback, active listening, judgments and biases, professional and ethical issues, termination, therapeutic boundaries, and observation skills.

Alpaugh and Haney (1978) have published a training manual for paraprofessionals and beginning counselors in the geriatric field. They introduce a nine-step counseling model. It is:

1. Understanding the client
2. Establishing rapport
3. Defining the problem
4. Setting a goal
5. Clarifying issues
6. Listing alternatives
7. Explaining alternatives
8. Supporting decisions
9. Providing closure

This training curriculum includes a section on the worker's feelings. It goes into detail on counseling issues such as using confrontation, learning how to make interpretations, developing a feeling vocabulary, and practicing self-disclosure.

Specific knowledge and skills also need to be incorporated. These may include newborn care, child development, nutrition, the diagnosis of mental illness, and chronic medical illness in the elderly. The issues addressed need to be program-specific and carefully selected to prepare home visitors for their work with particular groups of clients.

The following outlines describe content areas from published training programs for home visitors. They provide examples of the types of curricula being used.

Wasik et al.'s (1990) basic content of a home visitor training program includes:

1. History of home visiting
2. Philosophy of home visiting
3. Knowledge and skills of the helping process (basic and advanced clinical skills, professional and ethical issues)
4. Knowledge of families and children (prenatal/perinatal development, child development, child management, family systems therapy, health and safety, special issues, child abuse and neglect, alcoholism, drugs, spouse abuse, chronically ill child)
5. Knowledge and skills specific to programs (program goals and procedures, record-keeping and documentation, curriculum)
6. Knowledge and skills specific to communities (cultural characteristics, health and human service resources, other pertinent community resources, transportation issues)

The paraprofessional in home health and long-term care training modules for working with older adults by Cerventes, Heid-Grubman, and Schuerman (1995) is an especially comprehensive training curriculum. It includes:

• Principles of adult learning
• The process of normal aging
• Communicating effectively
• Understanding and identifying depression and recognizing the risk of suicide
• Understanding Alzheimer's Disease and other dementias and understanding and recognizing substance abuse and elder abuse
• Caring for confused older adults
• The effect of medication on older adults
• Ethical issues in caring for older adults
• Dealing with death and dying
• Managing caregiver stress

Musser-Granski and Carrillo (1997) outline a training program recommended for bilingual, bicultural paraprofessionals employed in mental health services. Included in the outline along with other topics are:

- Interpreting both words and affect
- English language and American cultural training
- Community organizing, outreach, education, prevention
- Personal boundaries, burn-out, overidentification with the client
- Community resources and referrals

I am currently the administrator of a home visiting program for first-time mothers who are at risk of difficulty in parenting. The home visitors are volunteers who are trained and supervised by the agency. The formal criteria for the selection of volunteers include that they have been parents themselves and must have children who are of adolescent age or older. We have found that because our clients need and respond to a mother figure rather than a peer, young volunteers are not accepted. The volunteers themselves are a rather diverse group. Some have previous work experience in related fields and others do not. They all wanted to contribute to the community in some way beyond writing a check for a donation. They all felt that parenting is the subject they know the most about. I have found that there are two important characteristics shared by successful volunteers. The first is that they can acknowledge that there are many paths to get to the same place. The second is that they do not feel that others need to make the same life choices they made. These two observations may seem simple or obvious, but over and over again I have witnessed these two "mind-sets" influence the ability of lay people to succeed in helping others.

At the Jewish Children's Bureau, the training curricula for volunteer home visitors in our program serving mothers of newborns who are at risk for difficulty in parenting is as follows:

- Program procedures—rules, note taking
- Confidentiality
- Prevention
- History of home visiting
- The high risk family
- Parenting in the '90s
- Abuse, neglect and violence
- Active listening/open ended questions
- Problem solving
- Judgments and biases
- Therapeutic friendships and boundaries
- Infant care
- Infant development
- Special parenting situations—adoptive parents, premature infants, infants with special needs, multiple births

- Postpartum issues
- When to call for back-up

In training lay people, we found the primary training challenge was the discussion of biases and having a nonjudgmental attitude. We found that this is the area that determines how successful volunteers will be in their placement. It was made clear that everyone has biases especially when it comes to parenting. It was explained that being aware of one's own biases and judgments is necessary in order to keep them from interfering with working with clients. During training, we use a decorated shoebox labeled a "bias box." All participants are asked to write their biases on slips of paper and put them in the box. The group leaders do the same to insure that common biases are included. When the task is completed, the papers are read aloud. Important biases such as "mothers should stay home with their babies," "all babies should be breast-fed," "all babies deserve to live in two-parent families," and "gays should not be parents" are discussed by the group. It is crucial that the volunteers gain understanding of their own biases before being matched with a client. For this activity to succeed there needs to be an atmosphere of trust between members of the training group and with the leader. Volunteers must not fear that having any biases will have them dismissed from the program. They need to understand the importance of being a nonjudgmental person in the life of their client. Trainers need this information to match each volunteer with the appropriate client.

In addition to designing the content of the training, the format of the training also needs to be determined. Green (1996), citing Jackson and Neighbors (1990), urges trainers to use the principles of adult learning in setting up the training program. They are:

- Learning is more effective when it is a response to a felt need of the learner.
- There should be active participation on the part of the learner.
- Learning is made easier when the material learned is related to what the learner already knows.
- Learning is facilitated when the material learned is meaningful to the learner.
- Learning is retained longer when it is put to immediate use.
- Period plateaus occur in learning.
- Learning must be reinforced.

Norris and Baker (1999) point out that, for paraprofessionals, the least effective training model is one that features a lecture by the trainer with minor support from printed materials. They recommend an interactive, hands-on approach to training. Robin and Wagenfeld (1981) add that "training that stresses the concrete and practical is most effective" (p. 301).

Obviously, in addition to appropriate content and format, training should be done in a comfortable setting, be given in reasonable time periods, and promote an atmosphere of trust and comfort. Norris and Baker (1999) recommend that supervisors do a learning needs assessment prior to training that will help them be aware of safety and comfort issues. Wasik et al. (1990) strongly recommended three interrelated training procedures. They are: (a) role-playing, (b) experiential learning, and (c) peer teaching. The majority of training models stress the use of role-playing. At the Jewish Children's Bureau we have also found this the most useful method of teaching skills and evaluating how the information is being integrated. In the training we do for volunteers, role-playing accounts for at least one third of the time spent in training. Volunteers pick from a hat filled with preprinted scenarios. A list of scenarios is included in the appendix. It is such an easy and effective way of determining whether the didactic material is being absorbed without any risk to clients. I've often been amazed at how poorly some volunteers have done in role-plays after I thought, due to their questions or body language, they understood the lesson.

What is picked up in role-plays most often is a subtly judgmental attitude or a volunteer giving her opinions too much instead of encouraging the client to find her own answers. Also apparent in the role-plays are ways that volunteers close off the conversation by asking "yes" or "no" questions instead of open-ended ones. A volunteer may ask "Are you worried about going back to work?" instead of "How do you feel about going back to work?" It is also important for the group members to be able to give and accept feedback from each other. Cervantes, Weid, Grubman, and Schuerman (1995) include difficult role-playing scenarios such as a client making sexual advances or a client trying to give the workers money. Many other models also include some form of practicing skills. This may include trying out skills on a friend or family member (Danish et al., 1978). Green (1996) discusses the arrangement for a clinical experience which tries to mirror the actual experience. She notes that inpatient settings with a similar population can be a common site to train home health care aide students. Peer teaching or a mentoring relationship is advocated by several programs. Gordon and Arbuthnot (1988) pair trainees with each other, with graduate students, or with others who have completed training and have received ongoing supervision.

Having two practitioners go on a home visit for the purpose of training can work if it is done very carefully. They must plan in advance how they will work together so they do not confuse or overwhelm the client. The novice home visitor needs to be clear as to whether he or she is expected to observe or lead the session. If the trainee actively participates and makes an error, there needs to be a clear plan with respect to whether the senior clinician will correct it in front of the client or wait until they have completed the session.

The use of videotaping as part of training has become popular in some settings. It is my belief that in a home setting it is intrusive and influences the outcome of the treatment. I feel it is a more useful tool in traditional office-based psychotherapy.

In all aspects of the helping professions there is increasing emphasis on assessment and accountability. No longer can we get by being a "soft science," feeling immune from proving that interventions truly work. The same is true for training. We need to be able to tell if our training programs have the desired outcomes. Danish et al. (1978) advocate a training program where each skill is taught in a structured systematic package that includes an explicitly stated goal and rationale, attainment level, guidelines for acquisition of responses and strategies, detailed procedures, and homework.

The model-training project for paraprofessionals, Home Care Providers to Rural Minority Elderly by Joan Wood (1985) is also based on very clear goals and objectives. In every topic, participants undergo pre- and posttests. Participants also complete an evaluation form of the training for each day of training and for the overall training program. Possibly most important is that this model includes a follow-up questionnaire received later in time after training has been completed. This allows participants time to put their training into practice and identify any topic areas in which they wish they were trained.

Chichin (1992) and others have received follow-up data directly from the families served and from the workers themselves. These satisfaction surveys also have implications for training. As she points out, workers who receive verbal abuse from their elderly clients can tolerate this treatment if they have been trained to understand behavior associated with dementia. The families who have received services can identify areas of knowledge lacking in their home visitors. Training programs should not be set in stone but should be routinely adjusted based on feedback from clients and workers.

Although the focus of this chapter is training, it is difficult to ignore the separate but related issue of supervision. It is clear from the literature that ongoing supervision from home visitors of all education levels is necessary. Wasik et al. (1990) state that all home visitors should have supervision. As mentioned earlier in this chapter, the complexity inherent in home visiting, the potential for isolation, and the lack of observed experience all call for intensive supervision of home visitors. Robin and Wagenfeld's (1981) work with Home Start home visitors notes that the lack of opportunity to observe, model, and receive direct and indirect feedback from co-workers regarding performance makes supervision of paramount importance. Home visitors also need to have the ability to evaluate their own practice which can come through the supervision process. Klass (1996) refers to this as "reflection-on-action" and views it as a critical skill in home visiting that parallels teaching skills to clients. Klass continues to point out that these parallels continue in the process of supervision. She states that "effective supervision parallels home visitors' relationships with the families that they serve because it is likewise a relationship of respect, support, collaboration, and mutuality" (p. 102).

Supervision differs greatly depending on the type of home visitors. When supervising volunteers one needs to take into consideration that the lay person needs to get his or her own needs met as well. It is often difficult to find the balance between feeling needed but not feeling overwhelmed. One volunteer told me weekly that she did not feel her client needed her until one week when the client broke down crying and disclosed her feelings of sadness and hopelessness. The volunteer then called me frantically saying that she was so worried about the client and didn't think she had the expertise to help her as she wasn't a therapist. Another issue concerning supervision of volunteers is that it can be difficult to enforce rules about paperwork and meeting attendance when they are unpaid and giving to their program "on their own time."

In supervising paraprofessionals from the same culture or community as the client, supervision needs to focus on boundary and transference issues. These relationships have the potential to be powerful and very therapeutic but supervision is critical.

Supervision of professional staff must include their feelings about their role as a home visitor especially if they work in a setting where other professional staff do traditional office-based psychotherapy. They will need more support from their supervisors than other therapists in order to do their best work.

CRITICAL COMPONENTS OF AN EFFECTIVE TRAINING PROGRAM

The following critical components can be used when establishing a new home visiting program or evaluating an existing one. Most of these components hold true regardless of educational level of the home visitor. These assume that a careful and systematic selection process had been done in the recruitment of home visitors. An effective training program:

- Begins with an assessment of the learning needs of participants including safety and comfort issues
- Incorporates what is known about adult learners
- Provides both initial and ongoing training sessions
- Includes a clear program philosophy which states the role home visitors have in that philosophy
- Provides clear expectations of the role of the home visitor, outlining procedures and policies
- Utilizes an interactive, hands-on approach focusing on what is concrete and practical
- Identifies objectives of each skill taught and formulates an assessment tool to determine whether objectives are met
- Is very clear on what skills (broken down if necessary) are necessary to perform the job
- Includes both interpersonal skills and program-specific skills equally in the curriculum and views them not as separate components but rather as an interrelated set of skills necessary to become a skilled home visitor
- Includes information about cultural differences, child and adult development, different family structures, and social systems
- Gives information on community resources
- Incorporates role-plays in training which mirror actual occurrences in practice and encourages group feedback on the role-plays which will also serve as a lesson on how to give feedback to clients
- Offers opportunities for trainees to practice skills within the agency or with outsiders
- Offers a trainee support system which may include mentorship with a more experienced home visitor
- Evaluates the training program upon completion
- Decreases long delays between completion of training and placement so skills will not be lost
- Provides individual supportive and insight-oriented supervision consistently throughout employment or placement
- Teaches home visitors to reflect on their own performance from the first day of training throughout their work in the field
- Evaluates training through feedback from former trainees after having had several home visiting experiences
- Makes sure that program supervisors also receive support and respect, which they will need in order to provide the same to home visitors who, in turn, must pass these along to the families served

In summary, the goal of this chapter was to clarify challenges involved in training home visitors, give characteristics of existing programs, and outline critical components of effective training programs. Home visiting involves innate skill and instincts which are enhanced by training and supervision. The goals for the home visits need to be thought out and clear regardless if it is a program utilizing home visits alone or if home visits are one approach in a continuum of services.

Not every good clinician is capable of being a successful home visitor. Potential home visitors regardless of educational level should be carefully selected. Home visitors need to be creative and flexible in their work with clients. They must have a heightened sense of boundaries. As mentioned earlier, they must be capable of controlling the interaction without having control of the environment.

This chapter emphasizes that both initial and ongoing training are important. Training programs must include information on both the techniques to be a successful home visitor and the skills related to the specific program such as infant care or care of the elderly. Including role-playing in training is an effective way to teach many skills. The training program must be continually evaluated. Home visitors need ongoing supervision and support in order to do their best work. In my experience, well-trained and closely supervised home visitors can make a tremendous difference in the lives of the people they serve.

APPENDIX: ROLE-PLAYING SCENARIOS

During your visit, the mom has the soap operas blaring and chats with a friend who drops by, excluding you from the conversation.

The new mother discusses with you her ambivalence about going back to work.

The new mom pleads with you to baby-sit for just 20 minutes while she drops by her boyfriend's to finish up a disagreement they had the night before.

The new mom shares her doubts about being a good mother and her fears that the baby doesn't love her.

The new mom tells you that her secret is that she is trying to get pregnant right away to keep her boyfriend in the relationship.

The new mom and you are eating a snack together in the kitchen and she begins feeding the baby a carrot and raisins.

You are with the new mom and baby at an ice cream store and run into a nosy neighbor of yours who asks a lot of questions.

You come into the house, which is a mess, and the baby is alone in the swing downstairs while mom is upstairs napping.

You are working with a pregnant women who is due next week who says that she may want to place her baby for adoption.

The new mom wants to talk about your marriage and how having a child affected your sex life.

The baby is sick with 104° temp and the mom says that the doctor wasn't helpful. She is anxious and upset.

REFERENCES

Alpaugh, P., & Haney, M. (1978). *Counseling the older adult: A training manual for paraprofessionals and beginning counselors.* Lexington, MA: Lexington Books.

Cervantes, E., Heig-Grubman, J., & Senverman, C. K. (1995). *The paraprofessional in home health and long term care: Training modules for working with older adults.* Baltimore, MD: Health Professions Press.

Chichin, E. R. (1992). Home care is where the heart is: The role of interpersonal relationships in paraprofessional home care. *Home Health Care Services Quarterly, 13,* 161–177.

Danish, S. J., D'augelli, A. R., Brock, G. W., Conter, K. R., & Meyer, R. J. (1978). A symposium on skill dissemination for paraprofessionals: Models of training, supervision and utilization. *Professional Psychology, 16,* 16–37.

Gordon, D. A., & Arbuthnot, J. (1988). The use of paraprofessionals to deliver home-based family therapy to juvenile delinquents. *Criminal Justice and Behavior, 15,* 364–378.

Gould, D., Pritikin, M., & Mork, N. (1995). *The Chavera Moms, one mother to another training manual.* Northbrook, IL: Jewish Children's Bureau.

Green, K. (1996). *Home health aide training manual.* Gaithersburg, MD: Aspen.

Jackson, J. E., & Neighbors, M. (1990). *Home care client assessment handbook.* Gaithersburg, MD: Aspen.

Kates, N., Webb, S., & LePage, P. (1991). Therapy begins at home: The psychiatric house call. *Canadian Journal of Psychiatry, 36,* 673–676.

Klass, C.A. (1996). *Home visiting: Promoting healthy parent and child development.* Baltimore, MD: Paul H. Brookes.

Musser-Granski, J. R., & Carrillo, D. F. (1997). Critical care update: The use of bilingual and bicultural paraprofessionals in mental health services: Issues for hiring, training, and supervision. *Community Mental Health Journal, 33,* 51–60.

Norris, J. A., & Baker, S. S. (1999). *Maximizing paraprofessional potential.* Malabar, FL: Keiger Publishing Co.

Robin, S. S., & Wagenfeld, M. O. (1981). *Paraprofessionals in the human services.* New York: Human Services Press.

Wasik, B. H., Bryant, D. M., & Lyons, C. M. (1990). *Home visiting: Procedures for helping families.* Newbury Park, CA: Sage.

Weissbound, B. (1987). Design, staffing, and funding of family support programs. In. S. L. Kajan, D. R. Powell, B. Weissbound, & R. E. F. Zigler (Eds.), *America's family support programs* (pp. 244–268). New Haven, CT: Yale University Press.

Wood, J. B. (1985). *Final Report for Model Training Project for Paraprofessional Home Care Providers to Rural Minority Elderly.* Alberta, VA: Southside Virginia Community College.

Zarski, J. J., Greenbank, M., Sand-Pringle, C., & Cibik, P. (1991). The invisible mirror: In-home family therapy and supervision. *Journal of Marital and Family Therapy, 17,* 133–143.

Home-Based Treatment Foster Care: Using Foster Parents As the Agent of Change

Charlene Rivette

In treatment foster care, the home is the treatment center. Char Rivette describes a model of treatment foster care that focuses on the foster parents as the agents of change. She developed the model from her experiences as a social worker in private treatment foster care agencies, and a public home-based mental health program.

Ms. Rivette is a licensed clinical social worker and for the past 10 years has provided therapy for children and families, in addition to working as a supervisor and administrator. She is currently the Director of Foster Care, Adoptions, and Families One at Little City Foundation.

THE STORY OF "ANGELA"

Angela is 14 years old and has been in foster care since she was 9. She was removed from her mother's care, along with her five siblings, due to their mother's being incarcerated for murdering Angela's father. Angela and her siblings were severely neglected while in the care of their mother, who was a drug addict, and Angela and her siblings were often left to fend for themselves. She and her two older siblings were responsible for taking care of their three younger siblings. She had little contact with her father before he was killed, and limited contact with relatives. Angela had several aunts and uncles, but since Angela and her family lived in Chicago and her aunts and uncles in a distant suburb, she was not able to see them very often. After the children were removed, relatives only agreed to take in the younger children. Angela and her older sister and brother were sent to separate foster homes.

Since being placed in foster care, Angela has lived in 14 different foster homes. As she moved from home to home, the private foster care agencies that were in charge of licensing and monitoring the foster home, supervising her care, and monitoring her health and welfare also changed. This was due to the privatization of foster care from a centralized regional system to a conglomeration of various sizes of private foster care agencies. As Angela's foster care placements were disrupted, the foster care agencies exhausted their own pool of foster homes. The agencies then looked to other agencies for placement, which would lead to a change in the provider responsible for her care and well-being. This led to poor continuity of care. Angela has continued to see her siblings and some of her aunts and uncles, but the visitation has been sporadic throughout the years due to the instability of her placements. She tends to idealize her family with whom she has never had consistent contact and longs to be in a home where she can stay.

Angela's many moves were primarily due to the foster families' unwillingness, and/or inability, to cope and intervene with Angela's behavioral problems. She has been accused of "corrupting" other children in the foster home by negatively influencing their behavior. Angela needs a lot of supervision and attention. She is learning disabled and emotionally immature. She often does not follow instructions and lacks motivation to change her behavior. Angela uses foul language, is vulgar, and has an "attitude." She has been known to get up in the middle of the night and make phone calls to people she has made acquaintances with or to previous foster homes.

Due to her learning disability, low self-esteem, and frequent school changes, Angela struggles in school, both academically and socially. In school, she lacks motivation and indicates that she "doesn't care" what the consequences are. Angela tends to get into trouble in school and was suspended several times for swearing at teachers and principals. Angela's school problems are exacerbated by her lack of maturity and social skills. Emotionally, she acts much more like a preteenager, and her interests lie in activities that younger children typically engage in. In addition, she is keenly aware of being different from other children her own age and struggles with wanting to fit in. Angela has never had a long-term relationship with anyone and has never learned how to form friendships. Because she is a foster child, she is already stigmatized among her peers, and since she moves often, she has little time to form friendships that can transcend this stigma. Often, Angela will misperceive the actions of other children and assume friendships when they don't exist, therefore setting herself up for more ridicule and rejection.

Twice Angela has been suicidal, expressing the desire to kill herself as a way of escaping her plight of being. On one of the occasions she became enraged when confronted by her foster mother for lying. She ran into the kitchen, grabbed a knife out of the drawer and threatened to stab her foster mother, then ran into her room with the knife. She did not hurt herself, but was distraught when the ambulance arrived and took her to the hospital. Her foster mother refused to allow her to return to her home when she was released from the hospital. On another occasion Angela threatened to jump out a window when her case worker informed her that she would have to move again to another foster home. This also resulted in a psychiatric hospitalization.

Due to the neglect Angela suffered while with her mother, along with the ongoing rejection and transfer from home to home since being placed in foster care, Angela has been diagnosed with reactive attachment disorder. Reactive attachment disorder is characterized by difficulty in forming an attachment or bond with caretakers. Reactive attachment disorder is a result of persistent disregard of the child's basic emotional or physical needs or repeated changes of primary caregivers that prevent formation of stable attachments (American Psychiatric Association, 1994). Children with reactive attachment disorder may respond to caregivers with a mixture of approach, avoidance, and resistance to comforting or may display frozen watchfulness. The child may also display excessive familiarity with relative strangers or lack of selectivity in choice of attachment figures (p. 118).

Given her history, Angela has little reason to trust that her caretaker may care for her or love her, let alone be willing to allow herself the hope that they may offer her a permanent home. Angela has come to expect rejection from those who are supposed to care for her. From early on, since her caretakers did not provide all she needed for her normal growth and development, Angela developed coping strategies to defend against eventual rejection. She exhibits defiant behavior to distance the caregiver or she runs away. Angela tends to form superficial attachments to most adults she comes in contact with, even with complete strangers. She appears to attach the same value to a stranger as to her primary caregiver. Since she does not trust that her caregiver will continue to care for her, she may be attempting to ensure that she has other adults in her life that could possibly fill this role.

Angela's tendency to push away parental figures created a self-fulfilling prophecy. Because Angela exhibits defiant behavior and tends to display the same level of affection to a stranger as to her caregiver, her foster parents have reacted by believing that Angela does not care for them and that it really doesn't matter to her if she moved to a new home. Her foster parents became discouraged with her behavior and

did not feel that they were making progress or developing a close relationship with her. In situations in which Angela's foster parents began
to earn her trust, Angela would be frightened by the unfamiliar relationship. She would display behavior that led to her being removed
from the home, such as suicidal threats, running away, or extreme defiance. Because Angela had come to expect that her foster parents
would eventually reject her, it was easier for her to lose a parent for
whom she had no close feelings than one for whom she felt an attachment. In other words, by exhibiting intolerable behavior, she forced
the parents to kick her out, as she felt they inevitably would, because
the wait for the inevitable loss was more than she could bear.

Angela is a typical example of a foster care child who is in need of
treatment foster care. Although foster parents in the traditional foster
care setting must attend basic training and should possess nurturing
and appropriate care-giving qualities, they are ill-prepared to meet the
needs of a child like Angela. The only alternative in the past has been
institutionalized care such as a group home or residential facility.

Treatment foster care allows children like Angela to receive intensive mental health treatment in a safe environment while gaining all
the benefits of building attachments in a family setting. Treatment
foster care utilizes home-based mental health treatment, well-trained foster parents, and a solid support system to provide a stable, long-lasting
home environment for severely emotionally disturbed children. This
chapter will describe treatment foster care, the use of home-based
treatment, and using the foster parents as the primary agents of change.
The rationale behind using treatment foster care rather than institutional care will be outlined as well as the components necessary to
make it successful. Angela's case will be used as an example throughout the chapter.

OVERVIEW OF TREATMENT FOSTER CARE

DEFINITION OF FOSTER CARE/POPULATION SERVED

Children who are unable to be cared for by their parents are in need of
substitute care, or foster care, either with a relative or with a licensed
foster parent. In the state of Illinois, the Department of Children and
Family Services (DCFS) becomes involved if the biological parent(s)
are accused of abuse or neglect. Foster care placement occurs when
the Juvenile Court orders that custody and guardianship be given to
DCFS due to the finding that the child(ren) are not safe in their home.
DCFS then becomes the legal guardian of the child, and the child is

placed either with family members or in a foster home. Since DCFS privatized its foster care system, the child is then referred to one of many private foster care agencies who contract with DCFS. DCFS retains legal guardianship while the private agency is contracted to manage the case and provide all services to the child, his or her parents, and the foster family or relative care provider. The foster parents or relatives are expected to provide the daily care of the child, including food, shelter, clothing, and nurturance.

TREATMENT FOSTER CARE

Treatment foster care is a provision of care which serves foster children who also need intensive mental health treatment. These children typically have experienced severe physical, emotional, and/or sexual abuse or neglect. Many experienced symptoms of mental illness prior to foster care placement. Many of the children in treatment foster care have experienced multiple foster care and/or residential placements as well as multiple psychiatric hospitalizations. It is likely that a majority of children in treatment foster care experience attachment disorders due to neglect by biological parents and movement from foster home to foster home.

Angela is an example of a child served in treatment foster care. Her negative and disruptive behavior patterns, lack of healthy coping skills, and inability to trust and attach, along with her past suicidal behavior, set her apart from a child that can be helped in a typical foster home. Foster parents who are unwilling and/or unprepared to work with a child like Angela would most likely not be able to tolerate the inability of the child to grow attached to them or to deal with the child's behavioral problems. This can often be the beginning of a pattern of failure, not only for the child but also for the foster parents. Foster parents who may be able to competently care for a traditional foster child can become disillusioned by a failed placement with a child who most likely should not have been placed there to begin with.

Treatment foster care is an ideal living environment and treatment setting for children with reactive attachment disorder for several reasons. A treatment foster family is prepared to accept the behavior of a child who has difficulty forming relationships and to be able to begin building a relationship with the child. A treatment foster care setting allows the child to live in an environment in which foster parents are able to tolerate negative behavior and address issues related to attachment difficulties, such as increased behavior problems, poor peer relations, and low self-esteem. Treatment foster care is a setting in which the focus of treatment is on building attachments between the child and his or her foster parents in addition to building positive and healthy friendships and relationships with peers and other adults. The relationship between the child and the treatment foster parent, as it is nurtured and developed, can then lead to a generalized ability for the child to make attachments and relationships with friends, teachers, and other adults.

Treatment foster care's success with this population of children is contingent upon two components: well-trained and prepared foster parents as the "agents of change" in a child's life and professional, home-based treatment by well-trained consultants and therapists. This "team" provides the core of treatment. This chapter will discuss how these two important components can work together to provide severely emotionally disturbed children with a stable home and effective mental health treatment.

RATIONALE FOR TREATMENT FOSTER CARE

In the past, children in the foster care system with mental illness or behavioral/emotional disorders were moved from foster home to foster home and eventually ended up in an institutional setting such as a group home or residential facility. The common wisdom was that these settings would provide a milieu that was safe and able to effectively address the child's mental health issues while providing a stable living environment. Children likely remained in the residential setting for many years and lost out on the opportunity to have a "family." The rationale for placing disturbed children in treatment foster care, as opposed to institutional or group-home style living, is based on the following basics beliefs:

1. Every child deserves a place to call "home," where he or she is raised into adulthood and can return throughout adult life.
2. Children should be raised and nurtured by parents, not staff. A person in a parenting role will be much more committed than paid staff, and there will be less turnover in caregivers.
3. A child is more likely to flourish in a home environment rather than an institutional setting.
4. A home environment will provide the child with more opportunities for appropriate modeling and development of a value system.
5. A child's mental health is directly related to the attachments he or she has made to significant others.

In a foster care setting, a child is cared for by a substitute parent rather than "staff," and the child is more likely to establish a long-term relationship leading to an attachment to a significant other. If that relationship is positive, it can form a basis from which a child can begin to build a positive self-image and begin to heal.

One of the keys to successful treatment foster care is intervention as early as possible after the child is removed from home. The child should be assessed quickly to determine the need for individual treatment and the possible need for treatment foster care rather than a traditional foster home. This allows the more disturbed child to immediately begin healing and learning appropriate social skills. In addition, placement in a competent treatment foster home reduces the likelihood of moving the child frequently, thus reducing the possibility of developing or exacerbating the symptoms of reactive attachment disorder. Reduction of movement from home to home is also key to successful care. If the child is able to return to his or her birth family, then the problems leading to removal should be addressed and remedied as quickly as possible. The treatment needs of the child and family should be assessed and coordinated before the child's return home, and follow up should be closely monitored. If the child cannot feasibly return home, then a life-long plan for the child must be developed.

The birth family should also be as closely involved as possible with the treatment of the foster child. If it is possible for foster children to return to their birth parents without risk of harm, this is their best chance at developing into a healthy adult. Foster children, with the possible exception of those removed at infancy, have a strong connection to their birth family. Although abused and/or neglected by their parents, most foster children want to return to them. Since the birth family was often key in the development of the child's emotional disturbance or was parenting the child at the onset of mental illness, they should be as involved as possible with the child's healing process. Often birth parents are in need of their own mental health treatment to help them understand and accept responsibility for their own harmful actions and to work toward remedying these issues. Often birth parents who abuse or neglect their children were also abused or neglected. It is quite common that the parent is identifying with his or her own parents who may have been abusive or neglectful. Therefore, the birth parents may have low self-image and self-respect and have no clear understanding of good parenting, let alone understand that their actions with their children caused the trauma they are now dealing with.

A MODEL OF TREATMENT FOSTER CARE

The model of treatment foster care that will be discussed includes the following components: well-trained, licensed foster parents; agency support in the form of consultation, respite care, and crisis intervention; home-based therapy for the child and the child's biological family if applicable; and intensive case management. Each child has a treatment team that includes the foster parents, the therapist, the case manager, the respite worker, and any other agency staff that may respond in a crisis. In addition, the child may have other ancillary service providers, such as a medical doctor, psychiatrist, teacher, tutor, school social worker, or volunteers.

With regard to the treatment of the child's mental health and attachment issues, the foster parents are considered to be the main agents of change. This means that the relationship between the child and the foster parent is seen as the key to the child's ability to form attachments and positive relationships and to learn coping skills. The other treatment components are in place to support the foster parents in this monumental task by providing them training, consultation, case management, and respite. Home-based therapists provide individual mental health treatment to the child, specifically to address past trauma and teach healthy coping skills. This treatment team is responsible for developing and implementing a plan of treatment which addresses the child's mental health needs as well as the permanency goal, such as return home or adoption. Each component will be looked at separately.

TREATMENT FOSTER PARENTS: THE MAIN AGENTS OF CHANGE

Licensed, well-trained foster parents are the primary agents of healing and change in the life of the treatment foster child. Treatment foster parents should be trained in specific strategies for teaching social skills and correcting severe behavior problems that could be displayed by the children in their home. The example that will be used in this chapter is training called "Rebuilding Children's Lives" (Baker, Burke, Herron, & Mott, 1996). Boys Town in Omaha, Nebraska developed this treatment intervention model. It is based on teaching social skills to emotionally and behaviorally disturbed children through the use of preventive teaching, corrective teaching, effective praise, and a "staying calm" plan. The strategies are based in social learning theory and behavior modification and focus on teaching children specific skills to decrease their negative behaviors and build on their strengths. Each of the four strategies will be discussed.

"Preventive teaching" (pp. 77–81) is a tool to give the child guidance and to prevent unwanted behaviors from occurring in the first place. Role-play and directives are used to prepare children for situations in which they have previously exhibited negative behavior. The child is clearly told the consequences of displaying the negative behavior and the rationale as to why it is in his or her best interest to display the alternative positive social skill. Parents are taught how to recognize negative behavior patterns and what motivates the child to display these behaviors in order to know when to use preventive teaching and what rationale to use. For example, a foster parent could use "preventive teaching" with her foster daughter who has a history of coming home late after school. The foster parents clearly states to her foster daughter before she leaves for school that she is expected to come home directly from school. The foster parent then indicates that if she does come home directly from school, she can go out with friends later in the afternoon. The foster parent and child then role-play the situation in which the child comes home on time and she is allowed to go out with friends later that afternoon.

Foster parents are taught to use "corrective teaching" (pp. 87–93) when the child is caught engaging in an unwanted behavior. The foster parent stops the child and points out that the behavior is not acceptable. The foster parent then identifies an acceptable alternative behavior and teaches it to the child. The foster parent uses role-play and gives the child reasons as to why he or she would benefit from displaying the appropriate behavior.

The foster parent is taught to use "effective praise" (pp. 71–75) whenever the child displays any positive behavior, whereas the negative behavior is corrected and the child is given a consequence. The foster parents are taught to use the "four-to-one rule" which is to give the child at least four positive comments for every one corrective action they must take. This may take work for the foster parents to look for and praise positive behavior in the child. It encourages the foster parents to focus more on the positive behavior, and it helps the foster parent feel more positive about the child. When the child is given positive feedback, the parents are taught to give rationales as to how this positive behavior will benefit the child.

"Staying calm" (pp. 83–86) is taught as a technique for helping children to remain calm when they feel as if they are having a temper tantrum or losing control of their emotions. During a calm period, the foster parent uses preventive teaching to prepare the child for situations in which he or she tends to feel out of control. The foster parent and child come up with a plan for the child to stay calm, such as going to his or her room, playing music, or going outside. The plan is role-played, and the child is told what the consequence would be if he or she does not follow it.

Following is an example of the use of the model. Before Angela came to their home, Angela's treatment foster parents were told that she had a history of threatening to harm herself when she didn't get what she wanted. They prepared for this situation by calmly talking with her before an incident occurred in their home. They let her know that this behavior could occur again and suggested that instead of threatening or attempting to hurt herself, they should develop a "staying calm" plan together. Their plan consisted of Angela going to a quiet place such as her room, taking several deep breaths, and playing her favorite CD. The foster mother assured Angela she would check on her frequently and that when she was calm they would discuss alternative ways Angela could get things she wanted. The foster parent also helped Angela come up with a rationale as to why she should use the plan rather than hurt herself. Both Angela and the foster parents agreed that by staying calm Angela could feel better faster, avoid hospitalization, and gain the trust of adults and peers in her life. She also would be more likely to get a "yes" answer from the foster parent the next time she asked for something. The foster parents also indicated that if Angela did not use her staying calm plan when she became upset and instead had a temper tantrum, threatened harm, or disrupted the home in other ways, she would lose a privilege for the evening. The specific privilege would be based on the severity of the acting out behavior.

Effective praise was used whenever Angela displayed a behavior the foster parents wanted to encourage, such as being polite, asking permission, accepting no for an answer, or following her staying calm plan. She was occasionally given rewards for spontaneous displays of positive behavior. When Angela displayed a behavior that was inappropriate, such as swearing, displaying a tantrum after she was told "no" by the foster parent, or using the phone without permission, the foster parents used corrective teaching to stop the behavior, indicate that it was wrong, give a consequence, and discuss what to do instead. For example, when Angela swore at the dinner table, her foster mother immediately informed her that swearing was not appropriate and that she should use another word to express her feelings the next time. She was given a consequence of helping with the dishes after dinner, a chore she was not already assigned to do that day. The foster parent also taught Angela to use another word and softer tone of voice when expressing anger. This new way of expressing anger was practiced with Angela through role-playing.

Other intervention techniques can be effective as long as the foster parents are well trained and the use of the model is monitored by the agency worker. Foster parents should be provided ongoing formal training on a variety of topics to educate them on the various emotional and behavioral disturbances their children may demonstrate, particularly sexually abused children. In addition, the foster parents should be taught to develop and use their own plan to stay calm when they are under extreme stress. It is extremely important that treatment foster parents be able to tolerate a great number of negative behaviors, especially at the beginning of placement. They must be willing to invest time and energy into teaching social skills and be able to adequately cope when it seems that no progress is being made. Foster parents need coping skills so they can hang in there for the long term with these children.

Treatment foster parents should also be expected to follow the child's treatment plan which addresses symptoms of mental illness and past trauma along with any attachment issues. In this role, the parents are expected to provide an environment in which the child feels safe, secure, and able to heal. The interaction between foster parents and their foster child is crucial. They are not only responsible for the care and well-being of the child but are also the most influential people in the child's life during foster placement. The treatment foster parents' skills must go beyond that of formal caretakers providing more than love and willingness to help a child. They must be willing to accept a child into their home who may be hard to love. They must be willing to work diligently with children to teach them the skills they need to become functional adults. In addition, this all must be done without the need to feel loved back.

AGENCY SUPPORT

In order for the treatment foster parents to function well in their role as the main agents of change for the child, the agency must provide strong supportive services. At minimum, the agency team should include a case manager, a therapist for the child, and a respite worker. Based on the needs of the child, the agency may need to add a nurse, psychiatrist, pediatrician, occupational therapist, speech therapist, and/or physical therapist. Agency staff need to have access to these professionals as well as consultation with various professionals to assess the need for ancillary services. Foster parents will be in need of a lot of support and direction from staff in order to carry out their task to teach social skills to the child and to assist the child in forming attachments.

The foster parents will also need someone to talk to in order to deal with their own feelings of insecurity, failure, and ongoing struggles of living with a child who may be disrupting the family and failing to attach to the parents. The potential for foster parent burn-out is high. The agency team should be available at all times for crisis intervention that includes telephone support, assessing the need for psychiatric hospitalization or emergency respite when the child needs extra supervision or the foster parent needs immediate time away from the child. Foster parents should be empowered to intervene successfully in most crisis situations, but there are clearly times when agency staff need to go to the home during a crisis. This includes times when the child is suicidal, homicidal, or so out of control that the foster parent cannot calm him or her down.

CASE MANAGEMENT

Contact by the case manager who is responsible for the overall plan for the child should occur frequently, at least twice per month, and once per week when increased contact is warranted by the needs of the child and foster parent. The case manager ensures that all the needs of the child are being met, that the overall treatment plan is properly developed and implemented, and that the foster parents are using the intervention strategies as prescribed by the child's treatment plan. A case manager functions as an advocate for the needs of the child and should focus on the child's best interests with regard to his or her permanency plan, treatment plan, and placement decisions. A case manager should consider himself or herself the supervisor of the foster parent's treatment of the child. The case manager also oversees the ongoing training of the foster parent. The case manager provides supervised visits between the child and his or her biological family and coordinates all services, such as psychiatric monitoring and therapy, while also ensuring the most appropriate school setting. The case manager is responsible for making all diligent efforts necessary to reach the permanency goal of the child, whether it be return home or adoption. The case manager should remain in contact with all parties involved with the child, especially the teacher and school social worker, so all providers can work together to help the child. Case managers should possess, at a minimum, a bachelor's degree in a human service field, preferably in social work, and have experience in the child welfare system. The ideal case manager would have a bachelor's degree in social work (BSW) or a master's degree in social work (MSW) with at least two years of experience in child welfare and a vested interest in working in the child welfare field.

RESPITE CARE

In treatment foster care, the respite worker takes on direct treatment tasks with the child. Respite care provides care for the foster child in order to relieve the foster parent for a specific length of time and provides one-on-one social skill development for the child above that which is provided by the foster parent. One-on-one respite for at least 8 to 15 hours per week is recommended for the most challenging children. The one-on-one respite should be provided by staff who either have a bachelor's degree in human service or a high school diploma and experience working with children. Respite workers should be trained in the same intervention techniques as the foster parents and have a working knowledge of the child's treatment plan. Respite workers, given the amount of time they spend with the child, can address the teaching of specific social skills, using role-play, discussion, and practice in the community. For example, the respite worker can work on the skill of making friends by role-playing, taking the child to areas where he or she is likely to meet kids of the same age, and helping him or her meet other children. Respite workers can also help children learn how to react appropriately when they don't get their way by teaching, role-playing, monitoring situations, and then giving them immediate feedback on their developing skills.

HOME-BASED THERAPY

Home-based psychotherapy is provided to the child to specifically address his or her psychiatric symptoms as prescribed by the mental health treatment plan. Therapy is also provided to the biological parents if the goal of the child is to return home and this service has been identified as a need. The therapy treatment plan should be developed with input from the other team members, along with the child and family members. Therapy serves three major functions: (1) decreasing the child's symptoms, developing coping skills, and encouraging positive interactions; (2) assisting the foster parents to understand the child's symptoms and teaching them intervention strategies; and (3) working with the birth parents, if the goal is reunification, to decrease their symptoms of mental illness or maladaptive coping skills, improve family functioning, and correct the problems that brought the child into placement.

Why home-based as opposed to office-based treatment?

When working with treatment foster families, home-based therapy may be more effective than office-based therapy for a variety of reasons:

1. Foster parents are typically under a great deal of stress. Many have their own children, and they are responsible for taking their children to medical and dental appointments, school activities, sports, and so on. Providing case management services and therapy in the home is a welcome relief to the parents.

2. Compliance with treatment increases when it is delivered in the home. Foster parents may resist therapy because they may not be as invested in the child as a biological parent would be or may feel that they have no part in helping to solve the child's "problems." Meeting with them in their home can cut through potential resistance and decrease the likelihood of canceled or no-show sessions.

3. Staff can model appropriate boundaries and professionalism by having a clear agenda for the session, asking that the session not be interrupted by phone, television, and so on, and by interacting with all family members in a calm, respectful manner.

4. Home-based treatment is more likely to reinforce the healing relationship between the child and foster parents and empower the foster parents as change agents.

5. The therapist can more accurately assess family dynamics by observing foster family members in their own environment. Staff has the opportunity to witness everyday interactions between family members, allowing them to acknowledge strengths and treatment gains as well as focus on problem areas.

6. Staff can introduce and model intervention techniques during natural situations, increasing the likelihood that families will implement them. As opportunities arise, they can provide foster parents with direct feedback regarding their use of the strategies. Working with family members at home increases the likelihood that generalization of new skills will occur.

7. Home-based services became popular in child welfare and foster care as a way to monitor the safety of the child. This is still a good reason for foster care agencies to prove home-based case management services and therapy. Staff will be more aware of potential youth rights and licensing violations and potential abusive situations.

POTENTIAL PROBLEMS OF HOME-BASED TREATMENT

1. Foster parents can come to rely on the presence of their counselor/ case manager in order to problem solve and resolve crises. Foster parents must be trained to use the techniques taught by their counselor and to resolve crises without direct intervention from the counselor.

2. Counselors who do not understand the treatment plan or their role in the home as teacher/consultant/supporter may misuse the "freedom" of not being in the office and closely supervised. In other words, going to the mall is not necessarily an effective treatment for a teenage child unless the treatment plan indicates that the child has a skill deficit in an area that shopping would present opportunities for teaching and feedback.

3. The therapist or case manager must have the ability to create strong, physical and emotional boundaries where they may not exist. It can be tempting for the therapy session to turn into a casual friendly "get-together." Foster parents may want to create a friendship rather than a professional relationship.

4. On the other hand, it may be tempting for the office-based therapist to recreate the office in the home. Keep in mind that home-based therapy, when used effectively, is effective *because* it is in the home, not just because it is more convenient for the family.

BARRIERS TO HOME-BASED TREATMENT

1. *Cost.* Although treatment foster care is much cheaper than institutional care, the cost of traveling must be taken into consideration. The productive home-based staff person must be a master planner in order to reduce travel times. While an office-based therapist can see three children in three hours in the office, a home-based therapist traveling to three different homes could easily spend an additional two hours.

2. *Boundaries.* When you travel to the home, parents "forget" that the therapist's time is precious, therefore, keeping to a schedule can be difficult. The family may be more likely to engage in typical "home behavior" such as turning on the television, answering the phone, or walking in and out of the meeting area. Boundaries and limits must be set by the clinician to minimize this behavior while also allowing for some "natural" time to observe family interactions.

3. *Clarity.* It must be clear to all family members what the purpose of the staff's visits are. It is also important that clinicians are clear on their role in the home, lest they tend to inadvertently encourage a casual relationship with the family.

4. *Responsibility.* When the staff person conducts home-based treatment, the foster parent may become more reliant on the staff and have expectations that the staff person will fulfill responsibilities that the parent should be fulfilling, such as teaching social skills or transporting the child to an appointment.

5. *Integration.* Integrating all the service components in home-based therapy, such as therapist, case manager, respite workers, and outside doctors, can be extremely difficult but crucial in the overall treatment of the child.

6. *Staff professionalism.* The freedom of home-based treatment, coupled with an inexperienced staff person, may lead to a lack of understanding of the task at hand. Clinicians must be clear on the differences between using play as a therapeutic intervention (Play Therapy) versus simply playing with the child. The treatment environment must be

conducive to the development of a therapeutic relationship between clinician and child and should enable confidential, meaningful treatment. Unless the clinician is observing a child in different environments, chaotic areas such as restaurants and areas with a lot of other activities should be avoided.

USING FOSTER PARENTS AS THE AGENTS OF CHANGE

In the treatment foster care model described here, the foster parents are considered to be the main agents of change. Their interactions with the child on a daily basis will have the most influence over their overall health status and healing from trauma. Treatment foster care draws on many of the behavior modification techniques used in the residential setting, but combines them with child and family therapy, respite care, intensive case management, and ongoing support for the foster parent. Services take place in the foster home or community, and all attempts are made to integrate the child into the family and surrounding community, such as school, church, camps, and neighborhood activities.

The keys to success are well-trained foster parents, supportive staff, and flexible services to provide:

1. ongoing treatment to address the mental health issues and symptomology of the child, to include individual and family therapy, and psychiatric monitoring if necessary;
2. ongoing training and supervision of foster parents;
3. respite for the foster family;
4. mentoring and social skill training for the child;
5. crisis intervention; and
6. the ongoing monitoring and integration of all the service components listed above in order to embrace the concept of the whole community (both professional and non-professional) caring for the needs of the child.

ANGELA IN TREATMENT FOSTER CARE

When Angela was referred for treatment foster care, her case was carefully assessed by the agency. The potential foster parents were given all the pertinent information in order to make a decision on whether or not to meet Angela. They were informed of Angela's past and given a summary of the types of inappropriate behavior she had exhibited in her previous foster homes. The treatment foster parents were also informed of Angela's strengths and the types of things that motivated her. They met with Angela several times before placement actually occurred. Both Angela and the foster parents were part of the placement process, with both being asked to make a long-term commitment to the placement.

After Angela moved in, the case manager worked with the foster parents to identify the areas to address. The foster parents chose to address the following problems first: (a) using foul language when angry, (b) making phone calls without permission, (c) suicidal ideation or attempts, and (d) being defiant when asked to do something she doesn't want to do. Over the first week, the foster parent discussed the four areas with Angela, gave her alternative social skills to use in these situations, and explained to her what the consequence would be if she chose to use the inappropriate behavior rather than the social skill.

In addition, the foster parents helped Angela become acclimated to her new environment by showing her the layout of the house, defining her personal space vs. family space, and explaining typical family patterns and rules along with making Angela feel comfortable in her new home. The foster parents identified the following social skills to teach: (a) expressing feelings appropriately, (b) following directions, (c) showing respect, and (d) developing and using a staying calm plan when upset. These skills were taught and role-played with Angela in an effort to prevent the display of aforementioned negative behaviors.

The foster parents worked hard to give Angela the message that they would not abandon her although she tested them again and again by breaking the rules. Each time Angela displayed an undesirable behavior, the foster parents consistently gave a consequence while teaching her the appropriate social skill. It took many months, but finally Angela began to understand that the foster parents would react consistently to all of her behaviors, both positive and negative. The foster parents gave her positive praise every day for her strengths and encouraged her to direct her energy into areas where she could excel. Angela found that she was good with young children and began to help babysit at church activities. She realized she could sing and joined the choir at school and church. She took swimming lessons and began to write her feelings in her journal. The increased praise and activities helped to raise her self-esteem and gave her more opportunities to make friends.

Angela's therapist worked with her on forming a more realistic relationship with her biological family and teaching her coping skills when her family let her down. She also helped Angela understand that what her birth parents did to her was not her fault and that not all parents behaved in this manner. They worked on ways to problem solve when Angela was upset about not making friends or was angry with her foster parents. Her therapist also gave information to the foster parents to help them understand that Angela would not attach easily and they would need to be tolerant and patient in order for Angela to make progress.

Respite staff spent one evening a week with Angela, along with occasional weekend days. Depending on the needs at the time, the respite worker either stayed in the home with Angela or took her out of the home to give some rest to the foster parents. The respite worker became a mentor to Angela and worked on social skills such as making friends and how to interpret the meanings of the actions of other kids. She worked on appropriate phone manners and reinforced the rules developed by the foster parents.

The foster parents struggled with Angela's defiance and seemingly endless "forgetting" of the rules of the house. Angela was full of excuses as to why she did not complete her chores, why she did not come home from school on time, why she swore, and so on. Angela would frequently have outbursts of anger and tell the foster parents she wanted to move out and that she hated them. By using corrective teaching, effective praise at a 4:1 ratio, and the staying calm plan, the foster parents were able to stay calm themselves and stick with their consequences. By being consistent, firm, loving, and simply hanging in there, the foster parents finally saw a reduction in negative behavior. They began to feel connected to Angela as she realized that this family would not kick her out. Angela began to give up her hard exterior, her defense against pain, and allowed herself to feel connected to the foster parents.

In treatment foster care, a child like Angela can be given the opportunity to develop healthy relationships, learn appropriate social skills, and eventually grow to be a mentally healthy adult. Treatment foster care can provide children like Angela with a family with whom a life-long relationship can be developed and a family that will demonstrate unconditional love while guiding and teaching. Treatment foster care can be the key to avoiding the cycle of foster home disruptions while also avoiding the need for the restrictive environment of a residential facility. Kids like Angela can have a healthy family life, develop relationships with adults and peers, and thus be armed with the abilities to cope and adapt to the world around them.

REFERENCES

American Psychiatric Association. (1994). *Diagnostic and statistical manual of mental disorders* (4th ed.). Washington, DC: American Psychiatric Press.
Baker C., Burke, R., Herron, R., & Mott, M. (1996). *Rebuilding children's lives, a blueprint for treatment foster parents.* Boys Town, NE: Boys Town Press.

Caring for Children: A Foster Parent's Perspective

Alice Farrell

Alice Farrell left a successful career as a special-education teacher to devote herself full time to fostering mentally ill children in her home. With warmth and humor, she here describes her experience as a foster mother. Reading her story, we were struck by the immensity of the tasks she and other foster parents take on.

My husband, Brad, and I were on the veritable verge of being "empty nesters" when I began to play around with the idea of doing foster care. I was teaching cognitively impaired adolescents in a local middle school, and he held a central office position in a nearby school district. After much discussion and considerable discouragement from friends, relations, and our family therapist, we decided that we would become licensed and then decide. We followed through on this plan and went through the 10-week training course, locked up our dangerous chemicals, installed a carbon monoxide detector, and had our fire extinguisher recharged. We filled out about a million forms, had our fingerprints taken, and gradually made our way through the bureaucracy of the Department of Children and Family Services (DCFS). Then one day, after we had dotted all of the I's and crossed all of the T's, our license arrived in the mail. Just 3 days later, our lives began to change forever.

I was out somewhere. I can't remember where, maybe dinner with Gina. I was writing curriculum with Peg, Joan, and Mary Kay. I think we worked until evening, and I met Gina and Sue for dinner. I came home and Brad said I should call Linda James about a possible foster child. The child was only 5 but he would probably be in school in the fall. Our age range was 6 to 12. We had been trying to avoid real teenagers. The memories of leaping each time you hear a siren, praying when the phone rings after 10:00 P.M., and wondering why the scotch is so very pale were all too fresh for us. Of course we weren't equipped for preschoolers. It wasn't just that we didn't have a crib or a high chair or toys. We both worked. I think we thought we could do foster care in our spare time. After all, we had nine children between us, and as they were all getting older, we had some time and lots of experience at parenting. My three boys were 17, 18, and 19, and Brad's children, who ranged from 13 to 23, were usually out of sight if seldom out of mind. I called Linda. It seemed that Michael Stanton, almost age 6, was currently residing at a local psychiatric hospital. Linda knew next to nothing about him except that there was to be a discharge staffing the next day and I should go if we were interested and available.

What harm could a staffing be? I said I would go. I remember arriving and meeting so many people who seemed to know that I was a Special Education teacher. This seemed so important to them. What difference did it make? My real credentials as far as I was concerned had to do with the three sons I had successfully raised with the help of a loving father and a pretty wonderful step-father. I taught mildly to severely mentally handicapped teenagers. That seemed a far cry from a 5-year-old in a psychiatric hospital.

I only vaguely remember what I learned about Michael at that meeting. I guess I heard that he sometimes got up in the night and that he had damaged some things in his parents' house. I know I heard that he was outside, naked at 6:00 in the morning attempting to drown the family's miniature dachshund. There was some suggestion that he may have been sexually abused but it was guardedly mentioned. He also was on lots of drugs: clonidine, Thorazine, and imipramine.

I listened while people talked about him. No one seemed to know very much or else they all knew a lot and didn't feel the need to discuss it for my benefit. At the conclusion of the meeting, I went with three people into a little room and someone brought Michael in to meet me. I remember being struck by how incredibly little he was. I teach in a middle school and my own children begin at 5'11". I had no memory of how little 5 can be. How little and how incredibly vulnerable. I stooped down to meet him at eye level. A woman from the group said, "This is Alice. In a few days you will be going to live with her and her family."

I'm not sure if I was more shocked by these words or the fact that he simply walked to me and put his arms around me. It would be fair to say that I was smitten. At that moment I knew that no matter what Brad said, this child would live in our home. I also knew that Brad would only need to meet this child to feel exactly the same as I did. I tried to focus on the fact that this kid did real damage to real property. I tried to remember that he attempted to kill an animal. I tried not to look into the most beautiful eyes I had ever seen. What color were they anyhow? Dark, dark hazel I guessed. His shorts and tee shirt were mismatched and I immediately began to conjure up the poor, drug-addicted, neglectful, dirty, disgusting criminals that had been so undeservedly blessed with this precious child. I found myself searching for the tell-tale cigarette burns and I imagined the welts on his back. I wondered if he had eaten dog food or lived in filth. Every report of child abuse that I had heard on the ten o'clock news rushed in at me. I was beginning to get a clear picture of the monsters who had so incredibly abused this child to force him to act out in these ways to get the help that we were more than capable of giving him. Act One of the play for control had begun.

Brad, with only minimal urging from me, stopped at the hospital on his way home from work that evening. I had to go and continue with my curriculum writing and it was not until I got home that I knew for sure that he was as smitten as I. Over the next few days we went to the hospital every day, sometimes together and sometimes separately depending on our schedules.

I was writing curriculum for the high school program in the evenings and tutoring a couple of mornings a week. We were having a high school graduation party for Andrew, my second son, and Patrick, my nephew from Ohio, on Saturday. This involved out-of-town company, a disc jockey, and a caterer for the 100-plus guests. Together with the case worker, we decided that Michael should come to our home on Sunday, the day after the party. Suddenly the party seemed to take care of itself. All I thought about was Michael. And my son Will.

On June 6, the first real day of summer to an educator, Will had come in an hour past curfew. I grounded him for a week. The next day he left our home and we had not seen or heard from him since. Through the teenage grapevine, I knew he was spending the nights with a close friend and working at 7-Eleven. He had left word that I could contact him if I wanted to talk about things. "Things" meant "rules," which actually meant changing the rules. Will was never one to simply accept the rules because they were there.

Well, I had no intention of changing the rules for him and nor did I feel the need to contact him. He was the one who left his home. I would be available when he wanted to contact me. Of course, all of this courage and steadfastness were the direct result of a few long, difficult sessions with Catherine, our family therapist. Will was not a new control issue for me, just one that I was finally learning to give up.

Thus it was that on July 2, 1995, we left the rubble of the previous night's party and drove to the psychiatric hospital to exchange our peaceful life for the experience of Michael.

We received our mini training session on how to care for this complicated little boy while standing in the lobby of the hospital. It was a Sunday. We were alone in the lobby of the hospital. No grandmas and grandpas waiting to bring a stuffed animal to their precious grandbaby. No husbands carrying flowers for their wives. We stood leaning through a window cut in the wall while a tall, thin, middle-aged nurse whom we had never met highlighted the discharge papers for us in rapid-fire style. Give him these drugs at these times. Give him time-outs like this. Keep an eye on your dog and good luck! Well, we were experienced parents. What did we need that these people could give anyway? So we drove home with a beautiful little boy and a garbage bag full of his possessions.

During our visits with Michael in the hospital, he had asked us one question repeatedly. Did we have a garage-door opener? We had assured him that indeed we did have a garage-door opener. When he climbed into our car he asked if he could hold the garage-door opener. There he sat in the back seat of our car clinging to the garage-door opener as if it were a teddy bear. The opener was held in his right hand. His left thumb was seldom out of his mouth.

Our home, a four-bedroom colonial, is located on a cul de sac, which our other children referred to as "the court." Oak Ridge Court to be precise. There were at that time no children under 17 living on the court. We were, in fact, the only family on the court with children who still lived at home. We were the only family on the court with more than one garbage can, a lawn that was not edged, a functional basketball net, and cars honking their horns in the driveway. The homes in the court were all approximately 30 years old, and many of them were occupied by the original owners. Our newest family member was soon to make an impression on each one of them.

Michael, on the other hand, was only impressed by a few things. Our ceiling fans, our dog, Sammy, and our garage-door openers—the ones in our cars and the one on the wall of the garage. We had borrowed a two-wheeler with training wheels from friends whose daughter had outgrown it. It was a girl's bike and it came equipped with a straw basket. I was concerned that Michael would object to the femininity of both bike and basket. On the contrary, his gross motor skills were so underdeveloped that I doubt if he could have ridden a boy's bike, and the basket was the perfect place to carry a garage-door opener.

We had been warned by the case worker that Michael was enthralled by garage-door openers and that this was probably related to his need to control his environment. We had decided to allow him freedom to use the opener until he lost interest. I had my master's degree in Special Education, after all. I knew about saturation. If allowed to use the garage-door opener with no restrictions, Michael would theoretically become bored with it and move on to some more interesting activity.

Unfortunately, no one had ever told Michael about saturation. Brad and I sat in lawn chairs in the driveway on Sunday, Monday, and Tuesday, July 2, 3, and 4, while Michael rode his bike around the cul de sac and back again. He opened the garage door, exited the garage, and closed the garage door. Then he rode to the end of the driveway and opened it again and closed it again. He rode around the circle until he was across the street from the garage and opened and closed the door again. He would then ride to the end of the cul de sac and turn around and return with all of the same stops to open and close the garage.

He did try the opener on each of the neighbors' garages just to be sure it wouldn't actually open them. When Brad returned to work on July 5, I tried leaving Michael outside for short periods so that I could do a few simple household tasks like making the bed and washing the breakfast dishes. On his own, Michael located every garage-door opener in the court. He was not too shy to enter cars in driveways. If a garage was left open, Michael entered it and used the wall button. He asked every person he saw if they had a garage-door opener and if they could show him how it worked. People were charmed by the inquisitive little boy who was curious about garage-door openers and often gave him information they would later regret. They were quickly irritated by the persistent little boy who was obsessed with garage-door openers.

After about 2 weeks with saturation nowhere in sight, we moved the garage door opener to reward status. Michael was allowed to use the garage door opener when it was necessary to open or close the garage door, if and only if he had been behaving himself. When we visited friends, we explained to Michael that he would be permitted to operate their garage door once when we were leaving if he had behaved appropriately while we were there. Our friends looked at us oddly, but cooperated.

Michael went to sleep with no difficulty. In fact, he was usually tired and ready to fall asleep by 8:00 P.M. He had no apparent bedtime routine and was not too sure about bedtime stories. I was, however, extremely sure about bedtime stories and determined that I would establish a warm, nurturing bedtime routine. I simply reached for a book with no real thought. It was *Grandpa's Slippers*. This is a pattern book and very good for beginning readers and so, I deduced, for beginning listeners. The sentence structure remains the same throughout the story with only a few words changing as the story progresses. Grandma keeps attempting to dispose of grandpa's slippers, and grandpa keeps finding them and scolding grandma. Michael half listened, interrupted with questions not pertaining to the story, and fell asleep before I finished.

The next night I again insisted on reading. He insisted that it be the same book. Fine with me. By the fourth night of reading *Grandpa's Slippers,* Michael was attentive and in fact knew the book by heart. On night five I asked that we try a new book. He declined. I finally got him to agree to one book of his choice and one book of my choice. Each night I would select a new story and each night Michael would select *Grandpa's Slippers.* Eventually he moved on to *The Very Quiet Cricket* and *How Many Bugs In A Box?* Michael would never select a book for his choice that I hadn't already read to him. He memorized many books and was able to quote from them when a word or phrase would trigger his memory.

This also made bedtime into a very calm, quiet time between us. No demands were placed on either of us to really communicate with our own words. Some nights I was so angry with Michael by bedtime that I would refuse to read to him. Some nights he was so angry with me that he would tell me that he didn't want any stories.

To allow this to happen was a big mistake on my part. I do believe that a bedtime routine should be a consistent part of every child's life. Too often, life circumstances will make this routine impossible to follow. Our anger and resentment should not be one of those circumstances. Forcing both of us to participate in this bedtime routine, I, as the adult, take control while allowing Michael, as the child, to maintain control. Not to mention that it is very hard to read a bedtime story or listen to a bedtime story and not let go of your anger.

It became apparent to us very quickly that Michael could not play outside without supervision. He also refused to be outside unless the weather was sunny and 80°. Michael had no tolerance for heat and quickly became "sweaty" on warmer days. This usually led to removal of clothing. As our neighborhood was one in which people had no real appreciation of nudity, it was best to keep Michael inside on the warmest days.

When inside, Michael could entertain himself for hours in the basement rec room. Our basement offers a wide variety of activities for children of all ages. There are sofas, a television, a VCR, Nintendo, Sega, a pool table, a computer and printer, a treadmill, and shelves filled with paper, envelopes, markers, crayons, tape, scissors, a stapler, a variety of hole punchers, and all manner of school and office supplies. As we are somewhat concerned with environmental issues, there is a trunk filled with boxes and tissue paper that we break down after each Christmas celebration to reuse the following year. There is also a bin filled with ribbons, bows, fancy bags, and rolls of wrapping paper.

Michael would write his name and many other letter-like symbols on pieces of paper. He called this "doing his paperwork"—perhaps a phrase he learned from Brad, who was constantly doing paperwork. Michael would then put his papers inside of envelopes, tape the envelopes shut, staple them on all four sides, place them in boxes, wrap the boxes, tie them with string, and occasionally put them in his bike basket and ride them around the cul de sac. On a few occasions, Michael offered these packages as gifts to people, however, they were not allowed to keep them. Eventually, to further save our earth, we banned the use of boxes and wrapping paper. At about this time Michael began to prepare for Fido's birthday. Fido and Pete were stuffed animals, and they were the only toys Michael had brought with him to our home. Pete did not have birthdays, however, Fido had so many that I guess poor Pete did not miss his.

Say "Fido's birthday" to us, say "full moon" to the parents of a werewolf—the effect is the same. When Michael began to prepare for Fido's birthday, he put on his Oshkosh overalls with a belt. He taped papers all over the basement walls and ceiling, stapled papers to things—anything—and tied string, ribbon, dog leashes, belts, and virtually anything that could be tied to anything it could be tied to. We never really understood why the occasion was called Fido's birthday. There was no cake or ice cream. No pin the tail on the donkey. Just this simulation of crepe paper streamers.

During these birthday-preparation periods it would not be unusual to enter Michael's bedroom at 5:30 in the morning and find that something was strung from the door knob to the ceiling fan to the curtain rod to the bed post to the closet door. Various stuffed toys would be dangling from belts, ribbons, and even shoelaces from the ceiling fan or curtain rods. You could then look into Michael's eyes and see that he was "gone." He would not answer you when you spoke. He would work with a vengeance and occasionally he would scream at himself and begin to cry. He would actually break down and sob but was resistive to any assistance or comfort we would offer. As time went on, he began to do things that were destructive and even dangerous. He used cords from lamps, clocks, and telephones and just let the items dangle. He also refused to clean up and consequently the area became unusable by anyone else.

While Michael was in his "Fido's birthday" personality, he was unwilling to do anything else and he became violent if he was physically forced to leave what he was doing. He shared with us the full range of his vocabulary, bit, scratched, and kicked. Michael was very little and pretty easy to carry around; however, he did manage to give me a black eye simply by moving quickly and when I least expected it.

Never, never did he show remorse. He would let me know that it was too bad that I got hurt and advise me to leave him alone. We may have been slow learners but learn we did. We quickly let go of the idea that Michael was extremely creative and that this creativity would one day be channeled into his brilliant career in engineering. It eventually became clear to us that Michael would never be able to have a relationship with another person let alone work with people if he was allowed to continue in this fashion. We banned Michael from playing with anything that could be tied. We finally removed even his belts from his room. Tape and staples and even scissors became items that were only used with supervision. All overalls were packed up. Michael was very clever and, I guess, driven to find things that could be tied. He removed the strap from his camera, string from his windbreaker, and even the bows from his stuffed animals. We became vigilant and shuddered when he was given a stop watch as a gift. Michael commented that it could be worn around his neck, however, we feared that he had other plans. Within 4 hours, we removed the stuffed animal that was hanging from the ceiling fan in his bedroom. Michael learned to leave his shoelaces in his shoes only when we told him he would not be able to go out of the house unless his shoes were tied.

There were many battles that were quickly won with natural consequences. These are the consequences that will naturally occur if we can just be patient. Because Michael was such a bright, articulate child, he was quickly able to see the relationship between his behavior and the natural consequence. Table manners were among the first of these battles. We eat dinner in the dining room whenever there are more than three people for dinner. In the summer when our college students are home, this is almost every night. Brad does most of the cooking and in those last critical minutes everyone pitches in. Consequently, when Michael was served apple sauce and had no spoon, it was difficult to say whose fault it actually was. I doubt that his response would have been appropriate in any home. He simply began to scream. For a moment we all looked at him. He stopped to let us know that he needed a spoon. No one moved. I suggested that he either ask for one politely or get up and get one for himself. He chose to continue screaming. We chose to continue eating. At one point he threw himself from his chair onto the floor. One of the boys lifted him back to his chair and reminded him that he needed to ask to be excused. After about 5 minutes—which can seem an eternity when you are ignoring screams—Michael went to the kitchen and got himself a spoon. Michael learned to say "please pass," "no thank you," and "may I be excused" in much the same manner. The unpredictability of these little learning experiences led to a temporary reduction in our dinner guests, but eventually Michael adapted to our culture.

Michael was extremely afraid of water or perhaps it would be more correct to say that he was afraid of being wet. One evening shortly after Michael came into our home, I was finishing the dinner dishes and he was doing "paperwork" on the kitchen floor. After the last pot was washed I turned with a grin and playfully flicked Michael with my wet fingers. This was something I had done a million times over the years with my own children. I was completely unprepared for Michael's response.

He began to scream as though I had poured acid on his face. He pulled his T-shirt off as though it were on fire and ran into the bath-room to wipe the nonexistent drops from his chest. He then went and got a "dry" shirt from his dresser and refused to even touch the "wet" shirt on the kitchen floor. His only explanation was that he did NOT like to be wet.

Michael would not touch wet things nor would he leave on any wet clothing. If he spilled on his shorts, off they came. If his underwear had also gotten wet, his phobia was far stronger than his modesty. (His modesty for that matter was just about nonexistent.) He would not touch the car door after rain or snow. He would simply stand outside of the car and scream. After opening the door for him a few times, we threatened to leave him. He would then open the door and scream for the next few minutes until his hands dried.

As luck would have it, the summer did begin to draw to a close and we were faced with the hard cold fact that Michael would have to be subjected to the American public school system. I called our local grade school and they told me I needed to begin the registration process by completing about 5,000 forms and sending some of them off to DCFS so that records could be released and exchanged and all of that. I remembered some of this from our Foster Parent Training class-es and, of course, I am a cog in this wheel when I am in my teacher role, so some of this was familiar to me. At any rate, we did get through the paperwork and Michael was appropriately registered for first grade.

Next we had to face the issue of child care, as I would also be returning to teach school. We needed day care for both before and after school as well as for the occasional evening meeting. We were assured that there were a few spots for foster children in each of the local chain-type day care centers. I called around and found that all of these spots were indeed filled. Next we moved on to the list of day care homes that had agreed to take children through DCFS. This list was very short and after visiting some of the homes it was clearly evident why they would agree to take the very minimal rate that DCFS offers for child care. The homes were often dirty, located on extremely busy streets, lacking toys or play equipment, and already filled with the children who actually lived there. We ultimately, and extremely hesitantly, placed Michael in a private daycare home down the street from his school. The Good Housekeeping stamp of approval had been denied to this home and the primary caretaker was, more often than not, minus her teeth. It seemed that the contrast to our home was exciting for Michael and he loved going there. In fact, he may actually have continued going there if he had not done extensive damage to the plumbing by shoving enough Legos far enough down each drain to pass the elbow. He found himself incapable of walking from one location to another without body slamming several toddlers as they attempted their first steps. He taught the older kids how to tie all of their clothing and bed sheets together and connect the door knob to the curtain rod to the dresser drawer, thus creating a chain reaction when slamming the door. Michael was given several "one last chances" in this home. They may have desperately needed the money, minimal as it was.

Finally, at Thanksgiving, Brad and I made the decision that Michael could not return to this home for everyone's sake. There was a serious risk that Michael would harm another child, the caretaker seemed on the verge of a breakdown, and we were exhausted from listening to the litany of his crimes each day when we picked him up. We told DCFS that they would have to place a child care worker in our home or remove Michael from our home. Facing finding a new home for Michael was such a prospect that a respite worker was immediately placed in our home.

Michael was placed in Mrs. Ward's first-grade classroom along with 24 other bright, shining 6-year-olds. Mrs. Ward is just what every parent and every first-grader hopes for in a teacher. She is bright eyed, enthusiastic, soft spoken, gentle, and knows how to make 6-year-olds love school.

It became immediately evident that Michael had missed picking up those "school routine" skills in kindergarten. He NEVER raised his hand. He simply spoke out or got out of his seat and wandered around the classroom. He only agreed to do what the class was doing when it was of great interest to him. Most of what the class was doing was of

NO interest to him. He preferred to do his "paperwork" and wander around. When asked or required to participate in an activity with the class, he simply said no or began to kick and scream. On September 5, Michael ran from his aide, climbed on top of the monkey bars, and refused to come down. When the principal attempted to assist, he bit her and called her a "butt-sniffer."

At home, however, we saw changes in Michael's paperwork. He had quickly learned to write all the letters of the alphabet and was intrigued with putting them together to form words. He was thrilled that he could actually write words like "butt," "fart," and "fat." He copied words from the newspaper, magazines, books, and even the junk mail. He used pencils, pens, crayons, markers and he even carved the word "pee" into his dresser top with a fork. A boy in his class brought a dream catcher to school and Mrs. Ward explained to the children how people made dream catchers and hung them over their beds to catch the bad dreams and allow only the good dreams through the netting. Michael made dream catchers out of every conceivable material, and we each had one hanging in our bedrooms so we could all sleep more peacefully.

It was quickly determined that Michael would need some special education services and a one-on-one aide. We were informed that District 45 was a full-inclusion district, and this meant that all services were to be delivered in the regular classroom. Mrs. Atherton, the Learning Disabilities/Behavior Disorders teacher, began to work with Michael in the classroom. Other first-graders, however, are not accustomed to working quietly while another student is kicking and biting teachers and screaming obscenities.

A time-out area was constructed in another area of the school where Michael could regain control of his emotions before returning to the classroom to work. It soon became the place where Michael and his aide spent much of the day. On one occasion when Michael was particularly verbally abusive to his aide, she threatened to spray him with water. When she returned to the time-out area with the squirt bottle, Michael was completely naked with his clothes folded next to him. He told her that he did not want his clothes to get wet.

After many parent conferences and multidisciplinary meetings it was suggested that we look into placing Michael in a segregated facility. A school for behaviorally disturbed children. A therapeutic day school. A school designed to meet the individual needs of students who impede teaching and learning in the regular public school.

From the moment we entered the school I hated it. Teachers were wearing sweatpants and kids were milling around. I couldn't believe that any real learning went on in a place like this. I know that kids can learn without the formality of regular school. It was not the formality that was lacking. It was the starkness of the environment. No learning center, no computers, no bulletin boards, no bright colors, nothing to draw your attention. Nothing said this is a place where children are stretching and growing. But maybe Michael needed this. Can all the hours and minutes of therapy make up for the environment? Will those carpeted walls in the time-out room help him to control his anger? Will all these one-way mirrors enable someone to unlock Michael's secret pain? Will he ever have another dream catcher experience?

Brad and I shared our concerns with the staff at Michael's regular school and something wonderful happened. They would create a self-contained classroom for Michael. Jennifer Atherton would be the teacher and they would hire an aide. It seemed that Michael's last aide had all but run screaming from the building. Jennifer would continue to work with a few other children and, during these periods, Michael would be working with the aide. He would still use the learning center, go to assemblies, eat in the lunch room, and even occasionally visit Mrs. Ward's classroom for activities. Michael would complete the first-grade curriculum and participate in a program with appropriate consequences and rewards designed to shape his behavior.

Mrs. Atherton was everything we could hope for in a Special Education teacher. She was young enough to have the energy for the job and experienced enough to not be manipulated. She was gentle, demanding, consistent and, above all, she loved Michael. It began to seem like Michael could complete first grade in his home school in a program tailored to meet his needs. Brad, Michael, and I relaxed for the first time since the school year had begun.

Michael had no idea of boundaries. He simply could not understand that the whole world was not awaiting him with open arms. When we went into a restaurant, Michael commonly went behind the hostess counter to let her know that we had arrived. We quickly learned to censor what we said to him. When Michael asked when our food would be ready, I once told him that since I wasn't cooking it, I really couldn't tell him. In a flash, he was off to the kitchen to ask the chef. In grocery stores, he commonly disappeared to go watch the butcher carve meat or help the fish lady select the very best pieces of salmon. He often ducked under the counter to help at the check-out counter, and I was most surprised to see his face pop out at me when I selected my gallon of milk. He thought it best to sit with the receptionist in the doctor's office and take this opportunity to ask her for insurance forms, which would be helpful in his paperwork, and xerox a few of his other papers. He asked for and collected forms everywhere we went. Sales receipts, job applications, credit-card applications, warranty forms, insurance forms, and "how was our service?" forms were invaluable to Michael. His bedroom was filled with forms filled in with "dog bites" or "you are fat" or "yes" or "no."

His bedroom was indeed filled. Michael collected scraps of paper from everywhere. He was interested in all kinds of containers—bags, boxes, envelopes, anything that could contain something. His desk drawers, toy shelves, and closet floor were filled with his collections. Periodically, on a school day when Michael was gone, we would do a sweep of his bedroom. We would throw out everything but the top layer. He never seemed to notice or never complained if he did and, in this way, we were able to maintain space in his room for his bed, his clothing, and his fish.

On his first birthday in our home, we gave Michael a 10-gallon fish tank and all of the necessary apparatus to keep fish happy. Michael had a wonderful time setting the tank up and very impatiently waited until the water was ready to safely house fish. We took a trip to the pet store and purchased the recommended variety for a community tank. Michael fed his fish as part of his bedtime routine, rinsed the filter as part of his Saturday routine, and spent hours watching them swim around. He used the light from the tank as his night light and drifted off to sleep each night for a year sucking his thumb and watching his fish. Then he killed them.

I sensed that something was wrong when I walked into Michael's bedroom at 6:30 and he was still asleep. The chair from his desk was moved to the dresser and, as I walked over to put it back, I realized that my bare feet were getting wet. There was water all over the dresser top, around the fish tank as well. I then realized that the water level in the fish tank was down several inches. At first I didn't notice that there were no fish in the tank, just that the light and cover were askew and the gravel was lumpy. Michael woke up then and I asked him what had happened. He said he didn't know. I asked if he had played in his fish tank in the night and he replied that he guessed maybe he had. I was beginning to design a consequence for splashing water on the floor as I opened his drawer to get his school clothes out. There, amid T-shirts and sweat shirts, were two very dead fish. I continued to open drawers in the dresser. Each one held several dead fish mixed in with socks, underwear, pajamas, sweatpants, and jeans. I moved on to the desk where several other corpses were lying around in paperwork, paper clips, and crayons. I sat down on the floor and I cried. Michael comforted me and said that we could buy new fish. Indeed. And how could we help the little boy who so suddenly and so carelessly destroyed the things he loved?

The passing of the fish signaled the beginning of a downward spiral in Michael's behavior that ended with a psychotic episode that took him back into the hospital. Medication was changed and changed again as Michael continued to hear voices, sleep for 18 hours a day, and barely recognize us when we made our daily visits. Finally, as the result of efforts made by some excellent people in the field of mental health, Michael was diagnosed with Asperger's Syndrome as well as bipolar disorder. Asperger's is a pervasive developmental disorder on the same continuum as autism. Persons with Asperger's often become obsessed with things. Persons with Asperger's often are compulsive about things. Persons with Asperger's are often intellectually gifted. Persons with Asperger's often have difficulty with boundaries. Persons with Asperger's AND bipolar disorder have incredible mood swings with no apparent, precipitating event.

Michael is currently on a medication regimen that is meeting his needs. He is attending a school that specializes in meeting the needs of children with pervasive disorders. No one really knows what the prognosis is for Michael. Will he ever be able to live independently? Will he ever be competitively employed? Will he be able to go to college? For us, for now, for Michael, we are hoping that third grade goes well.

We have read lots of books on foster parenting, fact and fiction. Nothing could have prepared us for the experience of Michael in our lives. While we were struggling with the decision of whether or not to become foster parents, friends asked us many questions. The most common one was "Aren't you afraid of getting your hearts broken?" We thought about this and decided that life was all about getting your heart broken. Hadn't we ached as we watched our biological children struggle mightily, make poor choices, and waste potential? There are no words of wisdom, books, lectures, or videos to prepare you for the guilt, fear, and wonder of being a parent to any child, or anyone's child. Before Michael it would have been helpful for us to have known how to take really good care of ourselves. If only we had known we needed a massage before every muscle in our bodies ached. If only we had known that we needed a vacation before we found ourselves falling asleep driving home from work. If only we had known that we needed time alone before we put the bread in the refrigerator and tucked the ham and the mayonnaise in the bread box. Before Michael it would have been helpful for us to have gone to medical school, received doctorates in education, understood the intricacies of the child welfare system, and known the mind of God.

Sometimes we wonder about the life we could have had if we had never met Michael. If we had never crossed his path. If we had never fallen in love with him. Sometimes we wonder how we would have filled that enormous space in our lives. Mother Theresa said that God does not ask that we be successful, only that we be faithful. Michael has taught us the difference between being successful and being faithful. We have learned from our experience with him that the reward of perseverance is that you persevered, the reward of diligence is that you were diligent, and the reward of loving is that you loved. Words like "perfect," "fixed," and "finished" have vanished from our vocabulary. Words like "frustrated," "angry," and "exhausted" have taken on new meaning. Sometimes I still want my empty nest, and someday I'm sure I'll have it. I'll just be a little grayer than I would have been, my glasses will be a little stronger, my wrinkles will be a little deeper, and I will surely be a little wiser.

CHAPTER ELEVEN

Therapeutic Assistants: Cost-Effective In-Home Psychosocial Care

Nancy A. Newton

In the following chapter, Nancy Newton discusses a way of integrating paraprofessional home health workers into the treatment team as therapeutic assistants. As part of her discussion, she presents a case in which a certified nursing assistant plays a central role in the mental health treatment of a severely disturbed woman. This case illustrates how psychological symptoms can be an adaptive response to craziness in a person's daily life. By working closely with the client, the CNA discovered that her client's stolid resistance to returning to full functioning had roots in a long-standing conflict with her husband.

One of the challenges confronting in-home treatment programs for adults with severe psychiatric symptoms is providing high-intensity service in a cost-effective way. Often during periods of acute crisis, clients require more support than can realistically be provided in brief visits by mental health professionals, whether they are nurses, social workers, psychologists, or psychiatrists. Sometimes clients in crisis need assistance, such as help with personal care, meal preparation, errands, and structuring and maintenance of daily activities, that are not considered the domain of highly trained and credentialed staff. Some intensive, home-based treatment programs address this issue by involving family members and enlisting their support (Moy & Pigott, 1997), however, this solution is not always possible.

Within clinic, outpatient, and inpatient programs, therapeutic roles and responsibilities are assigned according to required level of professional expertise (and correlated) expense. Thus, when extensive staff time is required to provide treatment and/or monitor patient safety, paraprofessional roles, such as the mental health technician, are well-recognized and accepted. The home, however, is a more challenging treatment context in which to define acceptable and meaningful roles for paraprofessionals. They are inevitably working more independently and in a less controlled and predictable environment than their peers who work in inpatient or partial hospitalization programs. Thus, they are often called upon to use their own judgment to manage situations that might challenge even highly trained professionals. When paraprofessionals spend extended periods of time with clients and their families, they often possess more information about them and their experiences than does the supervising professional.

At the same time, home health care paraprofessionals are rarely viewed as respected members of the treatment team. Defining their work and role in a way that clarifies not only the importance of what they do but also how their interventions are relevant to the client's overall treatment goals and treatment plan is an important first step in legitimizing the paraprofessional role in treating psychiatric clients. This chapter describes the concept of "therapeutic assistant" as a way of addressing this issue. A case example of a woman with psychotic depression illustrates the potentially beneficial role that therapeutic assistants can play in home-based psychiatric treatment.

The case example is drawn from HomePsych, a program that addressed the needs of acutely and severely disturbed adult psychiatric clients. Interventions were based on a conceptual model that integrated ideas from Western and Eastern psychological traditions. A doctoral level psychologist (the author of this chapter) and paraprofessional caregivers constituted the treatment team. HomePsych drew on principles of Eastern psychology for conceptualizing the home as a therapeutic milieu (Newton & Brauer, 1999). The model of "therapeutic assistant" (Sinacola, 1998) captures the role of the paraprofessional caregiver.

HomePsych clients were primarily funded by managed health care organizations, although privately funded clients were served as well. Typically, managed care case managers referred clients who had a history of repeated psychiatric hospitalizations and who were experiencing an acute exacerbation of severe psychiatric symptoms. Often, the high risk and, thus, high cost status of the client made the case manager willing to consider innovative treatment strategies. Sometimes HomePsych served as an alternative to hospitalization. In other cases, HomePsych was contacted when clients were discharged after brief hospitalizations. Intensity of service varied according to client needs. When appropriate, a team of paraprofessional staff provided round-the-clock, 24-hour care for a few days or several weeks. When less intense assistance was needed, one paraprofessional care provider might work with the client once or twice a week for four hours. A doctoral-level clinical psychologist conducted the assessment, developed the treatment plan, trained and supervised paraprofessional staff, and sometimes provided in-home psychotherapy. Often, the in-home services complemented the work of the client's own psychiatrist. The majority of direct service was provided by specially screened and trained paraprofessional caregivers (Newton & Brauer, 1989). Caregivers included certified nursing assistants, graduate students, and young people from the arts community.

The roles of these caregivers were consistent with a "therapeutic assistant" model. A direct extension of the therapist, therapeutic assistants "assist the client, not only with goals and tasks agreed upon with the treating therapist, but with daily living skills and other behaviors found to be helpful and healthy" (Sinacola, 1998, p. 36). Arieti and Lorraine (1972) first described the role of the therapeutic assistant as a way of working with schizophrenic clients involved in psychoanalytic, outpatient treatment. They present a case in which Lorraine, a former client of Arieti, served as a therapeutic assistant for a young adult woman diagnosed as schizophrenic. Lorraine visited with the client one to three times a week (depending on the client's desires) in the client's home. Together, they organized their time—sometimes around shared interests and other times around conversation. Lorraine's patient and empathic companionship, shared interests with the client, acceptance of the client's freedom to exercise her own will, and willingness to discuss her own recovery experiences provided an active therapeutic experience for the client.

Arieti, an analyst, believed that therapeutic assistants both complement the therapist's work and provide their own unique help to the recovering schizophrenic client. By spending long stretches of time with clients in their ordinary worlds, therapeutic assistants help clients implement their new insights in that world, provide a reliable source of support, temper fears and perceived threats, and help clients overcome harmful habitual patterns for relating to the world. In this way, Arieti believed that therapeutic assistants were particularly useful during a specific period of recovery:

> When the patient, as a result of psychotherapy, has lost delusions and hallucinations, he may nevertheless retain a vague feeling of being threatened—an abstract, diffuse feeling, from which he tries to defend

himself by withdrawing. The therapeutic companion is there to dispel that feeling. The common exploration of the inner life by the patient and therapist is now complemented by an exploration of the external life by the patient and the therapeutic companion . . . the therapeutic assistant offers a concrete link between the psychodynamic understanding, the new relatedness with the therapist, and the external world. The assistant shows in an immediate way that many things that the patient fears do not exist or have power to hurt. (p. 8)

More recently, published case reports describe the use of therapeutic assistants in inpatient treatment of elderly psychiatric clients (Lichtenberg, Heck, & Turner, 1988), outpatient treatment of clients with severe obsessive-compulsive disorders (Pruitt, Miller, & Smith, 1989), treatment of substance-abuse clients (Woody, McLettan, Luborsky, & O'Brien, 1987), group therapy with parentally bereaved children (Levy & Zelman, 1997), and behaviorally oriented outpatient treatment with severely depressed clients (Sinacola, 1998). In each situation, therapeutic assistants carry out defined tasks and interventions that support the treatment plan and extend its implementation beyond clients' direct contact with the mental health professional. At the same time, less clearly definable aspects of the relationship between client and therapeutic assistant enrich the client's experience—whether this is as a role model or someone who can encouragingly give a "gentle push." As Arieti (1974) suggests, "Somebody is *there,* available, always ready to help. There is somebody the patient can rely on, somebody whom he trusts, somebody who could dispel many fears" (p. 600).

Arieti (1974) believed that capacity for empathy and understanding were crucial to the effectiveness of the therapeutic assistant. These qualities are at the foundation of the assistant's ability to establish a strong interpersonal connection with the client. It is this connection that is seen as fundamental to the healing process (Blechner, 1995). Arieti used former patients as therapeutic assistants, believing that their perspective on the analytic process made them a uniquely valuable resource to the client. Others (Benedetti, 1972; Blechner, 1995) argue that a previous client relationship with the therapist presents high potential for countertransference problems. The idea that assistants can bring valuable personal experiences to their work with clients, however, has been implemented in other ways. Levy and Zelman (1996) used assistants who themselves were bereaved adolescents. At HomePsych, we found that sociodemographic similarities between the caregiver and client in terms of gender, race, education, and age-facilitated therapeutic bonds and helped clients gravitate to the assistant as an important resource.

CASE EXAMPLE

At the time of her third hospitalization in fewer than 3 years, the hospital intake note described Betty in the following way:

> This is a 54-year-old married African American female who was brought in by her neighbors for emergency evaluation because of uncontrolled agitation, restlessness, severe confusion, and inability to carry out daily life routines. She had to have neighbors come over to watch her for the past few days so that she would not lose control on her grandchild. She was hearing voices that said that they would kill her and her family. She was very fearful that a gang was attempting to indoctrinate her 18-year-old son. She also reported depression, total insomnia for at least the past seven days, and complete loss of concentration.

HomePsych's relationship with Betty began following this hospitalization when discharge from the hospital's day treatment program was imminent. We received a telephone call from a case manager at Betty's insurance company. The repeated psychiatric hospitalizations had almost exhausted her $20,000 lifetime psychiatric benefits. Although her symptoms had abated during each hospitalization, Betty's pattern of repeated hospitalizations suggested that she would require more episodes of intensive treatment over her life than her insurance benefits would cover.

Lack of funds contributed to the case manager's willingness to look at innovative, creative interventions; clinical issues pointed to the nature of those interventions. Betty's inpatient and partial hospitalization treatment team suspected that family issues contributed to her psychiatric problems and repeated hospitalizations. Her symptoms of anxiety, depression, and paranoia had first emerged within a year after her husband's retirement and her mother's death. Prior to that time, Betty was, by all accounts, a competent wife and mother.

While respecting her therapists' concerns, Betty seemed at a loss to identify any connection between her symptoms and family relationships. She described an intact, middle-class family. She lived with her husband of 30 years and her 18-year-old son who was a full-time college student. Her husband, George, had been retired for three years; he was 66. Betty and George provided daytime child care for their 1½-year-old granddaughter while their daughter and her husband worked. There was no psychiatric history, drug or alcohol history, or physical/emotional abuse history in her family.

Betty's treatment team had been frustrated in their attempts to directly gather more information on the family dynamics. Betty's family did not have a telephone; her husband had not responded to their requests for meetings; her children could not be reached due to their work and school schedules. The only way to find out more would be a home visit. Thus, the case manager requested, and the partial hospitalization treatment team arranged, an in-home assessment to obtain a direct look at the family situation, assess the appropriateness of in-home support, and make treatment recommendations.

HOME ASSESSMENT

I conducted the assessment. It is difficult to capture the depressing and demoralizing quality of Betty's home. Despite their middle-class income, education, and occupation, the family resided in a deteriorating inner-city neighborhood. Their two-story, single-family home was surrounded by boarded-up buildings and weed-infested, overgrown yards. Many of the inhabited homes were in clear states of disrepair.

Inside Betty's home, the drapes and curtains were all drawn. The walls were freshly painted—bright green and psychedelic orange. There were no pictures. The dining room was cluttered with piles of papers and clothes; the refrigerator did not work. The living room furniture was old and worn; the room's centerpiece was a very large television tuned into a morning quiz show.

Betty's personal appearance, body language, and manner synchronized with her environment. She gave the appearance of a very chronic, long-institutionalized psychiatric patient—shuffling gait, flat affect, and vacant stare with little spontaneity in speech, behavior, or movement. In contrast, her husband George was quite animated, relating warmly and pleasantly to both me and his very active young granddaughter. He seemed genuinely pleased that a professional had come to their home, but also very frustrated by his wife's behavior, and skeptical that anything would help.

In contrast to Betty's stilted responses, George willingly elaborated his perspectives. He confessed that he had not met with the hospital staff because he felt blamed for Betty's illness. "Why should I go there to have them tell me it was all my fault?" He was confused, frustrated, and frightened by the changes in his wife's behavior. How could a competent woman just sit in front of the TV all day? Why didn't she just do what she had always done? Why wouldn't she leave the house? Why didn't she have any interest in their family anymore? He didn't understand how his previously very social and functional wife now spent her days staring at the television; he was angry that she wouldn't get up and do what she used to do. Her behavior changes had prevented the pleasant, travel-oriented retirement he had anticipated.

George had coped with Betty's withdrawal by taking over—assuming responsibility for the daily care of their granddaughter and for household chores. These were activities that he admitted he enjoyed— "I've always been busy; they keep me busy." It was Betty's passivity rather than her failure to carry out specific responsibilities that angered him. I spent much of the 2-hour meeting listening to George's frustration and providing him with information about depression. I encouraged him to conceptualize his wife's symptoms as an "illness." My goal was to give him a more informed and sympathetic framework for understanding Betty's mysterious behavior. Betty simply listened. As we talked, George's attitude toward her visibly softened. He seemed genuinely relieved not to be blamed and eager to be helpful. His initial skepticism dissipated.

As much as I could tell, Betty also seemed pleased by the meeting. Both George and Betty liked the idea of someone coming to their home to help. The couple agreed to have a certified nursing assistant visit three days a week, four hours each visit. The mutually agreed goals (although mutual as indicated by George's overt enthusiasm and Betty's passive agreement) were to: provide companionship to Betty, help her with personal care, support her re-involvement with household tasks, link her up with a local community mental health center, and pursue interests that Betty enjoyed. These goals seemed to balance the couple's differing agendas—Betty's desire for companionship and personal attention and George's desire that his wife return to productive activity. I explained that I would return with the caregiver to introduce her and finalize the treatment plan. I also indicated that I would maintain close contact with the caregiver and visit them periodically. I encouraged each of them to contact me directly at any time if they had questions, concerns, or any problems they wanted to discuss.

The assigned caregiver, Linda, was a married, African American woman in her early 50's. She was warm, friendly, enthusiastic, patient, and able to take charge of situations in a positive, nonthreatening way. Like Betty, she had been married for many years and had young adult children who often called on her to provide child care. Within a very short time, Betty became comfortable with Linda and accustomed to the routine of her visits. A pattern began to emerge. Betty liked the personal care—having her long, braided hair washed and styled and her fingernails manicured. And she liked going out—shopping, walking, going to the doctor. She increasingly used Linda's visits as opportunities for outings that she clearly enjoyed and eagerly anticipated. In contrast, Linda's efforts to get Betty interested in activities within her home were met with impassive acquiescence.

After about eight weeks, I returned to the home to meet with Betty, George, and Linda. The changes in Betty's mood, demeanor, and attitude were obvious. She was more energetic, alert, and engaged. She was happy about Linda's visits and their growing relationship. She reported that she felt much less depressed and was staying up to a more normal bedtime at night. She no longer felt so frightened and was willing to leave the house alone.

While acknowledging the obvious improvements, both George and Linda expressed frustration at Betty's continued passivity, particularly at home. They described Betty as continuing to show little initiative in taking charge of any area of her life. George was particularly angry at Betty's lack of initiative. He described himself as always busy and unable to stand how much time she still spent lying on the couch. "I don't care what she does, as long as she does something!" Although much more supportive and understanding of Betty, Linda shared George's frustration that Betty had resisted efforts to help her create a household routine and assume responsibility for preparing meals or doing the laundry.

With everyone's involvement, the initial treatment plan was modified. While the original goals remained the same, specific interventions changed. This time, Betty actively participated in the discussion. The revised plan included:

1. Improved personal hygiene. Betty wanted to retain this goal and agreed to be more proactive in assuming the responsibilities that her arthritis would allow her to handle, re-establishing a routine with a beauty parlor, and going through her clothes with Linda's help to get rid of things and reorganize what was wearable.

2. Reengagement in daily activities. We reframed this goal from assuming household maintenance activities (i.e., cooking and doing laundry) to creating a more inviting living environment. Betty's goals were to hang pictures and clean off the dining room table.

3. Identify and engage in activities that Betty enjoys. Shopping trips and other outings will continue.

Progress continued, with Betty beginning to take greater initiative in the areas identified in the treatment plan, particularly household chores. She also became increasingly open in sharing confidences with Linda. She described memories of her severe psychiatric symptoms—the hallucinations and delusions—and how frightened she had been.

She talked about her marriage—the long-standing lack of sexual intimacy, George's devotion to their children and lack of interest in her, his
unwillingness to re-establish telephone service after their son had run
up a large bill, his refusal to buy a refrigerator while generously giving
money to their children, and his unwillingness to set limits in response
to their daughter's requests for child care assistance. What Betty
found most distressing, however, was George's unwillingness to move
from their deteriorating neighborhood. Finally, she proclaimed, "I'm
on strike!"

When Linda and I discussed these direct revelations of marital conflicts and their apparent role in Betty's depression, I recommended
marital sessions in which Betty and George could focus on the issues
between them. The couple agreed. I met with them in their home three
times, without Linda. In these sessions, Betty came to life. She openly
and assertively stated her frustrations and desires. In response,
George's idiosyncrasies began to emerge. He promised outings for the
two of them, but did not follow through. When confronted on the need
to balance financial support for their adult children with basic purchases for their home, he balked, made excuses, set deadlines for the
purchases, and then never followed through. The couple did agree that
a joint goal was a family trip to Mississippi to visit Betty's family. They
set a tentative date for two months into the future.

About a month prior to the planned trip, a pivotal incident
occurred. Betty reported to Linda that she had gone out with a neighbor and the neighbor's boyfriend. The boyfriend had brought liquor,
and Betty had gotten drunk. While Betty herself seemed rather pleased
with the episode, George was very angry. Each of them described their
version of the event and their feelings to Linda. I returned to the home
for another marital session. This time, each spouse's frustration and
disappointment over long-standing marital problems was at a peak.
Each partner directly raised the question of whether he or she should
stay in the marriage. They agreed to continue with their vacation
plans, however, and to consider marital therapy when they returned.
In response to Betty's significant improvements, we began tapering
Linda's visits to twice and then once a week.

By all accounts, the trip was a success. Betty felt that she had been
"her old self" while in Mississippi. She renewed strong relationships
with family members, particularly a sister who invited her to return for
an extended visit. At home, Betty resumed many of her household
responsibilities and returned to active involvement in her children's
lives. Everyone agreed that she was her "old self."

While George was very positive about the trip and acknowledged
the positive changes in Betty, he became more insistent that maybe

the marriage should end. He refused to become involved in office-based therapy to directly address the marital issues. In response, Betty spent a number of months with her sister in Mississippi, coming home only for holidays and family occasions.

Shortly after the initial trip, we discontinued HomePsych services to Betty and George. The couple's insurance company had changed, and the new company would not pay for in-home service. Betty, however, occasionally called Linda. In this way, we were able to maintain follow-up for the next two years. At that point, Betty reported that she was spending more time in Chicago, she and George were on much better terms, and her life was going well.

DISCUSSION

Our work with Betty illustrates a number of the advantages of in-home mental health services. Some specific examples of these benefits are as follows:

1. *The first benefit is that in-home services allow the opportunity to gather information and to meet family members who are crucial to understanding the pathology and producing treatment gains* While suspecting the importance of family dynamics, the hospital treatment team could not pursue these hypotheses without Betty's ability (or willingness) to articulate the issues and without direct access to other key family members. Seeing them in their home seemed to communicate to both Betty and George an interest in their lives and commitment to helping them that provided a different basis for trust. In addition, the nature of her relationship with Linda allowed Betty to be much more open about her feelings and experiences than she had ever been in her more formally structured interactions with mental health professionals. Establishing this type of relationship took time as well as interpersonal skills. The therapeutic assistant was a cost-effective way of allowing confidences to emerge at a pace with which Betty was comfortable.

2. *In-home services provide a bridge to outpatient treatment* For the first time, Betty followed through with outpatient services. Linda set up Betty's appointments at the local community mental health center, went with her on the long bus ride to the center, and, at Betty's request, actually sat in on the sessions with her therapist. Linda's presence seemed to serve as a bridge to a world that Betty still found intimidating, enabling Betty to be more direct and forthcoming. Linda also served as an advocate, for example, getting the mental health center to pursue disability payments for Betty.

3. *An additional benefit involves medication compliance.* Linda arrived one day to discover that Betty had not been able to refill her psychotropic medication prescription because of a mix-up at the drugstore. Betty had resolved the problem by taking her neighbor's antidepressant medication. Linda intervened with the drug store and psychiatrist to get Betty's prescriptions renewed.

4. *In-home services allow one to model and support adaptive coping strategies in the client's natural environment.* In working with Betty, Linda balanced activities that supported Betty's self-esteem and sense of being special and important (personal care), re-established her self-confidence and sense of autonomy (leaving the house, taking public transportation), and encouraged her return to normal activities (household tasks). As issues emerged, Linda also provided education (i.e., on menopause, relaxation techniques). She became a respected and trusted confidante for both Betty and George.

In this case, Linda's presence had a much broader impact than was ever directly identified in the treatment plan. Whatever the factors that led to the onset of Betty's psychiatric symptoms, issues in the marital relationship were clearly key to her recovery. As Betty gained confidence, she emerged out of her withdrawn shell and increasingly took on George directly and assertively. She began voicing her complaints actively rather than passively. She created a lifestyle that she enjoyed, escaping from the home environment in which she felt controlled and stifled. As she returned to a more functional stance, George's pathology—his rigidity, obsessiveness, and paranoia—became more obvious. Long-standing marital conflicts came to the surface, and both members of the couple verbalized their anger and sadness. With support and validation, Betty was able to find her own solutions—spending long periods of time away. After many, many months in which George persistently denied that he did not miss his wife and was happy living his life without her, his attitude began to soften. The couple eventually reengaged on different terms that seemed to better accommodate both of their needs.

The success in this case supports the potentially valuable role of the "paraprofessional" therapeutic assistant in home-based psychiatric services. It is not difficult to make a pragmatic case for incorporating certified nursing assistants and other paraprofessional caregivers in home care programs. They cost less than master's, doctoral, or even bachelor's level professionals. HomePsych's work with Betty only became cost-effective when direct service could be provided primarily by a less expensive "therapeutic assistant."

The home health care literature, however, often gives little attention to the potentially therapeutic roles that less credentialed caregivers can provide for home care clients. In this case, Linda was a key therapeutic agent, not just a substitute for a too-expensive professional. The similarities in race, background, age, and gender, combined with the extended contact around daily activities in ordinary settings, allowed Linda to establish a strong relationship with Betty. With training and supervision, Linda was able to draw upon her natural personality style and interpersonal skills to become a therapeutic agent for Betty. She communicated a balance between professionalism and personal ease within Betty's world that many mental health professionals would envy. Linda understood and appreciated the therapeutic benefits of her relationship with Betty and thus took her role and responsibilities seriously.

In the process, Linda earned Betty's trust and respect. Betty talked to her in detail about all kinds of issues that she had only mentioned or vaguely alluded to in her meetings with therapists. At the same time, establishing that Linda and I were working as a team allowed me to step in periodically as a "therapist." It gave Linda the backup she needed to feel comfortable and provided a secure context for her interventions. It also allowed my more expensive sessions with the couple to be focused and timely.

A number of issues are key to the success of the therapeutic assistant model. Most crucial is the selection and training of the therapeutic assistant. My experiences in working with HomePsych staff supported Arieti's (1972) conclusion that caregivers' personal qualities and interpersonal skills are more important than their previous education, credentials, and professional experience. Empathy and interpersonal warmth, intuitive understanding of the concepts of personal and professional boundaries, common sense and judgment in unclear situations, ability to take charge without being controlling, and flexibility are personal attributes that cannot be taught but are essential to this work. Thus, it is crucial that hiring and selection processes screen for these qualities. The HomePsych screening process included personal interviews, written examination, and observation of new caregivers during orientation and training. Often paraprofessional staff members were assigned to HomePsych clients only after a period of working with nonpsychiatrically impaired elderly clients. We discovered that those who possesses these qualities and can implement them in home-based therapy is not predicted by professional background and training. Often, graduate students in social work or psychology had great difficulty while others with less formal training and skills seemed to naturally do well.

Training is also essential to provide therapeutic assistants, whatever their natural skills, with a basis for understanding their clients' strengths and vulnerabilities, conceptualizing the psychological meaning of their work, and developing intervention strategies. Our 12-hour training program included information on the psychiatric diagnoses, psychotropic medication, and psychological issues relevant to our client base. It also included role playing and discussion of cases to provide skills and confidence in handling the types of situations and problems staff would encounter. Training staff in small groups of five or six caregivers gave us the opportunity to get to know them well. We involved senior therapeutic assistants in the training program to insure that the "real" problems staff would encounter were addressed pragmatically rather than just conceptually and to provide role models with whom new staff could identify.

Supervision is also crucial to the success of the therapeutic assistant model. No matter how much training and ongoing support is provided, therapeutic assistants are inevitably working very independently in constantly changing, novel situations with highly disturbed clients. They must make judgment calls in real time, relying on their own knowledge and common sense. The supervisor's ongoing contact with both therapeutic assistant and client is essential. Linda turned in written notes of her sessions on a weekly basis. I reviewed these notes and generally talked with Linda by telephone each week. She also had at least weekly contact with a HomePsych social worker. Generally, the supervisor also maintained weekly telephone contact with the client, although this was not possible with Betty. In more intensive HomePsych cases involving more than one caregiver, a notebook was kept in the home in which caregivers kept their notes for review by each other. The supervisor maintained regular contact with all treatment team members; team meetings were held periodically to coordinate care and discuss issues specific to the client's needs.

Supervision of therapeutic assistants on home care cases differs in significant ways from more traditional supervision. Because therapeutic assistants work so independently, their relationships with clients can easily become stronger than their relationships with the agency. The supervisor must gain the assistants' respect and trust by demonstrating skill and confidence in working with clients in their homes and appreciation for the therapeutic nature of their work and the importance of their information and perspectives. Supervisors must develop and show understanding of the particular challenges that therapeutic assistants face. It is crucial that therapeutic assistants perceive the supervisor as accessible and approachable rather than available only through formal supervisory channels and contacts. Development of mutual trust and respect is also fundamental in empowering therapeutic assistants to carry out their responsibilities and to give the therapist confidence in the value of their work. Supervisors and staff must negotiate the same issues as a treatment team in any other setting, often without the built-in opportunities for direct collaboration that occur in inpatient and partial hospitalization settings. Because Linda and I had worked together on a number of cases, our relationship was well-established. In this case, I was able to play a minimal but useful role because the client and her husband accurately perceived Linda as a therapeutic agent and the two of us as a team.

In conclusion, this case illustrates one way of conceptualizing the role and services the paraprofessional level caregiver can provide in home-based psychiatric services. This model acknowledges the valuable and unique role of the paraprofessional caregiver in the client's psychiatric treatment. The therapeutic assistant model defines a role that complements and extends the work of the therapist and creates the basis for a team approach.

REFERENCES

Arieti, S. (1974). *Interpretation of schizophrenia* (2nd ed.). New York: Basic Books.

Arieti, S., & Lorraine, S. (1972). The therapeutic assistant in treating the psychotic. *International Journal of Psychiatry, 10,* 7–22.

Benedetti, G. (1972). On the use of the therapeutic assistant. *International Journal of Psychiatry, 10,* 27–30.

Blechner, M. J. (1995). Schizophrenia. In M. Lionelle (Ed.), *Handbook of interpersonal psychoanalysis* (pp. 375–396). Hillsdale, NJ: Analytic Press.

Levy, A., & Zelman, A. B. (1996). The use of parentally bereaved adolescents as therapeutic assistants in groups for parentally bereaved children. In A. B. Zelman (Ed.), *Early intervention with high-risk children: Freeing prisoners of circumstance* (pp. 173–188). Northvale, NJ: Jason Aronson.

Lichtenberg, P., Heck, G., & Turner, A. (1988). Medical psychotherapy with elderly psychiatric inpatients: Uses of paraprofessionals in treatment. *Medical Psychotherapy: An International Journal, 1,* 87–93.

Moy, S., & Pigott, H. E. (1997). Home-based services. In R. K. Schreter, S. S. Sharfstein, & C. A. Schreter (Eds.), *Managing care, not dollars: The continuum of mental health services.* Washington, DC: American Psychiatric Press.

Newton, N. & Brauer, W. (1989). In-home mental health services. *Caring, 6,* 16–19.

Newton, N., & Brauer, W. (1999). *Buddhist perspectives on in-home caregiving.* Unpublished manuscript.

Pruitt, S., Miller, W., & Smith, J. (1989). Outpatient behavioral treatment of severe obsessive-compulsive disorder using paraprofessional resources. *Journal of Anxiety Disorders, 3,* 179–186.

Schmidt, J. (1988). Evaluation of a short-term systematic training program for paraprofessional group facilitators in a psychiatric inpatient hospital. *Dissertation Abstracts International, 49,* 436.

Sinacola, R. (1998). The use of therapeutic assistants in outpatient psychotherapy. *Psychotherapy in Private Practice, 17,* 35–44.

Woody, G., McLellan, T., Luborsky, L., & O'Brien, C. (1987). Twelve month follow-up of psychotherapy for opiate dependence. *American Journal of Psychiatry, 144,* 590–596.

On the Front Line: The Respite Worker As Participant, Observer, and Consultant

Charles R. Barringer

Respite workers, like other support staff, may spend more time with a client than any other member of the treatment team. Yet they are likely not to be included in treatment planning, staffing, training, and clinical supervision. Attempts to integrate paraprofessionals into the larger treatment team are made more difficult by the current emphasis on cost cutting. As a result, in many programs, respite workers, housekeepers, transporters, and nursing assistants are isolated.

Charles Barringer, now a psychologist, was working as a respite worker when he became involved in the case that will be described. His report illustrates how respite workers can make a unique contribution to treatment.

As we were sitting in the car, the case worker made it very clear that Janet and Donald Stewart were approaching their limit. They were exhausted and discouraged after 7 years of trying to manage their 9-year-old adopted son, Damien. His behavior had become so disruptive and threatening to people around him that babysitters quit with alarming regularity, neighbors were hesitant to let their children play with him, clinical staff had become blaming and defeated, and Damien's mother feared for her own safety and the safety of her younger son, William. Both Janet and Donald felt that they had reached the end of their emotional and financial resources. They were in the process of considering whether to quit their jobs and move to the country or send Damien to a special residential school. The option of having someone work with Damien in the home was a last-ditch effort to turn things around. With this first impression of Damien, I somewhat anxiously entered the Stewart home as a respite worker. (I was to leave as a better psychologist.)

I found myself greeting Janet and Donald in a small, comfortable living room. While the case worker played with the boys upstairs, Janet, Donald, and I began the process of getting acquainted. They asked questions about my background and experience, and we briefly formulated the broad goals for the work ahead. The goals included: (a) to relieve Janet and Donald from the constant pressure of monitoring and managing Damien, (b) to explore and develop ways to manage Damien's volatile behavior and help him moderate his aggressive impulses in a variety of contexts, and (c) to model or suggest treatment approaches for Damien's parents and other key caregivers.

During our talk I also learned about some of the interventions that had been utilized in an effort to address Damien's behavioral and learning problems. They included cognitive-behavioral techniques such as setting limits, clarifying expectations, contracting, redirecting, time-outs, and token systems; private schooling in three different, highly structured educational programs; and individual and family therapy. Janet and Donald had clearly made a concerted effort to provide a happy and secure home environment in order to socialize Damien and build his self-esteem. Both maintained flexible schedules in order to meet Damien's and Williams's needs. In addition, six different medication trials had been tried, including Ritalin, Cylert, lithium, clonidine, and imipramine. Unfortunately, in each case positive results were short-term and accompanied by adverse side effects. Even though Damien received extensive state-of-the-art multimodal treatment and grew up in a healthy, committed, and intact family, he failed to show sufficient progress in academic or social areas and required continuous monitoring by people involved in his care.

As we talked, Janet and Donald were occasionally distracted by the noise upstairs. A couple of times they called up and asked the boys to calm down. At one point, Damien came down and in a demanding tone asked Janet, "Where's my plastic sword?" Janet patiently answered, "I don't know. You'll have to look for it." As he went off to search, Damien radiated a tense energy that seemed too high for the confines of the small, quiet home. Though an intimidating first exposure, I felt excited by the prospect of working with Damien. I looked forward to the challenge ahead and felt confident that I could find my way to an understanding of this wild boy.

After reassuring themselves that I was trustworthy, Janet, Donald, William, and the case worker left Damien and me alone for 4 hours. Damien quickly took advantage of his new freedom, pulling me into one activity after another. We played pool in the basement, frolicked with his pet ferret, Sneaky, engaged in board games, and threw darts. Toward the end of the dart game, Damien suddenly took off. I followed on his heels as he ran downstairs and into the study. He rummaged through his mother's desk, which I later learned was expressly forbidden, for some stick-on letters and then ran back upstairs. Using the letters, Damien quickly made a sign for the door to his room that read "no girls." I was in, for now. During the entire session, I had the sense that Damien was just released from a corral. Like a wild mustang, he played hard and vigorously, with a seemingly endless source of energy.

Understanding Damien was a complex enterprise, undertaken over the course of 17 4-hour, home-based sessions; every visit peeled back another layer of insight. What I knew about Damien indicated that his problems were long-standing, that the cards had been stacked against him from the very beginning. Both biological parents had a history of substance abuse and mood problems, suggesting that biological factors played a significant role in Damien's difficulties. By the age of 2, Damien was already behaving in an impulsive and aggressive manner. He received a formal diagnosis of attention deficit hyperactivity disorder (ADHD) at the age of 6, and, at 8, his clinical diagnosis included oppositional defiant disorder (ODD). Test results also revealed relative weaknesses in long-term memory, verbal reasoning and expression, written language, reading comprehension, and mathematics. Damien's difficulty in school and social functioning was consistent with a learning disability profile, and his behavioral patterns met the diagnostic criteria found in the *Diagnostic and Statistical Manual of Mental Disorders,* as well as other clinical descriptions of ADHD and ODD symptoms. He was indeed unpredictable and resisted daily routines or obligatory activities, and he usually failed to plan or anticipate the consequences of his actions or follow through on tasks. Damien's endless energy, assertiveness, and fearlessness were also typical of ADHD children, as were his intrusive manner and frequent displays of irritability that often quickly escalated into anger and hostility.

Working primarily from a humanistic perspective and methodology, I sought to engage Damien less as a "behavior disorder" and more as a boy struggling to live with a handicap. I set out to understand his subjective experience in the world and to forge a relationship. At the onset, I thought of Damien's foibles, troubles, and reactions as both symptomatic and adaptive, a complex psychological process by which he sought to maintain some equilibrium between his inner self and the outer world. Although his adaptation (and thus evolution) was often at odds with his social environment, many of his characteristic patterns seemed to express an underlying imperative to maintain some semblance of emotional cohesion. Thus, before I could identify adequate substitutes or ease Damien into other adaptive behaviors that he might accept and adopt over time, I had to understand the intrinsic order that must exist in this troubled, sensitive, sometimes charming, often baffling nine-year old. Guided by these assumptions, I embarked on a mission of discovery, experimentation, and friendship, the stuff of relationships.

As I considered my first experience with Damien, I wondered whether part of the problem might be that in more structured or confining circumstances Damien's willful pursuit of energetic outlets ran contrary to the restraints placed on him. When he encountered resistance and was asked to stop, move slowly, or reflectively take others into account, he experienced an acute disruption of his inner balance. Like a spinning top that was bumped, Damien wobbled from feelings of frustration and confusion.

That Damien grew restless and irritable when external demands and constraints interfered with his automatic way of being was confirmed in future sessions. It was perhaps most clearly evident at church on Sundays. During services, Damien couldn't sit still for a moment; he ran to the back of the church or crawled under the pews while the congregation faced the sanctuary, singing and listening to the minister or music. The highly structured nature of the service as well as the level of environmental stimulation, including the hymn singing, seemed to make it difficult for Damien to remain calm. Since he was by nature a highly energetic child, it was not surprising that an increase in environmental stimulation overwhelmed and disorganized him. His restlessness began to appear like a desperate search for a means to ground himself, to escape, to contain his emotional turmoil.

In Sunday school classes, Damien often became fidgety and disrupted the planned activities, even when only a few children and adults were present. He spoke out of turn and moved about the room doing his own thing. He appeared ill at ease in a closed setting with other children. In part this was because the classes, like the services preceding them, followed a fairly structured routine, with little room for improvisation. Another dynamic was at play here, however, one that was absent in the confines of the church. In the classroom setting, where children interacted primarily by talking to each other, Damien, with his difficulty in verbal expression, was forced to confront his deficits. Sunday School activities such as being read to or being asked questions precipitated similar self-doubts. From this perspective, Damien's disruptive antics clearly expressed emotional discomfort and served as a means of diverting attention away from feared activities.

I soon learned that Damien became agitated and acted up whenever verbal skills were required. Once I observed him and his friend Sam playing UNO followed by some games on the computer. UNO was easy for Damien, but the computer game required spelling simple four- and five-letter words in a limited time frame. I could see that Sam spelled much better and faster than Damien. Damien appeared embarrassed and attempted to conceal his weakness in spelling by switching back to simpler levels of the game or trying to claim credit for a correct spelling when Sam offered answers. After this and other observations, I was certain that some of the "acting out" in classroom settings could be explained as the anxiety Damien experienced when faced with his scholastic limitations and demands for verbal communication.

I practiced reading and writing with Damien now and then, but his discomfort was so evident that I did not press too hard for fear of arousing his self-doubt and undermining the safety of our relationship. I could not help wondering, however, about how stressful his school environment must be for him. If the impulsive, desperate coping behavior I observed in Sunday School and other social contexts resembled his days in the regular classroom, it was no wonder he had difficulty learning and was often sent to the "quiet room," isolated from other children. Under such conditions, Damien was probably depleted and discouraged at the end of each day.

Although Damien's verbal skills were limited, he was not an uncommunicative child. The difference was that, unlike most adults and other children his age, he communicated primarily through play and nonverbal language. His gestures communicated a range of emotions, including affection, regret, and anger. They were often touching in their directness and sincerity. During Sunday School on Palm Sunday, for example, when the class was baking flat bread, Damien suddenly left the room, bread in hand, and went up to the sanctuary. I watched him boldly walk down the aisle through the communion ceremony, locate Janet, and silently hand her a piece of the bread he had made. While Damien was often angry toward Janet, this incident revealed his natural impulse to make amends and solicit her affection. Another time, after a particularly volatile day during which Damien accidentally slammed the basement door into William's head, he spontaneously handed William the game Sorry as a way of apologizing.

Many of his gestures were subtler and less easy to interpret. Once, while we were in the kitchen snacking on some fruit, for example, Damien tossed some grapes at me. At first I was surprised, then thought, like an adult, that I should ask him to stop. Then it occurred to me that some of what we call "testing the limits" may actually have been his attempts to communicate with others in nonverbal ways. I was able to see the gesture for what it was—a sign of trust and familiarity, a way of playfully, teasingly connecting, not uncommon among friends.

While understanding Damien's language of gesture and play was important, being able to respond to and engage in it was equally so. It was through the play and antics of nonverbal communication that I was able to "reach through" to Damien on some level. Although at first I felt ambivalent about the physical contact that would inevitably be involved, I realized that I could not avoid such contact when playing with or restraining Damien without significantly compromising the quality of our communication. At times Damien and I playfully wrestled, and on several different occasions while playing in Damien's room, I picked him up and tossed him onto his bed. Bouncing and laughing, Damien inevitably asked me to do it again and again.

There were numerous occasions when our physical contact was not so playful, when I needed to hold Damien firmly until an aggressive impulse had passed. Once, while we explored things to do in the basement, Damien grabbed a can of insecticide and started running around the room randomly spraying different objects. I tried to stop him and retrieve the can with firm commands. When Damien did not heed my request, I chased him around the basement for a few minutes. Still unsuccessful, I escalated my efforts. I grabbed him quite firmly, took the can away, and placed it on a shelf out of his reach. To divert his attention away from this tempting game, I suggested going outside and engaging in another activity. By not taking a threatening and coercive approach, I avoided a power struggle and was able to gradually shift his focus in another direction.

Perhaps in part because I was becoming more proficient in speaking Damien's language, he was more willing to learn to speak mine. Over the course of the sessions, I saw Damien struggling with and succeeding in small ways with verbal communication. One such event occurred when Damien had gone back on an agreement we had made. I had agreed to be an accessory to Damien's wish—another visit to the corner grocery store, an activity that was typically reserved as a reward by his parents—if he would help me put away his toys in the back yard and spend time reading with me. Damien spontaneously honored my first request, but he avoided reading by starting a game on the computer. I set a time limit and tried coaxing him to read, but no amount of patient persuasion or negotiation could lure him away from the computer. With plenty of warning and appeals, I gradually became firmer in my request and eventually shut the computer off. Damien went into the dining room in a huff and sat in a corner. I followed in my usual shadow-like fashion and engaged him in a quiet, soothing dialogue. Damien apologized for being so stubborn, and I apologized for shutting the computer off. He also said that he was angry with me because we had not wrestled that night. I was surprised to hear this, so I suggested that, in the future, if he wanted something in particular, to let me know. While very few words were actually exchanged during our dialogue, and I had to remain incredibly patient to allow Damien time to speak his mind, it was our first real conversation. After this experience, I decided to continue to find ways to gently coax Damien onto the dance floor of conversation.

Another brief conversation occurred when I tried to get Damien to describe a fight that had just occurred between him and William. Damien had gotten angry with William for playing with one of his toys and struck him on the back. Janet severely reprimanded Damien and sent him to his room. I sat with him during this time-out and tried to engage him in talk. The whole time he squirmed on the floor and inched his way toward the door. When he started to crawl down the stairs, I gently and playfully called him back to finish our talk, adding that the sooner he returned, the sooner he could be released. Very, very slowly Damien crawled back up the stairs and came to rest at the threshold of his room. We sat silently this way for a few moments until I asked Damien for two reasons why he would not talk. He said, "I don't know how to talk, and I don't like to."

Risks having to do with verbal self-expression were not the only ones I encouraged. Like all children, Damien needed to perform competently in a range of activities. I supported his drive for competence by allowing him to engage in activities that might have been seen by others as too challenging or even dangerous. Once, when Damien and I were playing in the backyard of his home, he climbed to the top of the jungle gym, stood up, and threw a thin pole, like a spear, to the ground. I retrieved the pole and handed it up to him. Again, he threw it to the ground. We repeated this sequence over and over for at least 20 minutes. I was a little nervous about letting Damien stand on top of the jungle gym. Part of me knew that most adults, including his parents, would not approve of giving Damien such latitude. I decided, however, not to react with fear or restriction. I was confident of my ability to "spot" him and I could see that he maintained his balance very well. In fact, I was impressed by his physical coordination, his willingness to take risks, the inventiveness of the game, and his ability to stay with the activity for such an extended period of time. I praised his agility and courage, and I gently provided safety guidelines and suggestions to help improve his throwing.

Another time, after Janet, Donald, and William left for the afternoon, Damien and I made plans to go to the park with Bucky the dog. Damien found his way over the six-block walk with no interference from me. He showed good judgment by following landmarks, he safely crossed the streets with little input from me, and I was impressed that as a safety precaution he also took the initiative of handing Bucky to me before crossing at busy intersections. The walk to the park was significant because, despite his age, Damien was rarely given such a high degree of independence. Up to this point, Janet, and to a lesser extent Donald, had never let Damien travel on his own. They assumed he would get lost, or worse, get into trouble. While they were understandably cautious, I believe that in the process of restricting his natural desire to roam and explore, Janet and Donald unwittingly interrupted some of Damien's natural developmental attempts toward autonomy and competence. Thus, when he managed to escape restrictions, his enthusiasm was so great that he often exercised poor judgment and *did* place himself in harm's way.

I saw Damien's successful demonstrations of competence as positive developments and stressed his successes in my conversations with his parents, hoping that they would trust him a little more in the future. They were often pleased when I informed them of his accomplishments, but I was also aware that my behavior with Damien was sometimes viewed as overly permissive and lenient. During my time with Damien, I was considerably more flexible and imposed only mild "limit setting." I was trying to win him over so I could get close to him and thus understand him better. As soon as Janet and Donald returned home at the end of each shift, stricter patterns of limit setting were resumed, creating a contrast that was hard for Damien to accept. Janet informed me that Damien became more stubborn and harder to control for a short time after I left. I agreed to be more mindful of the contrast and to gradually incorporate some behavioral methods already in use to help structure and control Damien. I felt conflicted on this issue, however. On the one hand, I could see that the Stewarts' concern was founded in a desire for Damien's safety and well-being as well as anxiety that they not be seen as "the bad guys." On the other hand, it was clear to me that Damien responded positively when a more "relaxed," nonprescriptive approach was used. I gradually became convinced that he understood many of the expectations and rules he encountered, but he needed more opportunities to exercise them on his own.

During one session, I arrived moments before Damien came home from school. When Damien came in, he tossed down his coat and book bag, got an ice cream sandwich from the freezer, and sat down to watch TV. In response to this series of events, Janet asked Damien to put his things away properly, challenged him for getting an ice cream sandwich without permission, and reminded him that he could not watch violent cartoons on TV. Damien became sulky and annoyed, but he reluctantly complied with every request. As I observed Janet's interactions with Damien, it struck me, that at times, she seemed too determined to enforce rules or maintain a stringent behavioral program.

If this exchange represented some of the ongoing dynamics between Damien and Janet, it was not surprising that antagonism and conflict routinely manifested between them. I was getting the sense that because she was so eager to see improvement, after so many years of frustration, Janet had perhaps become overreactive. In addition, I was concerned that she had fallen into the pattern of seeing Damien as the trouble-maker, often absolving his younger brother of responsibility. On one occasion, I was talking with Janet and Donald when we were interrupted by the two boys feuding over a toy. Out of the corner of my eye, I saw William abruptly grab a toy from Damien. Damien responded by kicking William and calling him names. Janet and Donald immediately scolded Damien and sent him to his room. After a few minutes, I went in and tried to process the event with Damien. Janet followed a few minutes later. As I listened to Janet coach Damien on alternative reactions he should have considered, I noticed that Janet talked for Damien. She often answered her own questions and provided Damien with a list of options to consider in the future. During this 5- to 10-minute exchange, Damien squirmed and chewed on a small toy. He was noticeably uncomfortable and completely inarticulate.

As I acquired more and more experience with Damien I developed a growing need to share my observations and to supportively reach out to Janet and Donald. Likewise, Janet and Donald needed a means to inform me about the boundaries and customs of their family system and how they were experiencing my presence. In so doing, I hoped to have more input into Damien's family context and build a higher level of trust. Gradually, we devised a structure for regular exchange and began to explore a wide range of issues. For example, Janet and Donald talked extensively about changes they hoped to make in working with Damien: a different school, alternatives to medications, and ways to continue the kind of intervention I was providing as a respite worker. I, in turn, shared more about how I was coming to understand Damien and his patterns of behavior. Thus, just as I worked to resonate more accurately with Damien, I worked to establish harmony with the whole family. Janet and Donald began to see me as part of a team, along with them on yet a new path of trial and error. In this way, I began to introduce my ideas about a more relaxed approach.

During one particularly productive telephone conversation, Janet and Donald acknowledged that their attempts to control Damien were often overreactive. They sounded sad as they considered the times that their well-intentioned efforts led to conflict and stress rather than compliance and cooperation. The level of safety and trust during the conversation also allowed Janet and Donald to acknowledge that feelings of anger and frustration with Damien often interfered with their ability to differentiate between his "acting out" behavior and his natural and reasonable needs for attention. Using a developmental framework to explain my point, I suggested that their restrictive reactions to some of Damien's spontaneous behaviors interrupted some age-appropriate steps that he was trying to take, steps that would enhance his personal sense of competence and self-control. I was supportive during the exchange, and I praised them for their patience and the fact that they provided a loving and consistent structure for Damien. I encouraged them to gradually and selectively reduce the intensity of disciplinary measures, and except for minor adjustments here and there, let the structure do its slow work.

I believe that Janet and Donald would have seen considerable improvement with this approach. Unfortunately, the progress we were all making began to fall apart when the managed care company refused to extend respite services and Damien started to exhibit a dramatic change in his behavior. Apparently, Damien had become unmanageable in school, requiring extended time in the padded time-out room, and Janet and Donald were forced to chauffeur Damien to and from school because he was banned from traveling on the school bus. Janet informed me that his pediatrician and the case worker had recommended hospitalization again, and his psychiatrist was considering tranquilizers. Janet was very upset by the recommendations and very frustrated about what to do. She was tearful and despondent as she informed me about their depleted emotional and financial resources. I tried to reassure Janet and help her explore alternatives. I offered to come over more often or even accompany Damien to school, if she thought that would help. In addition, I encouraged Janet to continue investigating a diet-related treatment program that had been known to help hyperactive children. At the end of the conversation, Janet shared her confusion over the fact that in the midst of Damien's decline, he was better behaved at home. In fact, the next day she left me a phone message informing me that Damien was acting like an "angel."

Interpreting this behavioral language was a challenge to my growing sensitivity. I considered two possible contributing factors. First, with only one more approved session, I thought it might be related to the approaching end of my work with him, since the changes in Damien's behavior coincided with this inevitability. Symptoms often reoccur as therapeutic relationships terminate. I also wondered whether the dramatic change had anything to do with a conversation Damien had with his friend Peter a few sessions back. Peter innocently had told Damien that he would soon get out of school for the summer break. Damien appeared to be noticeably bothered by the news and changed the subject to avoid explaining his own school situation. Going to school through the summer while "normal" kids got time off may have deeply upset Damien. It was a harsh reminder of his special-student status and his frustrating deficiencies. With child-like concrete reasoning, he acted out at school in hopes of being dismissed and acted like an angel at home in hopes of winning his parents' sympathy. Sadly misunderstood, Damien was faced instead with the dilemma of either behaving in school or being hospitalized, a choice that only increased his agitation. My impending departure and no summer school break could easily have sent Damien into an emotional tailspin which he communicated nonverbally. The possibility that Damien was trying to let us know that he wanted, or needed, a break from the torment of school and some extra comforting was not considered. Unfortunately, I never had a chance to fully test my hypotheses or advocate on his behalf.

My last session with Damien before his hospitalization was at Donald's birthday party. While the adults were engaging in talk, Janet set up some organized party games for the children. The games were competitive in nature and aroused Damien's eagerness to perform and outdo other children. Eventually, however, he became so volatile that Janet brought the games to an end. Sensing his negative role in the turn of events and openly angry with Janet, Damien drifted off to an activity of his own. He went around to the back alley and started to pick through a pile of wooden doors, windows, and wall frames discarded from an old backyard shed. Damien decided to salvage some of the parts to use in his tree house. After hauling a half dozen sections of the old shed across the street, Damien went into the house, returned with a hammer and nails, and asked me to help him install some of the parts in his tree house.

Although I felt slightly self-conscious about my complicity in this display of trash-picking, I continued to support Damien's now familiar means of grounding himself through focused physical activity. Already distressed from a difficult week and by the threat of hospitalization, Damien was easily overloaded by the stimulation of the party crowd. While his mood and energy level was volatile during the party games, once he was on his own Damien managed to constructively discharge his feelings and energy through the building project. He remained obsessed with the project until it was time for me to leave.

I was disappointed at not having more private time with Damien, and I worried about what would become of him over the next few days. After I heard about his hospitalization, I wished I had been more assertive in arranging additional sessions or sharing my concerns directly with Janet and Donald that evening. Although I would never know whether a more assertive response on my part would have averted Damien's hospitalization, extended and responsive one-on-one sessions probably would have provided the additional support he needed during his precipitous decline.

I visited Damien in the hospital two times. Both visits began with play. Damien was quite manageable and he played very appropriately with Janet, Donald, and me. The lethargy I observed at the beginning of each visit seemed to lift somewhat when he was given the opportunity to express himself through the familiar nonverbal language of play. The hospital staff had a hard time bringing Damien under control during his first few days, leading me to wonder whether his symptoms had not been exacerbated when they prevented him from discharging his energy through his usual coping style of physical activity and relating to others through play. While the hospitalization successfully subdued the aggressive, hostile behavior that led to Damien's admission, it was at a great cost to his self-image.

Not wanting the hospital visit to be my last time with the Stewarts, I arranged to visit the house after Damien was discharged. Janet and Donald offered me lunch and for a short time we all played in the backyard with the water hose and a small pool. Damien related to me in a friendly manner, playfully spraying me as a way of establishing contact. In addition, when we were all sitting at the kitchen table eating lunch, he was attentive to me and made sure I got enough to eat. On several occasions, when Janet acknowledged this as my last visit, Damien chimed in with "yeah, I'll miss you."

Although Janet, Donald, and I had very little time to talk without the distraction of the boys, I learned that Damien had been moved to a different school, one they seemed happier with because of its 1:5 student/teacher ratio and a more child-centered approach. In addition, they informed me that in place of medications, Damien was now being treated with a regimen of vitamin and mineral supplements. Janet and Donald sounded optimistic and more comfortable with the new treatment measures.

Over the course of the 17 sessions, it had became clear to me that Damien's lack of progress and exaggerated and regressive behavior patterns reflected an internal emotional state that was easily overburdened by the growing demands in his life. Damien's pattern of difficulties was due to a complex interplay of inherited and environmental factors that compromised his emotional equilibrium. As his uncontrollable impulses and cognitive deficits (inherited factors) encountered social rejection and endless demands and expectations he could not fulfill (environmental factors), the development of his already fragile self was repeatedly interrupted, injured, or undermined. The stress and frustration created by this interplay alienated Damien and kept him in a chronic state of anxiety and fragmentation that seemed to necessitate vital, but often counterproductive coping patterns to maintain a semblance of psychological cohesion.

Although Damien's cohesion was always tenuous and transient, he was playful, clever, and quite enjoyable to be with when he was engaged in a nonthreatening activity and feeling safe and affirmed. As long as people refrained from harshly setting limits on self-enhancing and self-protective activity, and instead tried to match his energy and mood, Damien felt understood, contained, and connected. When he experienced this quality of external support and affirmation, it was much easier for an outside agent to moderate his behavior and ease him into a change of activity.

In my all-too-brief time with Damien, I found myself siding with Damien and I endeavored to build a relationship that facilitated guidance, rather than aroused resistance. I tried to identify and honor his natural process of self-organization and enhance or redirect it through strategies of negotiation and collaboration. I focused on supporting existing strengths and competencies rather than repeatedly highlighting and addressing deficits. I attempted to understand his way of communicating before asking him to engage in mine. As I became more accurate at interpreting his (behavioral) language, I became more effective at enhancing his sense of emotional strength and security across a wide range of conditions.

I believe we were misguided in expecting Damien to speak our language. We were asking him to do many things he was not ready or able to do. We would not insist that a paraplegic walk or a recently traumatized person act in a "normal" manner. Damien communicated through his actions. He tried repeatedly to inform us of how he felt, but we did not always understand. He strove to connect with us, but we did not always respond. It was only through clear and consistently safe relationships with others that Damien would establish a deeper trust in people and reconnect with "our" world. This could be achieved only by meeting him on his terms, not ours, and only then would he become receptive to the learning and guidance so crucial for his progress.

Helping Damien change would inevitably be a slow, delicate, and subtle process. The positive feedback I received from Damien and his parents, however, as well as my own assessment of the process, indicated that important steps were taken. Janet and Donald's stress levels were sufficiently reduced to renew their hope and restore some of their energy. Also much to their relief, I successfully built a relationship with Damien and moderated his volatile behavior across a variety of settings and conditions. In addition, the hundreds of interactions I had with Damien and members of the family and community provided Janet, Donald, and others with suggestions and alternative ways of dealing with Damien.

Even though home-based respite workers typically have limited input into treatment planning and are often viewed as "babysitters," my experience seemed to demonstrate the tremendous potential in this treatment modality. The homesetting proved to be a safer (and softer) treatment context for Damien since the verbal world of institutional settings such as schools and hospitals had been traumatic for him. In the home I had the opportunity to directly provide and reinforce the kind of emotionally positive experiences necessary for the delicate work of building Damien's self. That is, in the safety of his home environment and our relationship he found the flexibility to use physical expression and structured activity to express his emotions and improve his natural coping strategies. By participating in Damien's everyday life for extended periods, I acted as a translator and buffer that helped him adjust to the world, and I acquired some vital insight into his emotional process that promoted an understanding of him that would have been nearly impossible through indirect sources or from the isolation of an office.

PART FOUR

Home-Based Treatment Across the Life Span

CHAPTER THIRTEEN

The Home Setting for Perinatal Care

Karen Laing

As the length of hospital stays following childbirth decreased, many new mothers began to find themselves alone with their newborns shortly after the birth. Without the support of extended families, new mothers are often overwhelmed. Karen Laing describes how workers especially trained to help new mothers are performing an important service in the home, providing support so that the mother and child can focus on each other, and begin their life together.

This is an example of "well baby" psychological services. The purpose of the doula (as these workers are called) is to support and enhance the normal functioning of the mother-infant pair. The doula can particularly be of assistance when the mother experiences postpartum depression, as the case example illustrates.

The postpartum experience of new mothers is one filled with unfamiliar challenges. The following chapter shows how the needs of postpartum women, particularly women experiencing postpartum mood disorders, can be met in their homes by specially trained providers known as postpartum doulas. A number of studies have shown that the nurturing care and emotional/physical support of a professionally trained childbirth assistant during labor significantly impacts birth outcomes, mothering ability, and mother/baby attachment (Kennell, Klaus, McGrath, Robertson, & Hinkley, 1991). We believe research will show that the postpartum doula also makes a significant contribution to the quality of the experience of the first weeks and on mothering in general.[1]

This chapter explains who doulas are and what they offer women in the childbearing year. It will explore the unique role that the postpartum doula plays in the prevention and treatment of women at risk for or with postpartum mood disorders and present a case study of a first-time mother with newborn twins exhibiting attachment difficulties and symptoms of postpartum depression.

The chapter describes the work of Birthways. Birthways is a private-pay (with sliding scale) doula service in the Chicago area. Our clients are mostly two-partner, well-educated professional families with adequate financial resources and access to childbirth preparation and pregnancy related information. The majority of our clients are 30 to 40 years of age and have had planned pregnancies. The issues facing these women are becoming increasingly common with postponed childbearing and urban living. Their extended families are not in the area, and often, community support is minimal. Isolation is a recurring theme. As professional women, they often experience a sense of loss as their relationship to their career changes. Their unfamiliarity with newborns and new mothering creates a lack of confidence, and they often struggle with the dramatic changes that new motherhood brings. Some women experience caring for the infant as a series of suffocating tasks in an unstructured day. Many, unfortunately, are also recovering from a less than empowering birth experience. Quite a number of our clients, about 25%, went through treatment for infertility before becoming pregnant. Infertility treatments have a marked effect on both couple relationships and the woman's emotional reaction to motherhood (Edelmann & Connolly, 1998).

WHAT IS A DOULA?

The term "doula" was coined in 1976 by Dana Raphael, in her book *Tender Gift: Breastfeeding,* to describe the role of a woman helper to new mothers. The term is used interchangeably to describe both labor-support doulas who provide knowledgeable and nurturing support during the birth process and postpartum doulas who do the same

---

[1] Some studies have addressed a home-visiting model for intervention for at-risk families that include postpartum visits (Olds, 1997; Olds et al., 1998). They conclude that benefits include improved health behaviors and infant caregiving, and decreased instances of maltreatment.

in the homes of women after the birth of their babies. Throughout this chapter, we will be referring specifically to the postpartum doula unless noted otherwise.

The doula's goal is to ease the transition into parenting. She is knowledgeable and experienced in all aspects of the postpartum period. She answers the new family's questions about their newborn, breast-feeding, and postpartum adjustment. She prepares meals for the family, performs light housekeeping, laundry, and errands. She helps with sibling care. Doulas are advocates for new parents, often linking them with referrals or helping them get optimal information to and from other practitioners. Their experience and training equips them to alert a family to signs of problems with mother or baby; they are a reassuring presence with regard to normal newborn behavior and postpartum recovery.

Postpartum doulas can be certified through the National Association of Postpartum Care Services. Certification requires knowledge of postpartum health including women's postpartum physiology and health, nutritional requirements, birth outcomes and postpartum discomforts as well as a thorough understanding of the psychological changes of new parenthood. Knowledge and practical breast-feeding experience are required as is experience with newborn care and well-being.

Consistent with these requirements, Birthways requires new staff to complete a 16- to 20-hour training program that covers all aspects of women's postpartum wellness, newborn assessment and care, and childbirth outcomes, facilitating attachment and the role of the doula to nurture and assess the family as a functional unit. The training stresses a holistic model of care and prepares the doula for the range of experiences they may face supporting postpartum women and families. In addition, a six-hour workshop led by a lactation consultant gives them a foundation for providing breast-feeding support and resolving common complications of lactation. A clinical psychologist provides a workshop on postpartum mood disorders. The workshop also introduces our model of home-based psychosocial support which emphasizes skillful listening, teaching relaxation techniques, and modeling attachment behaviors.

Birthways requires and provides 16 hours a year of continuing education. Workshop presenters include midwives, nurses, a variety of holistic health practitioners (herbalists, massage therapists, etc.), and mothers sharing their experiences. Senior staff provide ongoing support and supervision, and monthly staff meetings provide a forum for discussing challenging cases or specific issues. When a doula is working with a woman experiencing mood disorders or other complications, the supervisor provides more structured support, and consultation with a psychologist or other appropriate professional is implemented as needed. The supervisor and doula recognize and set goals, track the progression of the mood disorder, and together take appropriate action to ensure the safety and well-being of the family. Support to the staff also includes discussing self-care while working with depressed and anxious women. The role that the doula takes in supporting women with postpartum mood disorders is often far too overwhelming for a family member.

THE MODEL OF CARE

Unlike the medical nursing visit, the doula visit is within the framework of a holistic model. It is a model that has advantages to healthy postpartum women and their newborns when there are no presenting problems and offers a myriad of benefits when complications arise. The average duration of postpartum care is 2 to 6 weeks. Some families have doulas for longer periods, frequently when multiple infants or mood disorders are involved, and some receive support for just a few days, to provide immediate postpartum guidance with newborn care and breast-feeding. At Birthways, each visit is a minimum of 4 hours and is structured to meet the individual family's needs.

Often, the first days of care are spent resolving immediate needs and establishing a relationship. The doula is a guide for the new mothering skills that are being established and for the mother's self care as she encounters postpartum discomforts and questions. The doula educates about the baby's needs in direct ways, such as teaching about specific newborn care tasks, and indirect ways, such as modeling and affirming mother-child interactions. Emergence of unanticipated feelings—about the child, the birth, the frustrations and anxieties of being a new parent, the changing relationship with the partner—may lead to a different focus than initially anticipated.

For instance, we often get a call from a mother citing a breast-feeding problem. The doula begins by answering her questions, acknowledging her concerns and guiding her if appropriate, and reassuring her if no suggestions are needed. Support involves educating her about the mechanisms involved with breast-feeding, assuring correct positioning and latch of the baby at the breast, and assessing problems such as inverted nipples or sucking problems in the newborn. The breast-feeding guidance is similar to the model of La Leche League where counselors are trained to support new mothers paraprofessionally and to refer to professional lactation consultants when appropriate. Most of the time, new mothers need simple guidance and much reassurance and affirmation as they and their baby gain confidence in the skill of breast-feeding.

In addition to addressing the breast-feeding and newborn issues, the doula is attentive to the mother's physical needs and offers information about self-care for her postpartum discomforts. Once the breast-feeding crisis that precipitated service is being addressed, the doula often notices other factors that are likely contributing to the mother's feelings of being overwhelmed.

The lifestyle changes that a new baby brings can leave new parents feeling overwhelmed very quickly. The house may be in a state of chaos and the phone ringing busily with friends and family wanting to congratulate the family. The doorbell is another constant chime as presents and flowers arrive. Laundry has piled up from several days before labor began and grew with the things unpacked from the hospital stay and the baby clothes and blankets that need to be prewashed before they can be used. New parents don't understand why it is so hard to do such simple tasks that, prior to the baby, rarely felt unmanageable. By fielding calls and visitors, doing the laundry, picking up clutter, and setting a nice table for a meal she has prepared, the doula creates a more orderly and peaceful environment. These more subtle aspects of creating a safe "nest" for the family are of paramount importance. By meeting the practical needs of the family and addressing the mother's individual uncertainties, the doula frees the mother and baby for the important work of attachment. Her presence is reassuring to the new mother and the guidance she offers can resolve the issues that undermine her confidence.

As the relationship develops, the mother often shares her experiences as a new mother more freely and openly with the doula. The nonjudgmental and reassuring presence of the doula in addition to the camaraderie that develops as mother and doula work side by side at the tasks of early motherhood fosters trust and intimacy. The doula is not a clinical visitor for whom the mother needs to prepare herself with a repartee of appropriate questions as she does when she prepares for the brief visits with other health care professionals. The mother often feels more willing to share the joys and the frustrations of her experience.

The doula is also there as witness to the challenging moments, such as the frustrating hour that it took to get the baby to latch on or the long unsoothable fussiness of the afternoons. The new mother can share her feelings and reactions while they happen. Honest dialogue about her experience often follows. Beyond the challenging moments that are to be expected with a new baby, the doula can also witness and track developing problems, such as escalating resentment toward the baby, attachment problems, anxiety, depression, and other symptoms of developing mood disorders. The doula in the home makes behavioral observations and asks questions about the mother's well-being that may not have been addressed by other health care providers. She is, as a part of the daily experience of the new mother, a witness to the whole life of the client and, thus, can help to support the mother in a holistic way.

CHILDBIRTH AND THE POSTPARTUM EXPERIENCE

To understand the mood disorders that affect 5% to 20% of all new mothers, it is essential to appreciate the context in which these occur. The childbearing year is one of tremendous change for all women. The experience of pregnancy and childbirth has a significant impact on the postpartum period and early motherhood.

It has become widely accepted that the birth experience, including the initial hours of life of the newborn, impact the mother/baby relationship. There is strong evidence that cesarean delivery and mother–baby separation negatively impacts newborns and their mothers. Today, approximately 20% of women deliver their babies by cesarean (Korte & Scaer, 1992). It is estimated that as many as 75% of these are avoidable.

The 1981 National Institute of Health Report on Cesarean Childbirth compiled the then-current research on the effects of cesareans. The report has been instrumental in encouraging practitioners and hospitals to track and actively reduce their c-section rates. Maternal responses to cesarean deliveries were studied. These included: "feelings of powerlessness; loss of autonomy; lowered self esteem; change in body image with feelings of being 'not whole'; difficulty in integrating the labor experience; difficulty in establishing feelings of closeness with the infant and in 'claiming' the infant as her own; blame of the infant; fears of another delivery; grieving behaviors, including denial, anger, self-blame, and depression; and finally, guilt at a time when the mother believes she is supposed to feel happiness at the birth of a healthy infant" (U.S. Department of Health & Human Services, 1981, pp. 419–420).

The report also cited the specific psychological impact of mother-baby separation after birth. Mothers separated from their newborns "displayed less self-confidence than either multiparas or primiparas with early infant contact . . . when the mother's ego is threatened, the baby becomes the locus of maternal self-doubts, and a threat to the mother" (U.S. Department of Health & Human Services, 1981, p. 422).

There are similar impacts on women who deliver vaginally, but in highly interventive and traumatic ways, involving such things as limited freedom of movement, narcotic medication, episiotomies, and forceps or instrumental delivery. In most hospitals some separation routinely occurs after delivery. At best, this separation involves 1 to 3 hours in the newborn nursery for assessment, bathing, measuring, etc. Some hospitals do these tasks prior to the initial nursing, which means babies are taken away from their mothers immediately after childbirth, leading to ill-established breast-feeding as well as attachment problems.

Certainly, mood disorders do not only effect women who have experienced difficult or traumatic births, nor does the experience of loss of power and control during childbirth constitute a mood disorder. At the same time, understanding an "average" birth and postpartum experience helps clarify what is normal. Many women experience unnecessary interventions during childbirth that can create challenges to their early mothering.

CULTURAL EXPERIENCES OF MOTHERHOOD

In our culture, an individual mother's attitudes are shaped by contradictory messages. At one extreme is the view of pregnancy, birth, and postpartum as a medical event. It is seen as a treacherous and risky journey that requires medical management. Women are seen as essentially vulnerable and in need of professional rescue. At the other extreme is the expectation that women should be productive until the last minute of pregnancy, have their babies as quickly and efficiently as possible, and resume functioning in their former roles without missing a beat (or at least not more than 6 weeks, the standard maternity leave.)

Regardless of changes in the workplace, women still feel the pressure of the superwoman myth. Even if not returning to work they expect to take care of everything, look great, and keep up their calendars of professional or social engagements, essentially denying that anything has changed with the birth of their baby. One woman that we supported exemplified the conflict of the professional woman expecting her first baby. She returned to work after 2 weeks (4 weeks less than the allotted maternity leave) in order to prove to her firm that she was determined to be as productive and dedicated as she was prior to having a child. It was even a struggle to "leave the briefcase" out of the birthing room. She illustrates what many women are faced with—integrating the always-in-control and composed professional identity with the laboring, sound-making, primal woman who gives birth to, breast-feeds, and nurtures an infant. The doula provides a model of woman-centered care that helps to place the experience of motherhood in an empowering light and assists with the integration of roles.

POSTPARTUM MOOD DISORDERS

Feelings of sadness, irritability, feeling overwhelmed or "oversensitive," crying spells, appetite changes, headaches, and disturbed sleep/lack of energy are common to new mothers. This experience, labeled "baby blues," affects 85% of new mothers. It is not identified as a disorder but a normal emotional adjustment most likely attributable to hormonal changes, the profound human experience of giving birth, and adjustment to a different sleep schedule and a new baby. Postpartum blues typically resolve 2 weeks to 3 months following the birth with little lasting impact on the mother or baby (Susman, 1996).

Postpartum mood disorders are distinguishable from the normal postpartum adjustment described above. They are estimated to affect 5% to 20% of new mothers (Susman, 1996). Sometimes baby blues may develop into postpartum depression as anxiety about oneself as a mother and negative feelings toward the baby and motherhood build. Symptoms of postpartum depression include: depressed mood; fearfulness and anxiety; ambivalent feelings about the baby; dramatic fluctuations in mood; feelings of shame and hopelessness; feelings of inadequacy; and loss of interest in activities and social connection. Difficulties in bonding with the baby are common. In severe cases, women experience suicidal thoughts and/or disturbing thoughts that often are about their baby. The mother may have feelings of blame or anger toward her child and/or guilt at not meeting the infant's needs in the ways that she hoped. She is often painfully aware that she is not experiencing the anticipated happiness of motherhood.

Postpartum depression is more common with the birth of the first baby. Clearly, it is with the first child that a woman experiences the most dramatic of shifts into motherhood. As was previously discussed, many first-time mothers struggle to gain confidence, and feelings of inadequacy are common. Many women are surprised to learn that babies cry as much as they do and are sometimes inconsolable. Without an understanding that such behavior is normal, she may blame herself or develop feelings of resentment toward the infant as the source of her anxiety.

Another factor is lack of support from her partner, family, and friends. Having a new baby can be tremendously isolating. Often, the time with her new baby is the first she has spent not working and participating in social activities. For the families we support, we see that community connection is often minimal or focused on professional relationships and distant family members. Jeffrey Susman (1996) identified withdrawal of social support (for example, when the mother leaves the hospital or when visiting relatives go home) as a potential precipitant for the development of postpartum depression. Isolation can escalate as the weeks go on. Partners return to work, as family and friends return to their lives and routines. When a new mother is home with her baby, her friends are at work. New mothers can feel overwhelmed at the practical planning involved in taking their new infant on outings. Winter weather makes outings even more difficult. Postpartum depression may increase during the winter months as a result of this increased isolation as well as the potential impact of seasonal affective disorder.

Lack of partner support and marital difficulties are risk factors for postpartum mood disorders. Pregnancy can escalate problems within a relationship; statistics show that domestic violence increases during pregnancy (Schornstein, 1997). New parenthood can itself put stress on partnerships. The first year of parenthood often challenges marital relationships as the infant takes priority within the relationship (Galinsky, 1987).

The birth of multiple infants is a contributing factor to postpartum depression. Not only is the pregnancy and delivery of multiple infants statistically more complicated, but the demands of caring for multiple infants is overwhelming. Guilt and anxiety about meeting the needs of not one, but two or more infants contributes to postpartum depression. Experiences of loss, including previous pregnancy loss or death of a child, or loss of a parent, particularly the mother of the woman, are also factors in postpartum mood disorders. Traumatic birth experiences contribute to postpartum distress. Sometimes the birth experience is so traumatic that it triggers post-traumatic stress disorder, the same disorder that is linked with survivors of violence, rape, and sexual abuse. Other studies correlate postpartum mood disorders to women with a history of depression or anxiety disorders (Steiner & Tam, 1999).

Postpartum psychosis, which affects about 1 or 2 mothers in 1,000 is a rare postpartum mood disorder. It is a more sudden and disturbing break that includes hallucination, extreme confusion, and manic behavior. Women who experience psychosis often have thoughts of harming themselves or their babies or have psychotic fantasies about the baby (such as the baby is not theirs, or is dead or dismembered). Predisposing factors for postpartum psychosis include a personal or family history of affective disorders, an experience of perinatal death, cesarean delivery, or isolation (Susman, 1996). Hospitalization and psychopharmaceutical management is required in most cases; prognosis is good with treatment.

There is significant controversy about the etiology of postpartum mood disorders. Hormonal changes have been implicated (Abou-Saleh, Ghubash, Krymski, & Bhai, 1998; Ploeckinger et al., 1996), although the aforementioned predisposing factors seem to play a stronger role. The hormonal changes specifically identified as potential contributors to postpartum mood changes involve estrogen and corticotropin-releasing hormone, known as CRH. Both estrogen and CRH levels are elevated during pregnancy. CRH is especially high in the last trimester. CRH, through a cascade of events, triggers the production of cortisol which affects blood sugar levels and blood pressure and assists the body in managing stress. Because the placenta had been producing CRH in magnified quantities, after delivery, the normal (pre-pregnancy) cycle of the production of CRH is compromised, and women have lower than normal levels of the hormone. These low levels of cortisol may contribute to development of mood disorders.

SEEKING TREATMENT FOR
POSTPARTUM MOOD DISORDERS

Treatment options are available for women experiencing postpartum mood disorders, yet many blocks to seeking support exist. Postpartum mood disorders often catch mothers and family members by surprise. Many women are likely to find their symptoms frightening and shameful. It is not easy to admit that one's own feelings do not fit the cultural image of the idealized new mother. Sharing her feelings with a partner can feel like a questioning of their mutual decision to become parents. The mother might have tried to reveal her feelings only to be told that she just needs sleep or that she'll snap out of it. Particularly if her feelings follow an interventive or traumatic birth, she is often reminded to be grateful that her baby is healthy. The mother who is courageous enough to seek professional support often encounters misinformation and lack of support from the medical community (Medow et al., 1993). It is not uncommon that a woman we identify as clearly depressed has her concerns dismissed or minimized by her physician.

Unless physicians and psychotherapists are familiar with the specific needs of postpartum women, their assistance can be misguided. New mothers have many needs that are distinct from other sufferers of depression or anxiety disorders. To begin with, they represent a "dual patient." Treatment, both psychotherapeutic and medical, needs to attend to mother and baby as a unit. Treatment should be focused on immediate stabilization of the depressed mother in order to lessen the impact on the parenting relationship. This immediacy may call for a postponement of work on deeper psychological issues (such as family of origin or early abuse experiences) even when these issues have been brought to the surface by the mother's birth experience. A therapist working with postpartum women must also be versed in newborn mental health, mother–infant attachment, childbirth, and breast-feeding-related issues.

Unless specializing in postpartum mood disorders, psychiatrists may not recognize the impact that terminating breast-feeding can have on women and their babies. Breast-feeding is an important part of the mother/baby relationship and attachment process and a source of competence for the new mother. Breast-feeding releases hormones that increase the new mother's sense of well-being. Without this awareness, psychiatrists are often less committed to researching alternatives to the medications that are incompatible with nursing. We have also seen many partners or family members suggest terminating the breast-feeding relationship: "You'll feel better if you weren't so tied down feeding the baby." If antidepressant therapies that are incompatible with nursing are unavoidable, the mother should be supported through her inevitable sense of loss and her likely feelings of failure in addition to the physical discomforts of weaning.

Mental health treatment for women with postpartum mood disorders includes psychotherapy, antidepressant medications, and/or support groups, such as Depression After Delivery. In severe cases, women may undergo psychiatric hospitalization. Often women feel like an anomaly in a hospital setting designed to address patients struggling with other psychiatric problems. One new mother described her experience of being in an inpatient group: "We went around the group and everyone described their problems. After other patients described horrendous issues with drugs, abusive families, and so on, I said, 'well, I just had a baby.' People stared at me. They couldn't understand why I was there . . . neither could I." Neither she nor they could see any common ground between their experiences. Even if special treatment facilities are available to meet their specific needs, hospitalization in the United States inevitably means that women are separated from their babies. As a result, fears and anxieties about parenting skills, infant bonding issues, and guilt about one's ambivalence about mothering are exacerbated. While the hospitalization may help stabilize the mother temporarily, she is distressed by what she has missed. In addition, the absence of the baby prevents treatment staff from directly facilitating the mother's confidence and parenting skills and bonding with her baby. At times, staff and family even discourage contact with the baby. At best, the mother sees her baby briefly in the unnatural setting of the hospital ward. For nursing mothers, the separation creates an abrupt weaning which is traumatic and difficult for mother and baby and carries with it increased feelings of failure and loss.

We briefly supported one mother before, during, and after psychiatric hospitalization, around the time of her fourth week postpartum.

In our first days of service before her hospitalization, we made progress in resolving breast-feeding problems and helped her rest by caring for the baby while she napped. We also handled a large number of extraneous things that she felt responsible for. Although we encouraged her to postpone such tasks, she felt a need to "wrap up" these things that were unfinished before the arrival of the baby.

Even though she was quite depressed. she was confident in her handling of her newborn, and attachment was good. She told us about her baby's patterns and behaviors with authority. We were not scheduled to see her for four days, and during that time, she was hospitalized. During hospitalization, her family decided to keep visits with the baby to a minimum and strongly rallied her to terminate breast-feeding. After a week of inpatient treatment, she returned home. The doula was there to greet her and support her for the first days home. When handed her infant, the woman tentatively and awkwardly held him with a pained look on her face. She asked repeatedly if she was holding him correctly and throughout the day asked about diapering, how to dress the baby, etc. Her confidence had been truly shattered, and the family responded by again withdrawing the infant. We unfortunately were not able to continue working with this mother, as the family preferred to retreat and handle the "problem" privately.

DOULA SUPPORT FOR WOMEN WITH POSTPARTUM MOOD DISORDERS

Although some women know the preventive value of postpartum care or seek in some way the role of emotional support that a doula offers, most families who hire postpartum care providers are not anticipating postpartum mood disorders. While their goal when setting up support is practical care, often as service progresses, the emotional support of the doula becomes key.

When unexpected postpartum emotions feel out of control, the client can access emotional support or guidance from the doula in a way that unfolds naturally. If she does experience symptoms that concern her, she might ask the doula what normal postpartum reactions are. Clients often ask: "Do other mothers feel this way?" The doula, as someone who has intimate knowledge of other new mothers' experiences and is often a mother herself, can talk about the more "nitty-gritty" aspects of the experience.

Often clients who are resistant to professional help are open to support from an in-home paraprofessional. The doula can manage symptoms and encourage her to seek professional support once a relationship of trust has been established. The doula can suggest treatment resources knowledgeable about postpartum mood disorders and generally help the mother to understand her options.

The postpartum doula's holistic approach complements the care the mother receives from mental health professionals. By addressing issues of isolation and inadequate emotional and practical support, she lessens the factors that contribute to depression. Her experience allows her to encourage and affirm the mother's involvement in treatment. The doula, with permission of the client, consults with her therapist or other professionals to discuss her observations and get their guidance for working with the client. And, as the following case study illustrates, the doula can make the best of the situation when a depressed mother resists other treatments.

CASE STUDY

Mary and her husband, Bob contacted Birthways in the 30th week of her first pregnancy. She was 37 years old and carrying twins. They sought support to guide them as new parents, provide breast-feeding information, help to establish a routine with the new babies, and assist with infant care. They requested three or four daytime shifts and three overnight shifts per week to allow them full nights of rest.

Two doulas, Diane and Lisa, were assigned to work with Mary and Bob, as their scheduling needs were more than one doula could fulfill. Each doula met with the family in Mary's 31st and 32nd weeks of pregnancy. Diane had extensive experience working with women with postpartum mood disorders and is a mother herself with grown children. Lisa's son was then 4 years old. Lisa had personal experience with postpartum depression after a cesarean delivery.

Diane and Lisa each came away from their prenatal visits with concerns about the family's preparedness for the arrival of their babies. Mary and Bob were very involved in their careers. Mary was planning a national job search 1 month after the full-term due date of her infants that would involve extensive travel. She also expressed common fears and concerns regarding the birth, a potential cesarean delivery, and breast-feeding. The doulas listened and acknowledged her concerns, provided suggestions for getting off to a good start with nursing while in the hospital, informed the couple of the availability of a professional labor support doula, and welcomed them to call at any time for support or resources. Mary and Bob planned to begin care immediately upon discharge from the hospital.

Mary delivered in her 40th week. She delivered vaginally with an induced but fast and uncomplicated delivery. She was unsuccessful with breast-feeding while in the hospital. A doula began working with the family on her fourth day postpartum. One of the twins, Susan, nursed more successfully within the first week, while the boy, Ben, continued to struggle with nursing. The problems were common for babies not nursed frequently in the first hours and days after birth. They exhibited nipple-confusion, which occurs when a newborn learns to suck on the artificial nipples of a bottle, and "forgets" how to nurse at a breast. They were generally fussy at the breast. There were no physiological problems with mother or baby.

The doulas assisted Mary with positioning, helped her understand the physiology of nursing and what was happening with the babies, and gave lots of encouragement. Breast-feeding sessions were stressful for Mary, but she did well when in the presence of a doula. By the end of the first week, Lisa reported that nursing was steadily improving. Bob, however, who had been very supportive of breast-feeding prenatally, was now telling the doulas that he was not sure if Mary could do it. In the hours when Mary was on her own, nursing was traumatizing and difficult. It was becoming the focus of her negative feelings about motherhood.

It soon became very obvious to the doulas that Mary was in trouble. She mechanically listed her symptoms and physical discomforts when they asked how she was feeling. She was easily frustrated with nursing and newborn care tasks, and responded with resentment to the repetitive nature of the babies' needs. During breast-feeding she rarely sought eye contact or showed stroking or connection with the babies. The moment they were done nursing, she would hand them to someone else and leave the room. Mary otherwise cared for the infants in a very mechanical way. Her interaction was limited to what tasks needed to be done; she was not interested in holding them. She had no interest in food, and even when the doulas prepared and offered meals, would often not eat until late in the afternoon. While the doulas saw the danger signs, it would be 6 weeks before Mary would begin to share her emotional experience with them and admit to feeling resentful toward the babies and frightened about being alone with them.

The doulas tried to engage Mary about her feelings. In the fourth week, when Mary abruptly weaned the babies, Lisa asked her about her decision. She explained that she "couldn't take it anymore . . . I was so angry that I almost shook (the baby)." Lisa shared this information with Diane and supervisory staff. Together a plan was developed to track Mary's moods and to encourage her to seek professional support. Mary had hired additional childcare help and so was rarely, if ever, alone with the babies. At the doula's insistence, Mary agreed to call someone if she ever felt at the end of her rope or that she might hurt the babies. She also agreed to discuss her feelings with her doctor at her 6-week checkup. She said she felt much better since she was no longer nursing. For a short time she could believe that breast-feeding was the source of her frustration and mood swings.

At her doctor visit, Mary did talk candidly with her physician. He told her to wait 2 to 3 weeks and "see how she felt then." He told her that she shouldn't be concerned and that her feelings were normal. The doulas were very concerned that their recommendations to seek professional help or at least attend postpartum depression support groups were not supported by the physician. They feared further denial would take root in Mary and her husband. Mary, however, said she felt invalidated by her physician. Although she was not willing to take steps to seek additional help, she began to share more of her feelings with the doulas, particularly Diane. Although Mary felt a slight lifting of her resentment for a few days after terminating breast-feeding, she quickly began to sink further into depression. She was even less attached to her babies now that she could leave feeding up to others. She often found reasons to be gone for much of the day, leaving the babies in the care of the doula or her other babysitters.

Bob worked full time and so did not have much opportunity to talk to the doulas. One day when he was home earlier than usual, he shared his concern about Mary to Lisa. He said she was "not herself" and was not enjoying motherhood. Another family member also spoke with the doulas about Mary's behavior. All were encouraging Mary to seek help, but Mary continued to evade the subject. Husband and family concurred that Mary was not the type of woman to talk about her feelings and that she was very resistant to counseling.

A breakthrough occurred shortly after the six-week doctor visit. Mary asked Diane if her feelings were normal, although she hesitated to describe those feelings in detail. Diane listened carefully and validated her feelings. She said that she could see that Mary was struggling. She shared her own experiences as a new mother and how hard it can be to be with a newborn. "We can sometimes have negative feelings about our children as infants if we felt that we, ourselves, as infants, were not liked." Mary took this in silently and Diane felt a connection had been made, although she was uncertain if Mary would accept her invitation to explore this further.

Two days later after Mary returned from a visit with her own mother and immediately upon Diane's arrival at her home, she said that she wanted to talk. Mary had asked her mother directly what she was like as a baby and how her mother felt about new motherhood. What her mother shared was that Mary had been very colicky and "miserable" and that they (Mary's parents) would put her in a room, close the door, and retreat to a distant part of the house. They would turn up the volume of the television or radio to shut out the sounds of Mary's cries. Obtaining this information allowed Mary to begin processing her own feelings about mothering. She began to discuss her grief and resentment with Diane.

In subsequent conversations, Mary began to pump Diane for information about the postpartum experiences of others, including Diane herself. She shared her fears more openly. Rather than handing off the babies and running out the door during Diane's shifts, she spent the shifts talking. Mary spoke of her feelings of loss of control, of loss of her career. One day Mary expressed her hopelessness. "I'll never travel again, never have a life."

Diane validated her feelings about "losing her life" while introducing new possibilities. She brought in a photograph that showed two children seated on a bluff overlooking the Swiss Alps. "I wanted to share this with you, as a reminder that you'll be able to have new adventures that you can share with your children. Your children are so fortunate to have you as a mother." The photograph moved Mary deeply and served also as a reminder that newborns become children . . . that this crisis of early infancy would change in time.

As Mary struggled with depression, the babies' needs were met by the doulas and by Bob after work and on weekends. Both doulas spent all available time holding and interacting with the babies, and noting their symptomatic withdrawal from the caregivers. Susan's behavior in particular concerned them. She did not seek and avoided eye contact. Once Mary's depression began to lift, attention was refocused on her tentative attachment with her babies. While the doulas were nurturing Mary and giving her opportunity to share her feelings, they modeled loving and blameless interaction with the babies. By responding to a hungry baby with "Is it time to eat . . . I know you must be very hungry," they showed an alternative to a statement that Mary might make, "Oh you are always hungry . . . greedy baby." They consistently reminded Mary of Susan and Ben's innocence and that they were reliant on the loving care of adults. Letting Mary know that she could voice her negative feelings about the babies, but that they are not to blame for her feelings and need her unconditional love represents the way in which both mother and baby, or babies, in this case, are our clients.

Diane's report at 12 weeks, the conclusion of her care with Mary, included the following: "I saw signs today that Mary is falling in love with her babies. Was able to see her just gently and lovingly stroking Ben's hair and looking at him with a mother's love . . . she is calling him 'sweet boy' and Susan 'sweet pea' and talks of having much more trouble shifting gears from babies to work . . . I think because she is finally bonding. She spends less time with her job search and more time with the babies. And . . . Susan and Ben are smiling and cooing."

Diane was working with a depressed and struggling mother who was resistant to outside help, a physician who denied her illness, and babies whose needs were not being met. She continued, even after the program ended, to encourage Mary to get professional help. Diane has, while acknowledging Mary's progress, reiterated her need for counseling, reminding Mary that "kindness and support do not heal depression . . . professional help does."

CONCLUSIONS

Postpartum mood disorders can have a profound impact on the entire family. Due to the limited purview of this chapter, the impact on partner and siblings was not addressed, let alone the long-term implications for the mother/baby and family members. Ideally, depressed mothers and their families will utilize the support of postpartum doulas and access quality professional care and support groups.

We are regularly referred clients with postpartum depression from professionals within the community. Optimally, we participate as team members who, along with other professionals, meet the families' needs. Recently, we provided care to a woman who had delivered a premature infant that required hospitalization for several weeks. The special care nurses encouraged her to get support when she came home with her baby and referred her to Birthways. We began care the day that the baby left the nursery and assisted with breast-feeding alongside the lactation consultant that visited her in her home. She was allowed lots of time to process with her doula the many feelings involved with the premature delivery, a complicated pregnancy and birth, breast-feeding problems, and the loss of an ideal experience with her baby. She was admittedly anxious caring for her baby who had been so fragile for such an extended period of time. She was tremendously encouraged by the affirmations of her doula while noting that she observed the doula carefully to learn how to care for her baby more confidently.

When her depression escalated, her lactation consultant and therapist contacted us to work together in supporting her. We report back and forth, and encourage our client to utilize all of her resources. Her services, with the exception of her therapy sessions, take place in her home where she feels safe and comfortable. After the long months in the hospital nursery, she is particularly grateful to be in her own environment. She and her baby are struggling, but each day brings some relief and she grows more confident all the time.

The first months of a child's life are an important yet challenging time for families. The doula, together with other professionals, can ease the journey.

REFERENCES

Abou-Saleh, M. T., Ghubash, R., Krymski, M., & Bhai, I. (1998). Hormonal aspects of postpartum depression. *Psychoneuroendocrinology, 23,* 465–475.

Edelmann, R. J., & Connolly, K. J. (1998). Psychological state and psychological strain in relation to infertility. *Journal of Community and Applied Social Psychology, 8,* 303–311.

Kennell, J., Klaus, M., McGrath, S., Robertson, S., & Hinkley, C. (1991). Continuous emotional support during labor in a US hospital. *Journal of the American Medical Association, 265,* 197–201.

Korte, D., & Scaer, R. (1992). *A good birth, a safe birth: Choosing and having the childbirth experience you want.* Boston: Harvard Common Press.

Medow, M., Borowsky, S. J., Dysken, S., Hillson, S. D., Woods, S., & Wilt, T. J. (1999). Internal medical residents' ability to diagnose and characterize major depression. *Western Journal of Medicine, 170,* 35–40.

Olds, D. (1997). The Prenatal/Early Infancy Project: Fifteen years later. Issues in children's and families' lives. In G. W. Albee, & T. P. Gullotta (Eds.), *Primary prevention works* (pp. 41–67). Thousand Oaks, CA: Sage.

Olds, D., Pettitt, L. M., Robinson, J., Henderson, C., Jr. Eckenrode, J., Kitzman, H., Cole, B., & Powers, J. (1998). Reducing risks for antisocial behavior with a program of prenatal and early childhood home visitation. *Journal of Community Psychology, 26,* 65–83.

Ploeckinger, D., Dantendorfer, K., Ulm, M., Baischer, W., Derfler, K., Musalek, M., & Dadak, C. (1996). Rapid decrease of serum cholesterol concentration and postpartum depression. *British Medical Journal,* 664.

Raphael, D. (1976) *Tender gift: Breast-feeding.* New York: Schocken Books.

Schornstein, S. (1997). *Domestic violence and health care: What every professional needs to know.* Thousand Oaks, CA: Sage.

Steiner, M., & Tam, W. Y. K. (1999). Postpartum depression in relation to other psychiatric disorders. In L. J. Miller (Ed.), *Postpartum mood disorders,* (pp. 47–63). Washington, DC: American Psychiatric Press.

Susman, J. L. (1996). Postpartum depressive disorders. *Journal of Family Practice, 43,* 17–24.

U.S. Department of Health and Human Services, Public Health Service, and National Institutes of Health. (1981). *Cesarean childbirth: Report of a Consensus Development Conference sponsored by the National Institute of Child Health and Human Development in conjunction with the National Center for Health Care Technology and assisted by the Office for Medical Applications of Research,* September 22–24, 1980 (NIH Publication No. 82-2067). Bethesda, MD: Author.

Treatment and Trauma: Shirley Temple's Nightmares

Julia M. Klco

This case study illustrates how the home setting can enrich treatment. A young girl was being adopted by her foster mother. By bringing the treatment into the home, the therapist was able to help the child and the family join together at the same time as she helped the child recover from abuse.

One of the first times I met with her, she dove under the kitchen table because she didn't want to talk to me. Knowing that it would do no good to ask her to come out, I joined her there. Our therapeutic relationship began right there, on the floor, under the kitchen table.

Kimberly is a very beautiful little girl. Her large, expressive, dark brown eyes, warm olive skin, dark wavy hair, and petite features reflect a most exquisite blend of her Caucasian mother and her African American father. Kimberly also has tell-tale signs of her mother's heavy drug and alcohol use during pregnancy. She has bilateral epicanthal folds (around her eyes) and a flattened philtrum (the ridges under the nose), physical features that are consistent with prenatal alcohol and drug exposure. In no way does this distract from her beauty; rather, to the professionals working with her, it is but one more reminder of Kimberly's history of abuse and neglect.

Kimberly's biological mother used heroin, cocaine, alcohol, tobacco and marijuana throughout her pregnancy. Kimberly was a full-term baby and weighed 6 lbs., 6 oz. She left the hospital with her mother but soon went through a series of placements with relatives because of her mother's inability to care for her because of drug and alcohol abuse. During the first 4 years of Kimberly's life, she lived with four different family members. In between moves she stayed with her mother for brief periods of time.

Kimberly was 8 at the time she was referred to our agency by her adoption caseworker. Even at 8 Kimberly understood only too well and complained that "life is not fair." At the time of referral she was in foster care (a preadoptive home), with her younger brother Lou, 6 years of age. An older half-brother, Darrin, who had previously lived there with them, had been placed in another foster home due to his uncontrollable behavior. Darrin's acts of violence and rage included smashing a kitten's head in the refrigerator door, killing it. Kimberly has not forgotten the killing, nor has she forgiven her brother.

Kimberly's case first came to the attention of the Child Welfare Department when she and her brother Lou went from neighbor to neighbor asking for food. Kimberly was almost 4 at the time and Lou was 2. Shortly thereafter, the State Child Welfare Department took custody of Kimberly and her brothers due to abuse and neglect. Kimberly's pre-school teachers had observed her foraging for food in the garbage. At the age of 4 she didn't know what a toothbrush was. Over the next 3½ years, Kimberly was in several foster placements. In one of these placements she and her younger brother Lou suffered further physical abuse. They were hit and beaten with coat hangers, purse straps, belts, extension cords, and shoes. Kimberly told me that she lived in 7 different foster homes because "nobody else wanted us."

When I met her, Kimberly and Lou lived with their foster mother Ms. Heart, her two biological daughters, Claudia, 12, and Cindy, 15, and two other foster children, Laura, 12, and Lupe, 10. The family had been receiving in-home services which included respite care and family psychotherapy from a community based agency. Kimberly was in need of individual therapy but could not handle the closeness of such a therapeutic relationship. The family therapist began individual sessions gradually with Kimberly, however, one-on-one Kimberly quickly became overwhelmed. At the slightest hint of any discussion involving her feelings or her behavior she became avoidant and defensive. She did better in a family setting, with her foster mother present. Even during family sessions, however, Kimberly would often run to her room, slamming her door.

The two other foster girls in the home, Laura and Lupe, were Hispanic immigrants with very special problems of their own. Laura presented as anorexic, and Lupe was suffering from trauma-specific psychotic episodes. The girls' biological father had been abusive and had recently

died in a fire. Lupe kept "seeing" him in her foster home in places
such as closets, her bedroom, and even saw his head in the toilet.
These episodes often resulted in Lupe hyperventilating and in several
trips to the emergency room. To say this home was chaotic was an
understatement.

Services from the community-based agency were coming to an end
as their contract was expiring. Kimberly and Lou were being adopted
and the agency I work with was taking over the pre- and postadoptive
counseling. I was fortunate enough to work alongside the previous
family therapist for several weeks. This greatly enhanced the transition of services and made this very difficult change easier for all.

Previous mental health professionals and therapists had diagnosed Kimberly with underlying depression and adjustment disorder
with mixed disturbance of emotions and conduct—chronic. Kimberly
had been evaluated in both inpatient and outpatient settings. A pedi-
atric psychiatrist unfamiliar with symptoms of trauma and neglect
diagnosed Kimberly with attention deficit hyperactivity disorder and
prescribed Ritalin. The Ritalin had no effect and it was discontinued.
I quickly concluded that the prior diagnoses did not accurately capture this little girl. My impression was that Kimberly was experiencing posttraumatic stress disorder in addition to the behavioral
effects of prenatal exposure to drugs and alcohol. Later evaluations
confirmed this.

Primary difficulties included problems with anger and violence.
Kimberly often directed her anger toward other foster children in the
home by screaming and striking out at them. Oppositional and defiant
behavior had also been documented.

Kimberly had a very low opinion of herself. She worked to change
the nature of her hair for over a year. She hated the coarse kinky tex-
ture and wanted it straightened. Her self-esteem was very poor and
school difficulties further contributed to her poor self-image. Kimberly's
lack of trust in adults added to her difficulties, as she would often
refuse their help. Kimberly was easily agitated and had poor impulse
control. Her play often reflected themes of abandonment and of children taking care of other children.

Much of Kimberly's anxiety and depression was revealed through
somatization and nightmares. Kimberly's nightmares contributed to
sleep difficulties. She frequently complained of headaches, stomach
aches, and vomiting. It was never clear if she actually experienced the
symptoms or if they were feigned. Physical examination failed to
reveal any reasons for the complaints.

Over the course of treatment, Kimberly has had several nightmares
with rape as the main theme. In one nightmare, she was saved by

Michael Jordan. According to the history, in Kimberly's early treatment she presented as provocative and flirtatious with no fear of strangers. After about the age of 6, a fear of men emerged.

Other nightmares included visions of "her two moms fighting." In one nightmare Kimberly saw her foster mom throw her biological mom in front of a car. Additional nightmares included murders and stabbings. In real life, Kimberly had witnessed the stabbing of her aunt by her biological mother.

In many ways, Kimberly was mature beyond her years. She had a very difficult time not being the in-charge "mom." She had taken on looking out for her brothers as her primary responsibility. Her need to be in control took precedence over anything else. Kimberly could not even accept comforting if it meant that she would feel vulnerable or would need to relinquish some control.

Kimberly's need to be in control made it difficult to establish a trusting therapeutic relationship with her. Once this was established, however, Kimberly often showed her disapproval of my departure after visits. She hid my shoes (they had been removed at the door) or my keys, or ran out ahead of me and hid in my car. After several appointments ended in this way, I learned to keep my shoes on, to lock my car, and to keep my keys deep in my pocket until I got to the car. Kimberly had had three different therapists in a short time span and she was very concerned that I would leave and not come back, as had others before me. Once Kimberly was convinced that there was no set time limit on our work, her fears were somewhat reduced. As she began to feel safe with me, we began the very slow process of increasing her tolerance for treatment. It took considerable time before she was able to talk about her previous abuse history.

When I first started working with Kimberly, she was unwilling to discuss emotions. She often covered up her sadness with socially appropriate or desirable behavior. Kimberly could be quite creative in her avoidance strategies. Kimberly loves to sing, dance, and act, and she would literally go into a song and dance routine to avoid a painful discussion. We called this the Shirley Temple defense. She wanted very much to please those around her.

Kimberly suppressed her anger, which was later released in explosive episodes. These were episodes in which she couldn't control herself or her emotions. She would throw things, slam doors, scream, hit, and kick. After one of these episodes, it was extremely difficult for Kimberly to calm herself, and she resisted comforting or help from others.

When demands were placed on Kimberly at home or at school she was quickly overwhelmed. Her schoolwork was poor. She had no friends and had generally poor peer relations. Even at school she had to be the one in charge and she didn't know how to play with other children or how to make friends.

Kimberly hated the way she looked. She hated her hair and her face. She thought that she was ugly. This was only one of many distorted and faulty sets of cognition that needed to be altered. Pocahontas and face paints came to the rescue. Kimberly loved the Disney film *Pocahontas*. Ms. Heart had decorated Kimberly's room in a Pocahontas motif. Kimberly thought Pocahontas was beautiful and we talked about how many of Kimberly's features were just like those of Pocahontas. I pointed out how her skin tone and beautiful almond shaped brown eyes were just like Pochahontas'. At first she looked at me in disbelief but the idea began to grow on her, and she began to look at herself more in the mirror.

Kimberly had noticed how everyone in the family had a different skin tone. During one visit, I asked everyone in the family to line up at the kitchen table and put their arms out across it. No two arms looked the same. There were eight different variations and textures. We talked about how boring the world would be if there were only one color. The children themselves came up with problems like "How could you tell where the land ended and the sky began if the sky wasn't blue?"

To further illustrate the value of color, out came the face paints. Kimberly loved the face painting and spent considerable time admiring herself in the mirror. After I painted everyone's faces and arms, Kimberly painted me. She proceeded to virtually cover my face in bright blue and orange. This was the beginning of Kimberly's appreciation of herself. It was also a lesson in trust.

Kimberly's schoolwork was another problem. At one point, prior to her adoption, Kimberly simply stopped turning in any homework. Sometimes she would do it but not turn it in. At other times she would forget homework papers at school or not have the assignment written down. The solution was a behavior modification program that Kimberly and Ms. Heart helped design. I brought her an empty plastic peanut butter jar, stickers, paints, and colored pony beads. She decorated the jar with all the trimmings and the beads were given to her foster mother.

Together we decided that every day Kimberly turned in all her homework she would get a bead. Each bead was worth five points (we were also working on her math skills). When she earned 25, 50, 75, or 100 points she received a reward chosen ahead of time by her and agreed on by all. If Kimberly failed to turn in a homework assignment, her foster mother gave her an additional homework assignment. This often involved having Kimberly type a page from one of her reading books onto the family computer. Kimberly's teacher was very cooperative and helped Ms. Heart by staying in close phone contact and helping Kimberly to organize her work.

Kimberly's academic work improved almost immediately. To date, more than 1 year later, she rarely has difficulty in turning in homework assignments. The motivational rewards are no longer needed. Occasionally, when homework problems do surface, it is usually a cue that something is bothering Kimberly and a sign that she needs others to help her through it.

Another school issue to be addressed was other children's teasing and taunting of Kimberly. Although she went to a culturally and racially mixed school, she was called "Blackie." Kimberly was ecstatic about her pending adoption and thought that everyone else had a family therapist, an individual therapist, and dealt with all the crazy issues she had to deal with. Her openness about her experiences contributed to kids making her a target for teasing.

Kimberly had not lived in environments where there were clear boundaries, or where social skills were taught or modeled. More than a year after the adoption, when friends would get angry at her, they would say things like "At least I'm not adopted."

School projects about Mother's Day, Father's Day, and family trees confused her and almost always resulted in "acting-out" behavior the week following the project. Kimberly knew she had a biological mother, another mother who had adopted her, and a biological father who had given up his rights. What she didn't know was which family or person she should report on or which alliance she should protect.

Kimberly had not only chosen to take her adopted mother's last name but also chose to change her middle name to Ms. Heart's first name. We began to discuss how she would explain her name change in school. Together, we decided to create a book that she could read to her class about being adopted. I presented her with a hardbound journal book and together we went to work. Week after week during our sessions Kimberly spent time carefully writing and illustrating her book while we talked about what it meant to be adopted. She later used the remaining pages in the book to journal.

During the adoption process, I realized that all the children in Ms. Heart's home were confused about what a family was. Their ideas ranged from Ozzie and Harriet to chaos. The children had lived in chaotic homes and the families they had seen on TV were what they thought represented a real family. To further evaluate expectations and thoughts from the children's perspective, we started yet another project.

I brought a multitude of magazines to the children and asked them to begin cutting out pictures that represented a family. We would then make a collage of what they had collected. The pictures they chose were somewhat surprising. There were lots of appliances, refrigerators, furniture, and other material things. There were also pictures of food. It is of interest to note that much of our work was done around the kitchen table, and many of the pictures they had chosen were from a kitchen. There were no pictures of children, but Lou cut out one picture of a dog. His adopted family had two dogs and a multitude of cats. The pictures of people were all of Caucasian individuals. They selected no pictures of people in a relationship. There were no men in the pictures. This helped me considerably in understanding the children's limited view of what a family was. It became clear that there was no concept of relationship and that fathers had been absent. We went ahead and made the collage, the whole time discussing options, alternatives, and enhancements to the items they had chosen to represent a family. Family sessions provided further insight into how the children, particularly Kimberly functioned in a family.

During some of the family sessions, Kimberly had trouble following directions and letting others have a turn talking. One of the first interventions to address this was to have Kimberly and other family members reverse roles and pretend to be each other. One of the best and most productive sessions occurred when Kimberly and her adoptive mother changed roles. Ms. Heart pretended to be Kimberly and did a beautiful job of whining, crying, screaming, and overall not listening. Kimberly, who was pretending to be her mother, quickly became frustrated, and was at a loss as to how to get the situation under control (however, she also wasn't very anxious to give up the mother role!). Kimberly had a hard time believing that she really acted that way, stating "I don't do that, do I?"

Other interventions to assist Kimberly with relinquishing control involved playing games of catch, taking turns, playing Simon Says, Follow the Leader, and the Ungame. The Ungame is a family board game where nobody wins or loses but everybody gets a chance to speak about feelings, wishes, dreams, and so on and everyone has an opportunity to comment, but only in turn.

Another favorite was a game of mirroring in which Kimberly and I sat face to face. We would take turns "mirroring" each other's hand movements which became increasingly more complex. This was one of Kimberly's first formal lessons in following an adult and one she truly enjoyed.

All the children in Ms. Heart's care had special needs. When they all needed something at once, chaos reigned. When chaos in the home increased, Kimberly's sometime frantic efforts to manage her own anxiety and behavior increased. She became increasingly defiant. In an effort to reduce the chaos, much consultation and case management was done with other treatment providers and with Ms. Heart.

It wasn't long before I suggested that Ms. Heart consider terminating Laura and Lupe's placement with her. Before she was able to consider this, however, she wanted to make sure she had exhausted all resources in trying to stabilize the family and make the placement work.

I began to work closely with the other treatment providers, sometimes assisting them with sessions or co-leading a family group. Several interventions were effective during sessions with the family. They were usually short-lived, however. All the children had high needs for affection and attention. Competition to get their needs met disrupted family communication. Family sessions almost always required two therapists.

An effective intervention in getting the family to listen to each other and to take turns speaking involved a Beanie Baby. Only the therapist(s) or the person holding the Beanie Baby was allowed to speak. When someone spoke out of turn, s/he was reminded in a gentle but firm way to wait until s/he had the Beanie. This proved to be a very difficult task for all. Even Ms. Heart needed reminders. This helped everyone realize how often they interrupted each other. The family began using the Beanie Baby in the therapist's absence when things got out of control.

After a particularly difficult family session, I introduced visualization and progressive muscle relaxation. While this was highly effective for some family members, Lupe had great difficulty with it and she was allowed to entertain herself in the next room. During this first attempt, two of the children even fell asleep! For the next several sessions the family asked to do it again and it did prove effective in reducing tension and hostility.

Since listening to each other was proving so very difficult, the "telephone game" was introduced. We all sat in a circle and the person starting would whisper something to the person next to them and so on. The first and last person would then report on what was said. The family was clearly shocked at how a story changed after being repeated by only eight or nine people. We did this several times until their skill improved.

Finally, we did cooperative games designed to help the family work as a team. For example, everyone stood in a circle holding hands and a hula-hoop was passed around the circle. The rule was that you couldn't let go of your neighbor's hand. This clearly took cooperation and even the older siblings enjoyed the challenge. The children quickly learned that by helping each other we could make the hula hoop go around the circle much faster.

Another favorite of mine that this family had great difficulty with was to "make rain." In this task everyone sits on the floor in a circle with their eyes closed. It requires that you listen to the person to your left and follow their cue. One person begins by snapping their fingers and continues until this "sound" is passed to their right and all around the circle. The person who started then begins to rub their palms together (as if warming them), and passes this sound around the circle. The lead person then begins to pat their legs or the floor in a rapid drumming motion. When this sound/activity has gone around the circle, they rub their palms again, and then snap their fingers for the last round. When done correctly this really does sound like a rain storm coming and then leaving.

During family therapy sessions it was obvious that each child required slightly different behavioral interventions. Claudia and Cindy, Ms. Heart's biological daughters, had a hard time understanding why everybody needed to be treated a little differently and why everybody didn't have the same rules/punishments. In an effort to help Claudia and Cindy understand Kimberly's special needs (as well as Lupe's and Laura's), it was first necessary to help them (and Kimberly) understand the effects of trauma. So, one day while Lupe and Laura were visiting a biological aunt, Ms. Heart, Kimberly, Claudia, Cindy, and I sat down to discuss it.

I read out loud the *Diagnostic and Statistical Manual of Mental Disorders* (American Psychiatric Association, 1994) diagnostic criteria of posttraumatic stress disorder, interjecting examples of Kimberly's behavior. As I did this everyone's eyes grew larger and their mouths opened. Kimberly even said "Hey, that's me!" This helped Kimberly and her family understand the nature of trauma and the effects that it has on those who experience it. It gave them a way to understand and accept her behavior. There was subsequently less complaining about why Kimberly was treated differently or got a different punishment.

While all of the family interventions were somewhat effective in improving communication and interaction in the family, they were not effective in mediating the symptoms of each individual. Four of the six children in the family were also receiving individual therapy. Because their needs were so great, however, especially for a single mother, the family failed to stabilize as the treatment team had hoped.

It was eventually decided to remove Laura and Lupe from Ms. Heart's home and place them with their maternal aunt. The removal of Laura and Lupe was particularly helpful to Kimberly in reducing the intensity and frequency of cues that were upsetting to her. Each time Lupe had experienced a psychotic episode involving her father, Kimberly had been reminded of her own father and of her own traumatic history.

Kimberly also felt less threatened and more secure in her adoptive home when Laura and Lupe were placed elsewhere. Confronted with yet another loss, however, Kimberly became even more creative in some of her avoidance strategies. Shirley Temple was on stage again. When I tried to discuss how Kimberly felt about Laura and Lupe leaving, she asked me if she could show me a new song and dance she learned in school.

Kimberly's avoidance behaviors were effective in reducing her anxiety and were thus reinforcing. Although Kimberly's defense mechanisms were maladaptive in regards to long term solutions, they brought her temporary and almost instant relief. Kimberly's "Shirley Temple" defense helped her move away from both physically and psychologically distressing cues, served to reduce tension, and offset her anxious feelings. As she improved, Kimberly's problem behaviors such as anger, avoidance, and agitation occurred most often when she was caught off guard, when there was no time for her to implement healthier tension reduction behaviors.

One day while discussing Kimberly's behavior with her and Ms. Heart, Ms. Heart described an incident in which she said, "Kimberly was screaming bloody murder." Kimberly suddenly began crying. She desperately and emphatically pleaded "I wasn't screaming bloody murder!" Almost as suddenly as Kimberly had reacted, I realized that she was responding to the phraseology and not the complaint. Kimberly had seen her mother stab her aunt in a bloody scene. The words bloody murder had been a cue which was generalized from what was simply an idiom to an emotionally distressing event. I quickly explained to Kimberly that what her mother had meant was simply that she had been screaming very loudly and uncontrollably. The moral of this story is "be careful what you say!"

Much work has been done with Kimberly in helping her to recognize and label her feelings. It is still often necessary to explore affective issues at a distance. This is accomplished with the use of multiple distractions and therapeutic aids, such as symbolic play with Barbies, physical activity, writing, and drawing.

After working together for about a year, Kimberly and I began working on a picture book and story of her life. Ms. Heart had been given several packages of pictures by a girlfriend of Kimberly's biological father. We used these pictures to make a diary of Kimberly's early life. This resulted in fairly dramatic revelations by Kimberly about her past. In some of the pictures Kimberly was a baby sleeping in the corner, on the floor, with beer cans visible everywhere. Adults partied around her. With the aid of the photographs she has been able to openly discuss past trauma and painful feelings. More importantly perhaps is that she is also developing the ability to say "I don't think I can talk about this today," identify when she is avoiding things, and calm herself when she becomes overwhelmed. By exploring affective issues with a distracter or through another medium, Kimberly is able to process her traumatic history and then rehearse learned coping strategies as she discusses it.

Kimberly's biological father is serving an extended prison sentence. Prior to the adoption, he voluntarily terminated his parental rights. He continues to write to Kimberly, however, and occasionally calls her. Her biological mother, still drinking, occasionally drives by Kimberly's adoptive home.

Ms. Heart struggles with trying to protect Kimberly, respecting her needs, and recognizing that Kimberly has ambivalent feelings toward her biological parents. Recently, Kimberly has expressed fears of becoming like her biological parents. Last year, she would have beat up her brother and would have had no clue what was really bothering her rather than express these concerns. Kimberly can now identify and self-correct when she is using avoidance strategies and behaviors. She no longer runs to her room during difficult conversations.

Kimberly rarely has nightmares anymore and when Shirley Temple visits, it's to tease me and not to avoid talking about a difficult issue. Kimberly still often feels more comfortable discussing sensitive issues with Ms. Heart present. This is significant in that Kimberly has been able to develop trust as well as a secure attachment to her adoptive mother.

Almost all my work with Kimberly took place in the family home. Home-based therapy had originally been requested due to Ms. Heart's difficulty in transporting the children to the office. To date, I strongly believe that home-based therapy has been a key to Kimberly's fairly dramatic improvement. Kimberly is now comfortable enough, however, to come to my office once a week. I continue to meet with her in her home once a week as well.

Kimberly always wanted to please me and was hesitant to discuss anything that she feared might put her in a bad light. Often when I came into the home, other children or Kimberly's foster mother brought up problems the family was having, particularly when they involved Kimberly. Despite these discussions, Kimberly felt safe at home and especially safe in her room where we often ended up. Home-based therapy, however, came with its own set of problems. The home being as chaotic as it was, it was often necessary to attend to a multitude of problematic family dynamics when I was present. Kimberly often made it very difficult for me to leave (i.e., hiding my keys, shoes, etc.). There was often a multitude of distractions and more than once I was late for my next appointment.

Overall, the safety and richness of the environment in Kimberly's home made home-based therapy a key element in her treatment. She is blossoming in a warm, caring and supportive family. Thanks to her adoption case worker, her adoptive mother, and a dedicated treatment team, Kimberly is growing up in a family who puts her first. Three years ago Kimberly was given a poor prognosis. Today Kimberly is beating the odds.

REFERENCE

American Psychiatric Association. (1994). *Diagnostic and statistical manual of mental disorders* (4th ed.). Washington, DC: American Psychiatric Press.

Sanity Recovered

David Stark

David Stark has written a moving description of his experience with mental illness and of his attempts to make sense of the world. Especially helpful are the poignant and humorous stories of his evolving relationship with his therapist. At first he idealized both his therapist and the program and expected the magic of a cure. But over time he strengthened his ability to see the world around him, including his therapist, more clearly. He was able to make use of the therapeutic relationship to become more independent and gain increasing confidence in his own decisions.

His description of his rediscovery of both his therapist and himself is a testimony to his own honest courage. It also demonstrates the benefits of home-based therapy, even imperfect therapy without the promise of a cure, to people struggling with severe mental illness.

I would like to step back to November of 1993, the month in which my Windhorse treatment began. I was living in an apartment in my parents' home, shared by a housemate who was trying to impose her views on me about everything from religion to romance. I was overmedicated on Haldol (and antidepressants with unpleasant side effects), sleeping past noon and dreading the day because it illustrated the tremendous chasm between the condition of my life and the life I had hoped for and failed to attain. Simply, I lacked the skills, health, and personal resources necessary to make my own decisions and adjust my life conditions in a constructive fashion.

My professional supports consisted of a psychiatrist 50 miles away, a psychotherapist in town, and an orthomolecular clinic 200 miles away. While each of these treatments had its own merits, I was unable to attempt and sustain employment, to separate from my parents or enlist their participation in my recovery without undergoing criticism, to find a community of friends that was mature, healthy, and able to foster my own recovery, and to approach mental health care with inside information and outside support so that I would not be so naïve or vulnerable in facing my providers.

My treatments were all localized in offices. None of my providers visited my home; nor did I visit theirs. I sat on a chair or a couch, directly facing a provider in an opposite chair and recited my soliloquy of life events, current calamities, historical handicaps, and planned projects. The recitations left me fatigued, hungry, and with a sense that speech itself enacted a process of self-violation. The dosages of medicine rose and fell with the tides of my discourse, but usually increased. I learned gradually, through a circular, destabilizing process of physical discomfort, hour-long sessions of monotonous self-disclosure, anger, guilt, dread, dependency, and despair how to become a mental patient.

My life revolved around the taking of medication and the making of appointments. To soothe the sickness and satiate the soul, there was food. I was in every restaurant within a 20-mile radius of home, looking not just for nourishment, but for a sense of belonging, of economic participation, of having my needs met on demand, and of confronting the strangers who brought such fear and fascination to my fantasy life. I had learned to position myself as a consumer before I knew that term had psychological currency. So I journeyed from home to office to restaurant in a perpetual cycle of confusion and frustration, finding supernatural significance in random, trivial encounters and imbuing every moment and movement with more meaning than it merited. I had, quite simply, no perspective—on illness, on health, or on myself.

Then one day my mother read an article in the local newspaper about Windhorse. The article said that a new mental health organization with considerable success in treating psychosis had begun operating in Northampton. Windhorse aimed to restore a person's physical, social, psychological, and spiritual connections and balances within a sane environment—a milieu of compassion extended by a team of trained healers. About a week later, we were both in the small Windhorse office meeting Jeff Fortuna, Executive Director, and Eric Chapin, Assistant Director. They explained that Eric had just arrived from Boulder, Colorado and was available to see clients. Jeff seemed to me more sensitive, quieter, and somehow more representative of a typical therapist. Eric seemed boisterous, and I feared him a little because of his size and manner. It was decided, however, that I would work with Eric. Although I found them both to have slightly odd personalities (as if I myself were anything near normal), what I was mostly puzzled by was the name "Windhorse." They explained that "Windhorse" was the name of a legendary creature famous throughout Central Asia for its capacity to give people strength in healing illness or overcoming depression. The horse energy expresses power and the wind energy lifts people up; the symbol conveys discipline as well.

On my first shift with Eric, he asked me if there was any place that I wanted to go or anything that I needed to do. The only place I could think of visiting was a scenic overlook on the side of the interstate highway several miles south of Northampton. I had driven past it many times, but had never stopped because I felt uncomfortable doing so alone. Eric had no qualms about heading for the site or stepping out from the car onto the earth with cars whizzing by, a slippery slope ahead, a view of the vast unknown beyond, and strangers straggling astride the embankment.

We stood there together—or I should say, I stood and he crouched. Dressed in rugged men's work overalls (Eric was the first therapist I had ever met who dressed like a ranch hand), Eric knelt down to the ground on his haunches, as an aboriginal tribesman might. He explained that he had learned this posture while living in Saudi Arabia as a youth and communing with the Bedouins. I was uncomfortable socially, yet Eric didn't seem to notice. He just started to talk—about life, his own life, the earth, mind, and spirit. He didn't say all that much, yet he seemed to believe what he said (though I tended to doubt some of it), and seemed to know that he had arrived at some understanding of human existence that suited his purposes rather well. I had a burning question which I then posed to Eric: "Why do people do what they do?"

Years of unsuccessful living had etched the question into my consciousness. Why do I do what I do . . . why does anybody do what he or she does—because they want to, have to, are allowed to? My experience of life had so deteriorated from my youthful hoping and coping into a sickly moping and groping; my memories of prior joys so transfigured into patterns of purposeless pain; my habituation into the role of mental patient so engrained and debilitating . . . that I was emblazoned with a senseless anger, a haughty hostility, a de facto dependency, and a dangerous tendency toward self-destruction. I could scarcely fathom what or why anyone else on the planet did, what they thought or felt about their own situation and the larger human condition.

Eric seemed to respect the question and enjoyed contemplating its indefinite possibilities. In this brief, brave, benign meeting between our two minds, we found the seed of a friendship. The psychologist in overalls whose overall concern was to achieve peace of mind for himself and others and the mental patient who had lost pieces of his mind through illness, dormancy, and senseless judgment formed a link based on shared interest in understanding the mind and the world it inhabits and mutual concern in improving my health.

So I was relieved, startled, and simply seduced by Eric's calm and nurturing nature. For all of my universal questions about the human condition now had an objective reference in the person of Eric: Who was Eric? Why did he do what he did? What did he intend toward me and toward himself and others? Would he please or disappoint, cajole or control, speak truth or misinformation, help or hurt? When it was time for the shift to end and Eric suggested we meet again later in the week, I felt the joy of newfound friendship, the fear of the unknown, the responsibility of committing myself to this relationship and its requisite tasks, and the hope of having a hold on a useful truth, a higher level of health, and a wholeness of being.

Eric and I soon fell into the habit of two 3-hour shifts per week. On each shift, we would first go to the Northampton YMCA for a brisk swim in the big, cold pool, shower, and change clothes, then drive to a Mexican restaurant for two bean tostadas each and glasses of water. We ate Mexican food because it was inexpensive, mostly vegetarian, familiar to us both as former Texans, and the restaurant provided a quiet but open atmosphere for us to converse. The meals became rather festive, and we alternated buying a basket of totopos chips for the two of us to share.

Eric told stories about his life and asked me questions about mine. His stories were colorful and genuine, painful and promising. He had survived most of the things I had spent my life fearing and avoiding: separation from family, beatings, economic stress, short jail sentences, cigarettes, alcohol, car accidents, injuries, and sexual antics. Yet he seemed so placid about it all. Perhaps this was because he trusted his body: his size and strength, his like for physical labor, and his "grounded" connection to the earth. He clearly also trusted his mind; his anger was more than manageable, his fears all but dissolved, his love of humanity abundant, his spirituality meditative, and his psychology contemplative.

Faced with such a formidable friend, I could not help but hold him up to the heights of heroism. He had faced the world, found a place, and endured. Through sheer force of energy, will and grit, he had survived and prospered. Here was a therapist not of credentials but of essentials. He was schooled in the streets and in the school of hard knocks, so as a therapist he offered not merely insight but determination and the method to do right. Eric's speech, sensitivity, strength, and stamina gave him a sometimes magical aura. He seemed to care about things that I cared about and to not care about things not worth caring about. In short, he offered a compassionate alternative to the set of rules, feelings, and beliefs I had acquired about my own life and the lives of others. The not yet apparent difficulties with this scenario were that I believed our speech itself would have a magical healing power, that I expected he would overlook no detail in my recovery, and that I assumed the relationship would endure eternally.

SCHEDULE

Early in treatment, Eric began discussing the importance of schedule. He alluded to it while explaining the significance of a 3-hour shift (sufficient time for dinner and a movie), in asking about the timing and sequence of my activities throughout the day and week (from biological processes to social activities to work and leisure) and in philosophical preachings on how best to utilize one's time. He seemed genuinely curious about what I was doing when, in order not simply to raise my consciousness about my activity level and my potential, but to inculcate an awareness of the reactions connecting events and of the sense of structure, discipline, and spirituality resulting from a well-ordered life. As I have since read, one consequence of schizophrenic-type illness is impairment in the ability to judge the passage of time, with attendant limitations such as procrastination. I think Eric was trying to demonstrate that I could counter this debilitating tendency by making my use of time explicit.

One day Eric brought a written schedule to my home: one sheet of paper with spaces indicated for the days of the week and three time slots per day—morning, afternoon, and evening. He inquired about the upcoming week and wrote my responses in brief form on the schedule paper. I felt honored that he found my life's events worthy of transcribing, indulged by his attendance to my needs, concerned that it might or might not happen again, reluctant to comply with a formality I had previously not needed, puzzled as to the source of Eric's abiding wisdom, and uncertain as to the meaning of it all.

Eric then suggested I buy an appointment calendar to keep all my upcoming events organized. As I barely had but a few events per week to remember. I thought this too would be a superfluous waste. I relented and purchased the date book. My overwhelming sentiment was that the purchase signified a transition from non-conventional methods of organizing my life toward use of mainstream materials. It further signified that I need not rely exclusively on my own mental resources to remember my life's business but could enlist supplemental help. I needn't do things the hard way. This simple suggestion illustrated that

Windhorse had techniques for simplifying and structuring my life that might be obvious to the healthy person but forgotten by the sickly.

MIND–BODY SYNCHRONIZATION

Eric and Jeff explained to me that I needed a mind–body synchronization practice and that rigorous exercise would fill this need. The goal of the practice was to make the mind and the body establish unifying patterns and rhythms for a sustained period, relieve the mind from its incessant burden of psychotic thinking, and animate and liberate the body from its psychotropic medicine yoke and medicinal side effects. Eric suggested that we swim at the YMCA, an activity he gravitated toward. I consented because I had enjoyed the sport as a lifeguard and instructor in my teens. I had not swum much in the preceding five years, however, due to the neuro-muscular side effects of medicine, had avoided health clubs out of anti-social tendencies, and minimized exercise in general due to fatigue. Eric seemed convinced that we were doing the right thing and persuaded me to purchase a 1-year membership at the YMCA rather than rely on chance occasional visits. He was enthusiastic and spoke glowingly about the value of what we were doing. I naturally assumed that Windhorse had discovered a miraculous "swimming cure."

Eric and I swam together for several months and I began to notice several things: (a) Eric enjoyed the swimming more than I did, (b) I enjoyed talking to Eric and eating with him more than swimming with him, (c) several months of swimming had not cured my illness, and (d) I was under Eric's sway and needed to rebel and assert my wishes. I mentioned to Eric's wife, Janelli, at a course we were both taking at Windhorse that I was "kind of sick of doing what Eric wanted to do." She responded: "Yeah. So am I." This affirmation gave me the courage to ask Eric if we could do other things together or just talk, as I had become somewhat enchanted with our conversations. Eric said that would be fine; all I needed to do was ask. This sequence of events created in me an awareness that Windhorse treatment was not written in stone, that the model as presented to me might have shortcomings or lack efficacy, and that at some level, I had autonomy and could request improvements in my treatment interventions.

If Windhorse didn't offer a miraculous swimming cure and was partly determined by the exercise of my preferences and was not immutable, then just what exactly was it? Was I right or wrong to try to shape my treatment? Would my healers encourage it or resent it? Would they inform me of the implications and consequences of these decisions?

Was my assertiveness a mature expression of autonomy that signified new found friendship with myself or a childish rebelliousness that would make me my own enemy?

PSYCHOSOCIAL TECHNIQUES

Eric and Jeff employed a variety of techniques to get me to verbalize and transcend those elements of my personal history that thwarted my emotional development. First among these was the genogram. The genogram was simply a diagram of my family tree on a large sheet of paper. Eric himself inscribed most of it after questioning me extensively to identify all the members of my extended family, their relationships between each other, and their brief biographies. I was fascinated by the notion of the genogram. It seemed to capture and express so much of who I was. I had been born into a particular family. I had learned its rules, beliefs, attitudes, customs, preferences, feelings, strategies, suffering, and so much more. To give voice to this familial context of my psychological inheritance was to express something essential to my identity and elemental to my character.

Furthermore, to tell this grand plan of the family inside a man to my caretakers, Eric and Jeff, in a formal team meeting was to link the family dynamic to the therapeutic context and, consequently, to the wider society and world. I couldn't believe two strangers could generate that much interest and enthusiasm in knowing about another person's relatives. It demonstrated that Windhorse had specific, psychosocial tools that I had not previously encountered and that attracted my fascination, that I would enjoy using and ultimately find helpful and healing.

The second technique Eric employed to get me beyond my past and toward living in the present world was "processing." In this approach, Eric would simply get me to start talking about my past and, when I broached a painful topic, he would simply face it calmly and squarely, with curiosity and interest, briefly frame it in the language of transpersonal psychology or Buddhist thought, then suggest that I simply "let go" of the whole package as it no longer had any authority to rule my life but was merely a drama or "storyline." It was, in effect, no longer real. As Eric had told stories from his past to me, I began to recite stories to Eric—in restaurants, on park benches, in my home. No matter the story, he seemed able to cast it in an acceptable light. When I told of trying to hurt myself but recanting, he said, "Well, there are the thinkers and the doers." When I told of how my mother's words had humiliated me, he said, "How unskillful of her." When I described the intensity of emotion in my family and the patterns of conflict typically aroused, he said, "Can you imagine trying to bring this down one class level?" (in other words, what might these explosive energies have engendered in a family of less financial means?)

Eric was concerned not simply that I articulate these stories. He wanted me to transcend them by letting them go. He knew people whose lives consisted of little more than futile and endless self-psychoanalyzing—rehashing the past verbally and thus condemning themselves to live within it. He wanted me to be out of the whole syndrome, free and clear. He did, however, feel that it was important to achieve internal clarity about one's feelings and experiences in order to be able to live happily in the present. He himself had spent three years in therapy and shared insights not simply of his own recovery but of his therapists' and teachers' teachings about the process of recovery.

One of these insights was the need to summon total compassion for oneself. In order to fully recover, Eric said, I shouldn't continue to judge or suppress unpleasant emotions or shut down my compassionate responses, but should open my heart fully and with total compassion for myself and all beings. I should forgive others and myself, help others and myself, trust others and myself, know others and myself. It would take time to learn, but to become happy, or even recovered, would require, in Eric's view, cultivating tremendous self-acceptance. I was of course very relieved to hear these words. They gave me permission to continue on this path of recovery as long as necessary and to continue hoping that my quality of emotional life would improve and the future would be brighter and healthier. At the same time, however, Eric seemed a little judgmental of certain of my lifestyle choices—such as how much to work, whether or not to live at home, on what to spend money—and I had to reconcile these criticisms with his compassionate character and philosophy.

The third way in which Eric and Jeff assisted my psychosocial recovery was by providing a structure and focus that supported my venturing out into the community for recovery-promoting activities, such as support groups, workshops, alternative healers, and courses. Team meetings and family meetings provided opportunities for reflection and evaluation as well as scheduled points of reference in the life of my recovery. Eric and Jeff positioned themselves as mentors, friends, and healers who were assuming responsibility for keeping my recovery on track, my life in progress, and my support steady. With these resources in place, I felt the courage and drive to step out into the community to meet new people, learn what I could learn, attend to both daily business and unconventional projects, and see what this grand enterprise of living could be like in a new mode.

Specifically, I began attending the Starpoint Clubhouse. For people with a diagnosis of major mental illness, it offered an alternative community of volunteer activities, support groups, and informal classes. The focus was on health, cooperation and civility, empowerment, and recovery. I joined an eating disorders workshop for two 10-week periods and learned much about the connection between food and feelings. I attended several workshops in "transformational breath" and a workshop in "shadow work." I continued my participation in a class in the Alexander technique and supplemented it with a brief course in Tai Chi. I attended an ongoing writer's workshop and a several session workshop in writing about "My True Self." I continued writing poetry.

These diverse activities, many of them unconventional and certainly unprecedented in my own life, might seem digressive from or peripheral to life's main concerns (such as employment) but, in my case, were both necessary and extremely helpful. They enabled me to attain a sense of physical recuperation, mental awareness, and the possibility of these two realms achieving balance and harmony. These few years of feeding my mind and body with anything that might possibly encourage me to resonate with a healthier vibration internally and externally were an essential journey that I sought, sensed, secured, and subscribed to. It supplemented my Windhorse treatment and soothed my soul. These programs would not have been nearly as accessible without my ongoing Windhorse treatment to mold, manage, and make them materialize meaningfully. My only regrets are that, at times, the Windhorse treatment seemed at odds with what I was learning elsewhere; at times Eric and Jeff did not seem to regard these supplemental treatments as highly as I did and, in time, the Windhorse treatment itself gradually withdrew, thus forcing me to straighten out a large portion of the resulting confusion by myself or elsewhere.

COMMUNITY

The Windhorse community consists of clients and their families, and staff and their families. These members gather approximately once a month for parties in people's homes to celebrate housewarmings, holidays, Windhorse occasions, graduations, and goodbyes. Most of the parties are potluck, with offerings arranged by telephone, sign-up sheet, or alphabetical guidelines. The parties tend to be festive, calm, and harmonious—unlike college beer parties or stuffy status-seeking events. Children are welcome, and often there are speeches, toasts, or performances. Other ongoing community events include a hiking group, gardening project, staff meetings, a course in the skills of recovery, book readings, guest speakers, theater project, client newsletter, retreats, and an assortment of ad hoc groups that meet briefly around a variety of issues.

The Windhorse community is welcoming, accepting, educated, mindful, reflective, caring, and not a cult. It consists of surprisingly functional families; its members include both children and seniors. This community will treat anybody, no matter how ill or atypical, with dignity and respect. All persons are treated like persons, not patients. I find this community to be far more accepting than the local community (where I experienced some social mishaps), and far warmer than its New England locale might suggest. Working relationships and friendships between men and women are surprisingly harmonious, based on mutual like and respect, and rarely sexist. Indeed, my connection to the women of Windhorse has helped me to overcome many misogynistic attitudes. There is a special quality of closeness at Windhorse because people help each other. Client insight is valued and to be a client is a respectable role.

As my involvement at Windhorse continued, a chief benefit was having somewhere to go, to show up and be noticed, so that I would actually get on foot and into the car, be in motion and face the world—at times with a joyful optimism and pride that I could actually be doing something that I enjoyed and was good at, was learning from, and felt surrounded by people for whom I cared. My experience of community, on a fundamental level, consists just of people expressing an interest in me, and me expressing an interest in other people. In these elemental exchanges, however, remarkable transformations can occur over time. Fear, anxiety, and worry can be reduced, loneliness and alienation prevented, bad attitudes and hopelessness corrected, bitterness and hostility abandoned, apathy and irritability untied, low self-esteem lifted, and behavioral problems averted. Who wouldn't benefit from such a closing of Pandora's box?

EMPLOYMENT

In the few years prior to my Windhorse treatment, I had been relieved of duties as a teaching assistant in a graduate program at a major university, following academic incompletes and a growing gulf between me and my colleagues and students. After moving back across the country to be with my parents, I found part-time work as a Sunday school teacher, but was unable to contain the unruly students. I worked part-time on the telephone in a market research firm, but failed to complete a sufficient number of calls. I tried door-to-door soliciting for an environmental organization, but was promptly fired after failing to bring in enough cash. My experiences of work were disappointing and demoralizing, degrading and destructive. The world it seemed did not want to let me earn a living or even participate. I began to loathe the very notion that I would ever return to work, preferring to hibernate at home and venture out only to eat.

Half a year after my Windhorse treatment began, I felt sufficiently revitalized and hopeful to seek another job. I knew that I could not work full-time, could not handle stress, would have difficulty relating to employers and colleagues, and was not likely to obtain and maintain employment in any event. As luck would have it, I went to the Starpoint Clubhouse one day to pursue job leads. That very evening they were interviewing for part-time positions as telephone counselors in a program funded by the Department of Mental Health and a DMH consumer initiative grant. The confidential, noncrisis telephone support service was staffed and managed by recovering consumers. I applied and was hired, perhaps in part because the supervisor was a classmate of mine at the skills-of-recovery course being taught at Windhorse. Not only that, the local newspaper interviewed the new hires and took photographs that were published the following day. I had risen from sick and cruel obscurity to quick and cool celebrity in 24 hours. More important, I had secured a position where my illness was regarded as an asset, not a liability; I had entered a job environment where my needs would be not only respected but also rehabilitated; I had joined a community that would provide collegiality and companionship.

This warmline job provided many occasions for fun and learning as well as a focus on the more serious issues facing many people. It brought me into the world in a new capacity—that of healer and server—and helped to rekindle my interest in psychology which I had not studied since college. Finally, it was simply a leg up, a step toward the adult world of responsibility, and a foundation from which to continue this tremendous process of healing, growth, and awareness.

TERMINATION

Although Windhorse made a pivotal contribution to my recovery through support, education, and community, in some ways it fell short of my expectations. After I had been seeing Eric for a brief period, Windhorse began acquiring other clients. My schedule with Eric had to be rearranged to accommodate his new demands, and he even suggested that I consider seeing a different Windhorse therapist. This indicated to me that, on some level, Eric did not really enjoy or was not fully committed to working with me. The Windhorse image of ideal, perfect treatment generating dramatic, unprecedented outcomes, soon began to fade in my mind.

Eric's will was monumental at times, and I kept trying to maneuver myself around and within it in such a way that it might diminish, and its impact on me recede. But I was unable to attain this feat within the treatment period. Toward the end of treatment, Eric remarked to Jeff in a team meeting that he felt the only thing I might still need would be to return to the YMCA for more swimming, but that he didn't want to be the one to force me to go. It seemed that his huge will, to which I had become so accustomed, was thus withdrawing from my life, yet I had not been able to resolve my feelings about it. I concluded that Eric's will existed primarily in the service of his own wishes.

As treatment began to withdraw, Eric himself reduced the number of contact hours between us, virtually without my consent. He kept telling me that I did not require any more treatment, that I was, in effect, sane though extremely neurotic. Eric harbored a view that psychiatric patients might have no greater ongoing need for psychotherapy than ordinary people do. (How to reconcile this with his no medication, no vitamins, etc. approach is a problem—just what exactly do mental patients need in Eric's view, a shrine and a cushion?). I had become so accustomed to facing life with him—though this relationship was far from perfect—that I did not see how I could face life without him. And then, on one of our final shifts, when I asked Eric what my next step could be, he counseled that since I had spent several years learning how to be a mental patient, it should take approximately the same amount of time to unlearn these roles and learn productive citizenship. I had followed Eric's tutelage for a few years, paying close attention to everything he said, in the hopes that he would say those things that would enable me to overcome my illness. And now, at the close of the treatment, he was telling me that those 2 years themselves would have to be unlearned, on my own, in order for me to become well. What in the hell was going on?

After a year and a half of working at the warmline, I left, exhausted from the continual focus on people's suffering. Shortly thereafter, I graduated from Windhorse. To graduate from Windhorse is to cease formal treatment, though one might still receive "aftercare" and certainly everyone is invited to maintain affiliation with the community. Graduating is regarded with some pride, as it indicates that, in principle, a client has learned a great deal, overcome many obstacles, and has the means by which to advance his or her own life. While graduation is usually a joint client–team decision, in my case it was precipitated by Eric telling Jeff that he had taught me everything he knew about recovery.

Since there was no relevant material remaining to be taught, there was no reason for me to continue treatment.

Needless to say, the ending of my treatment, with its implication that wondrous Windhorse had served me well (presumably any remaining psychological difficulties were entirely my fault and responsibility, not theirs) and that I should sever myself from this community I had never fully belonged to provoked a long period of suicidality. I felt not only abandoned but cheated. I had extended hope and trust that had, at times, been met with criticism, apathy, or evasiveness. Though my treatment had effectively turned my life in many new directions, I had not enjoyed it very much because there were too many unresolved questions and too many personalities whose proper role in my life I could not determine. Yet the bulk of the disillusion was having to face the fact that so much work on my health still needed to be done, and I did not know when, where, how, or if it would occur.

Fortunately, I changed psychiatrists (again) around the time of my graduating, and my new doctor took my suicidality seriously, reaching out to me by telephone, offering the hope of new medications, and somehow establishing in my mind that he was genuinely on my side. It was a new start with a therapist whose gentle, mild, protective approach contrasted greatly with Eric's. A year later, I began orthomolecular treatment at a clinic near New York and started to learn an entirely different way of approaching mental health and treatment.

WINDHORSE LITERATURE

The Windhorse literature is already sizable and continues to grow; its centerpiece is *The Seduction of Madness,* by Dr. Edward Podvoll (1990). I will here focus on a few of the concepts appearing in the literature, and try to illustrate their applicability to my case. To me, much of the Windhorse literature has a peculiar quality of being recognizably true, yet difficult to invent; its authors have made simple and at times obvious observations on complicated and abstract matters in language that is both surprisingly concrete and illustratively metaphorical. It expresses generalizations and universalisms that do not discredit the authenticity of individual experience.

The inclusion of the Windhorse literature into treatment gives it a certain pedagogical quality. Through taking courses, such as the "Skills of Recovery," clients are expected to understand and appreciate these concepts and apply them to their own lives when needed. The writings are canonical; they are quoted and discussed, consulted, and disseminated. This scholarly emphasis in treatment has both positive and negative consequences. When one begins treatment, typically rational thought is at a low ebb, and sensation and feeling are suppressed. It is therefore difficult to concentrate on or understand new ideas, so making any meaningful connection with the literature is unlikely. The benefit to a tutorial approach is that, just as many clients may lack the inclination to study the abstruse, so too they may need to be informed of the obvious. In my own case, by gradually accumulating obvious information about ordinary matters that I somehow lacked, I was able to teach myself how to feel healthier and behave more constructively.

Dr. Podvoll (1990) identifies the "psychotic predicament" and the resulting "stages of psychotic transformation." The predicament itself occurs when personal character meets the force of circumstance; someone faces a situation that he or she cannot resolve with his/her own resources and is not willing to adapt. A battle within the self ensues that echoes this outer conflict. With groundlessness, switching out, loss of doubt and self-surrender, and wild identification, the stage is set for psychotic transformation which includes speed of mind, desynchronization of mind and body, absorption states, insight and power, thinking or acting beyond the law, conflicting commands, and death and rebirth. While such stages may seem too abstract or symbolic to capture someone's actual experience, I feel that they are more than mere metaphors; they have a factual basis in my own psychological phenomena. The stages of transformation I experienced occurred while I was a graduate student on the west coast and began a decline from harmony and connection toward total alienation and withdrawal.

The stages of transformation can and should be unwound if one is properly supported in a therapeutic milieu. I cannot imagine how I ever could have accomplished this lengthy and laborious task of restoration without the Windhorse community. Physically, I needed to learn to hold my head up, to breathe, and to guard, not risk my physical safety. Emotionally, I needed to choose feeling over not feeling, compassion over hostility, and kindness over contempt. Socially, I needed to choose independence over dependence, peace with authority over rebelliousness. Intellectually, I needed to choose awareness over ignorance. Every one of these choices needed to be considered and contemplated, tried and applied, sustained and ingrained.

Constance Packard, MSW, a long-time Windhorse board member and the mother of a former client, has written a set of guidelines for family members to help them face the challenge of caring for an ill relative without disrupting their own lives (1993). The five guidelines she articulates are: (a) cultivate an attitude of acceptance and respect; (b) choose happiness as an orientation; (c) set limits and boundaries; give space; (d) show full expression and appreciation; be honest; and (e) find community in the social environment. My own parents read this document. Its effect on them, and subsequently on me, was profound. My parents started treating me with more awareness, compassion, and sensitivity. They become more able to support and encourage me. The intensity of their emotions toward me reduced, and a more calm nurturing manner of engaging me arose. I began to see them as less threatening and fearful. In short, my parents became in some way my healers, or at least became more apparent as allies in the struggle I faced.

Perhaps an example would illustrate these developments. My father has a side that can be angry and cynical. If my father showed this side in my presence, I could conclude either that he was angry at me, in which case I became fearful, or that he was angry at something else in the world and I should share his sentiment. In either case, I internalized some anger. After reading Connie's guidelines, my father began to show me a more compassionate side. I then conclude that he is neither angry with me nor with anything else in the world, so there is no need for me to be angry or fearful. I begin to feel more joyful, to release old baggage, and my recovery grows in leaps and bounds.

Clearly, there is much information clients and their families need to acquire in the course of treatment, whether through therapy itself or reading materials or attending seminars. Not all of this information will be useful at the time it is acquired. Some may seem tangential, odd, or mistaken. What seems silly or digressive today, however, might have great use tomorrow after one has made a step in a new direction or resolved some intermediate difficulty. Having a body of literature to consult with open-minded critical awareness can be a liberating and comforting adjunct to the therapeutic process. It may even prove easier to tolerate than actual interventions in which personalities must play an important role.

CONCLUSIONS

About $1\frac{1}{2}$ years ago, Windhorse staff approached me and asked me to consider joining their board of directors. Here was the opportunity I had been waiting for. It would be intellectually challenging yet avoid the dangers of senseless intellectualizing. It would use my business skills, yet toward a socially valuable end. It would expand my world socially, yet safely and soundly. It would allow me to give much back to the community that had given me so much, yet without sacrificing personal needs or compromising political purposes. It was fitting and fantastic; I felt uniquely honored.

I have served on the Windhorse board for over 1 year, learning about how a small nonprofit organization handles its business matters and how a cohort of conscientious clinicians evaluate services to clients. I have written and spoken at the meetings about many topics that strike chords in me and enjoy articulating my personal experience. I have become, at long last, an insider in a small world I understand and appreciate, free of the painful pressures and senseless strivings that prompted my original descent into the morass of madness a decade ago. Today, I still visit restaurants and therapists, and enjoy monologues, meals, and meandering. I do so, however, with comfort and awareness, knowing that if I open my heart, people might embrace me, yet we will each continue to lead independent lives. If I open my mind, I will find its contents not too horrific to bear. A journey out into the world has become not a trip of alienation and defiance, but of integration and self-reliance.

I learned many obvious but important truths about the human condition and my own situation from Eric and others. I learned that I had a body and that this body had both needs and wisdom that could, would, and should override my mental attempts to dominate it. This body requires not simply nourishment, but exercise and hygiene.

I needed to be told that I had an obsession about food. Food had become so important in my life that it defined many of my choices (Where to eat? What to eat?) and limited my availability for other realms of activity. When choosing between dinner and a movie, I always chose the dinner. When trying to live on a budget, I did not know how to economize on food. Between meals, most thoughts were about food. Eric's strategy for addressing this tendency was to "cut through" my excessive appetites by suggesting that we take a walk or have a talk before dining so that I might relieve the emotion that was fueling the appetite before trying to feed the appetite. This was not only a reasonable and helpful approach, it inculcated an awareness that perhaps the force of many emotions could be mitigated by releasing their energy during a period of waiting. In any event, it was a safe strategy for striving toward health.

I needed to learn that I could and should live within my means. I had always depended financially on my parents. I knew very little about how to spend, save, or invest on my own. Eric told me stories about how he had been forced into financial independence at the age of 18, how he had lived in a trailer in graduate school, and how he and his wife watched their spending "like a hawk." When Eric and I went on shifts together, I watched how he watched his money. He ordered food carefully, noting the price. He gravitated toward thrift shops and secondhand stores. Although I had perhaps briefly entered one or two thrift

shops in my life, I was now exposed to and instructed in the art of buying from every thrift shop in the region on a regular basis. Eric took me
shopping for clothes at Army Navy stores. He told me about local auc-
tions. He encouraged me to subscribe to a frugality newsletter. When I
asked his opinion about whether to enroll in a 3-day workshop in
group psychological and symbolic healing, he said it was mostly a
question of money—whether I had the tuition and didn't mind losing it
for a novel experience. Yet, when Eric lost a $100 deposit for an item
he was unable to purchase, he seemed unusually calm about the
occurrence. "Oh well," he said, "there it goes."

The result of all of this consciousness-raising about money was that
I began to think more economically and weigh purchases more carefully.
If one could live on very little money, then why spend a lot of money? If
most other people were budgeting and economizing, then why could-
n't I budget and economize? If money would always have to be a part
of my life, then why shouldn't I start paying some serious attention to
how to make it, save it, spend it, or invest it? An understanding and
experience of money could further my mind and perhaps shift my
struggle away from madness. If I understood the game of living in a
monetary society, then perhaps I could learn to play it and even enjoy it.

I needed to be told that I should try to differentiate myself emotionally from my parents. Differentiation can be a puzzling concept and
requires both skill and health to learn. Initially, I assumed that I should
simply avoid my parents in order to establish myself as different from
them. This went on for some time, leading to a feeling of estrangement
that seemed to benefit no one. It left me alone much of the time, and at
times facing difficult situations with just my own resources. I began
avoiding many people and situations out of a newfound habit, and the
conviction that at some level my avoidance was a prerequisite to
accomplishing the noble task of "differentiation." It was only after I
graduated that my parents came back more fully into my life, and it was
only after I changed neuroleptic medicines and resumed orthomolecular treatment that I found the strength and confidence to manage a
healthy process of differentiation. I also needed ongoing Windhorse
involvement, successful work experiences, and close friendship to
assist my goal of differentiation. Eric was absolutely right that much differentiation was needed, but many conditions were not in place at the
time to support it.

I also needed to be told that I needed community and how to live in
one. I had acquired many distorted and dysfunctional habits for social
relationships and saw community as something that I could not have
and did not understand, and so I resented or belittled it. Eric seemed to
prize the opportunity for having communal relationships and managed

them with considerable skill. I realized that community was something I might want and would need to learn how to have. I felt that community might provide a touchstone or an anchor that I had been woefully missing. Eric offered a number of guidelines, such as "What you tell one person isn't what you tell another." This discrepancy is not a form of dishonesty, but arises naturally as we stand in differing relationships to each other.

I needed to learn a better way to treat other people (including myself) with sensitivity, concern, and respect. I needed to see that no harm is done when one errs on the side of compassion. I needed to try to do good, be good, and feel good—to realize that I am a good person, or if not yet, I can become one. I needed to know that it feels better to have the genuine compassion, respect, and camaraderie of a small therapeutic community than to megalomaniacally seek the glory of recognition in the world theater. I needed to experience that life can get easier as you go along, but that you must first start somewhere to attack the inertia. I needed to realize that some people, and by extension maybe even many people, really do want what's best for me.

Affiliating with a mental health organization that cultivates a kind, compassionate whole person view of healing necessarily promotes changing one's world view and one's view of oneself. In its idealism and social values, the Windhorse culture opposes the cynical world view. It gives its members an opportunity to shed the bitter and bilious baggage of previous life experience in the outer world. Personally, I had in the course of my young life reached many convictions about the intentions of others that needed to be revised. Windhorse provided a safe and skillful setting in which to unlearn past prejudices and learn new ways of understanding and approaching the world.

REFERENCES

Packard, C. (1993). *Windhorse guide for families.* Unpublished manuscript.
Podvall, E. M. (1990). *The seduction of madness.* New York: HarperCollins.

In-Home Assessment and Counseling of the Elderly

Nancy Flowers

Nancy Flowers serves as ombudsman for residents of Evanston, Illinois who are in long-term care facilities. In that capacity she advocates for older adults and trains volunteers to provide visits to nursing-home and retirement-community residents. She spent several years developing and administering home-based programs for the elderly and was involved in geriatric rehabilitation programs at Rush-Presbyterian-St. Luke's Medical Center in Chicago. In the following chapter, Ms. Flowers provides a guide for assessing the needs of the elderly in their homes.

THE ARGUMENT FOR IN-HOME COUNSELING

It has been repeatedly documented that the elderly utilize fewer mental health services than other segments of the population (Buckwalter, 1988; Butler, Lewis, & Sunderland, 1991; Turner, 1992). There are a number of factors that affect the use of mental health services for the elderly. These include lack of identification or minimization of the significance of symptoms, minimization of the effectiveness of mental health treatment in the elderly, unwillingness to seek treatment, the cost of treatment, and inability to get to the treatment setting (Bumagin & Hirn, 1990). Elders may not wish to seek mental health services because of the false perception that depression is a normal part of aging. This is a perception that, unfortunately, many medical professionals, family members, and friends share. Elders may also be reluctant to seek or accept treatment due to the stigma that can be associated with mental health services, psychiatry, and the mentally ill. Cost and lack of transportation can adversely affect involvement in treatment as well. Fear or distrust of medications, mental health practitioners, and the possibility of psychiatric hospitalization are other factors that can affect an elder's willingness to accept psychiatric care.

Elders who are reluctant or unable to see a mental health practitioner in an office or clinic setting may be willing to see that same clinician in their home. It can be argued that the home is the ideal and most effective setting in which to assess and counsel elders and their families. An elder's home will tell a clinician a great deal about the elder's history and functional status and provide information about the elder and his or her relationships with others that he or she might not immediately share with the clinician in an office setting. If the clinician has been requested to evaluate an elder's capacity for independent living, an in-home evaluation will provide a much more accurate picture of the elder's functional capabilities than an in-office assessment would provide (Cohen, 1993).

GETTING IN THE DOOR

Many elders are understandably reluctant to allow a stranger access to their homes. If the elder was not the person who requested the clinician's involvement, an introduction or a referral from a person trusted by the elder may be needed to facilitate access to the elder's home. Phone contact should be made to establish the date and time of the interview, with a follow-up reminder call on the day of the interview. This is particularly important when working with elders who may have cognitive deficits. The clinician should wear a name badge with his or her name and the name of the agency clearly marked and easily legible from a short distance. The clinician should knock loudly on the door and allow sufficient time for the elder to reach the door. The clinician may need to ring the doorbell or knock several times; if the elder is hard of hearing, the clinician may need to call by telephone to alert the elder that the clinician is at the home (cellular phones are particularly useful when making home visits). If the elder seems reluctant to allow the clinician access to the home, sharing the name of the person who referred the elder may help to decrease any apprehension that the elder might be feeling. If the elder remains reluctant to allow entrance, the clinician may wish to return at another time, perhaps with a friend, relative, or another person trusted by the elder who could assist the clinician to gain access to the home.

OBTAINING CONSENT FOR CLINICAL INTERVENTIONS

The clinician should always remember that he or she is a guest in the elder's home. Any interventions or actions need to be made with the elder's permission or at the elder's direction. The clinician should ask for permission prior to walking through the home or moving anything within the home even if the clinician feels that these actions will increase the clinician's knowledge about the elder or enhance the elder's function. The purpose of the home visit should be clearly stated at the onset of the interview and intervention plans and goals clearly established with the elder prior to clinician intervention. As with any adult client, consent should be obtained from the elder prior to communication with family members, friends, medical professionals, or community agencies. The fact that the elder has advance directives and has designated an individual, or agent, to carry out these directives does not negate the elder's right to direct his or her care or the clinician's responsibility to establish the treatment plan with the elder. The clinician can only contact the agent with the permission of the elder, unless the elder has been determined by the clinician to be unable to give informed consent.

ASSESSING THE ELDER'S HOME ENVIRONMENT

Counseling an elder in the home enables the clinician to observe the elder within his or her surroundings and to assess the elder's ability to function within those surroundings. The clinician should observe the condition of the elder's physical environment including the presence of extensive clutter or garbage, infestations of bugs or rodents, undone household tasks such as dishes or laundry, spoiled food, and the odor of urine or feces. Other environmental observations to make include:

- Are there stairs to enter the home? Are there firm rails on the stairs?
- Are there clear pathways for the resident to maneuver in the house? Are pathways clear of electrical or telephone cords and throw rugs?
- Is there evidence of physical deterioration of the home including peeling paint, holes in the walls, loose tiles or torn carpeting?
- Is the home multilevel? If so, is there an accessible bathroom on each level of the home?
- Is there evidence of devices to enhance resident function such as a walker, cane, commode, or tub bench? What condition are these devices in? Do these items appear to be used by the resident?

- Are the refrigerated food items fresh?
- Is the household set up so that the elder can reach necessary items such as the telephone, food items, and cooking and eating utensils?
- Is the home adequately heated or cooled for the season? Is there evidence of a working furnace, air conditioners, or fans?
- Does the resident smoke? Is there evidence of cigarette burns on the furniture or carpeting?
- Does the resident abuse alcohol? Is there evidence of a quantity of empty wine or liquor bottles? The clinician needs to observe for the impact of alcohol abuse on the elder's function and not base an assessment of abuse solely on the presence of alcohol bottles in the home.
- If the resident uses a medication box, do the medications appear to have been taken for that day?
- Is there evidence of misuse of medications? Is there evidence of multiple or duplicative bottles of prescribed medications from multiple physicians? Are the medications expired?
- Is there evidence of street drug use in the home? Is there evidence of syringes in the home when the elder is not taking injectable medications or a disappearance of the elder's syringes at a higher than normal rate? The clinician needs to determine whether the user may be a relative or friend who may be living with or visiting the elder.

DEVELOPING AND ENHANCING THE
THERAPEUTIC RELATIONSHIP

The elder may be fearful and distrustful of the clinician's reason for the home visit. It is important that the clinician do everything possible to make the elder comfortable in the session. Several interventions may enhance the elder's ability to participate in the interview. These include:

- Ask the elder where she or he would like the clinician to be seated during the interview. If the elder has hearing loss, the clinician should suggest that he or she sit close to the elder during the interview. The inability to hear conversations can result in social isolation for many elders. The clinician should take a chair facing the elder, close enough that the elder is able to hear the clinician clearly and read the clinician's lips if necessary. If the elder has but does not use hearing aids, you may want to determine the reason. The batteries may need replacing or the elder may not know how to properly insert the hearing aids or batteries. If the elder does not seem to hear the clinician, the clinician should move closer and speak slowly and distinctly. Yelling will cause the clinician to look angry and distort the clinician's speech. If the elder does not understand a particular phrase, the clinician should restate it using different words. If the elder continues to experience difficulty understanding, the phrase or sentence should be written and given to the elder.

• Sit facing the elder, with any natural light on the clinician's face. This seating arrangement will enable the elder to see the clinician's face most clearly. Glare from the sun should be minimized, as it will affect the elder's vision.

• If the elder becomes agitated during the interview or states that she or he does not wish to answer a particular question, the clinician may need to change the focus of the interview to subjects with which the elder may be more comfortable, in order to engage the elder. The clinician can attempt to clarify the reasons for the discomfort but should understand that the elder might not be aware of the cause of the agitation. The clinician can look at the decorations within the home for cues to possible topics ("Tell me about those photographs on the wall" or "I see that you have a thimble collection. Tell me about your collection"). Anxiety related to memory loss or the interview process itself may affect the elder's cooperation.

• Do not initially confront or dismiss any fears that the elder may present in the interview, even if these fears appear to be delusions. Listen to the elder's concerns in an attempt to determine if there is any basis in fact for the elder's fears. This will encourage the elder to continue to share concerns and participate in treatment.

• Provide encouragement, support and education as a part of the treatment process. For example, providing tips on memory enhancement or on ways to more effectively interview a potential caregiver provide the elder with the tools needed to function more independently and to self-advocate.

OBTAINING THE ELDER'S PSYCHOSOCIAL HISTORY

In order to develop an effective treatment plan, the clinician needs to obtain information about the elder's history. This history includes information about the elder's family and support systems, ability to meet daily care needs, and medical and psychiatric history. The value of psychosocial and biographical information cannot be overstated. The psychosocial history provides the clinician with key information about the elder, including significant past life events that may influence his or her response to current life events. This information may help the clinician support and build on the elder's strengths in adapting to the current situation. The following lists questions that should be asked.

EARLY FAMILY HISTORY

1. "Tell me about your childhood. Did you have any brothers and sisters? Tell me about them. Tell me about your parents." The composition of the family and the elder's birth order may provide information about the structure of the family and the elder's role in the family. It can be helpful to obtain information about the type of environment that the elder was raised in and about the work that family members did to support the family system.

2. Did the elder experience any significant early losses related to physical or psychiatric illness, disability, abuse, neglect, separation or death? What was the impact of these losses on the family system? How the elder adapted to these early losses may indicate how he or she will cope with current and future losses.

WORK AND LEISURE HISTORY

1. Inquire about educational background, the importance of work in the elder's life and the impact of retirement. The clinician might ask: "How far did you go in school? What type of work did you do? Did you work outside of the home (for older women of this generation)?" The clinician might also want to ask: "It sounds like your work was important to you. What kind of activities are you involved with now that you are retired?" A question about the elder's literacy and his or her primary language should be included. The elder's ability to read and communicate can affect his or her ability to self-advocate.

2. Obtain information about the elder's leisure history. What activities or hobbies does the elder enjoy? Has there been a change or loss of interest in previously pleasurable activities? If there has been a change in the ability to pursue certain activities due to disability or finances, has the elder found a satisfactory replacement for the previous activities?

MARITAL AND RELATIONSHIP HISTORY

Obtain information about the elder's marital and relationship history. Is the elder married or with a partner? Does the elder have children? Does the elder have friends? What is the quality of these relationships? Did the elder experience any significant losses in these adult relationships? If so, how did the elder respond to these losses? The clinician should attempt to clarify where friends and family live, how they maintain contact with the elder and their role in the elder's life.

Family and friends frequently are actively involved in the care and support of elders who live in the community. These significant contacts may provide important historical information and observations about the elders for whom they provide support. The clinician should obtain permission from the elder to speak with family and friends. When appropriate, key family members and friends should be involved in aspects of the elder's treatment. These individuals may benefit from counseling to support them in their role as caregivers and to assist them with decision-making related to the elder's care.

MEDICAL AND PSYCHIATRIC HISTORY

Obtain information about the elder's medical and psychiatric history. Note any history of medical or psychiatric treatment, whether in a hospital or on an outpatient basis. Obtain information about the elder's physicians and the hospital at which the elder prefers to receive treatment. Request permission to contact involved physicians or other medical staff when additional medical or psychiatric information would facilitate the clinician's treatment of the elder or when the clinician notes changes in client function that might require medical or psychiatric intervention.

Sleep

Changes in sleep patterns can be an indication of depression. The clinician should ask: "If you wake up at night, are you able to get back to sleep easily?"

Nutrition

Changes in appetite or weight can be indications of depression. Determine if the elder is experiencing any difficulty obtaining, preparing, and eating or swallowing food.

Smoking

If the elder smokes cigarettes, ask the following questions: "How long have you smoked? How much do you smoke? Where and when do you usually smoke? Do you ever fall asleep smoking? Have you noted any changes in your smoking habits?" An increase in smoking can be an indication of depression or anxiety.

Alcohol

Include questions related to alcohol intake: "When did you first use alcohol? How much do you drink? What and when do you usually drink? Have you noted any changes in your drinking?" If the elder takes prescription medications for medical or psychiatric conditions, inquire if he or she is aware of the consequences of combining alcohol and medications. An increase in alcohol use can be an indication of depression.

Ability to Meet Care Needs

Ask the elder if there are any aspects of care or community living with which he or she experiences difficulty. Is the elder's description consistent with the clinician's observations? If the elder could benefit from assistance with aspects of care, is he or she willing to accept this assistance? If the elder is receiving assistance, is this due to a recent change in function? Does the assistance appear to meet the elder's needs? If the elder is receiving assistance from others, how is she or he adapting to this?

Are the elder's financial resources adequate to cover the cost of household expenses, including the cost of housing, meals, medical care, and medications? If not, is the elder willing to consider some of the community resources that might assist with some of these expenses?

Ask the elder if he or she has noted any changes in memory. The elder should be asked to describe what types of changes he or she has experienced and how he or she compensates for these changes. The clinician could use the Folstein Mini Mental Status Exam to obtain additional information about the elder's ability to recall information. Should the clinician feel that additional testing is required to determine the elder's decision-making capacity, the elder's physician should be contacted to request a referral to a neuropsychologist.

PERCEPTIONS OF HEALTH AND AGING

Ask about the elder's expectations of aging. Is the way in which the elder has aged consistent with his or her expectations? If not, how is the elder responding to this discrepancy?

How does the elder describe his or her overall health? Is the elder's description consistent with the clinician's observations?

How does the elder describe his or her mood? The elder may not respond to the question "Do you feel depressed?" but may respond to questions that use the words "sad," "blue," or "low" to describe depressed mood. The clinician may want to include questions about changes in appetite, sleep and involvement in activities when assessing mood. The clinician should watch for changes in these areas, as they can be indicators of depression.

PERCEPTIONS OF RELATIONSHIPS WITH OTHERS

Ask the elder to describe the overall health or capabilities of his or her family and friends. Is the elder's description consistent with the clinician's observations?

Has the way in which significant others have responded to the elder's needs met her or his expectations? If not, how is the elder responding to this discrepancy?

What is the elder's ability to express his or her needs and feelings to others? Is the elder able to express appreciation for the assistance of others? If the elder experiences difficulty expressing needs, feelings, and appreciation to others, what impact does this appear to have on the elder's situation and on any involved caregivers or significant others?

COMMUNITY SUPPORTS

Ask the elder what community agencies or professionals are working with him or her and try to determine their role in the elder's care. This can be difficult information to obtain at times. The elder may not recall the name of the home health care or social service agency whose staff is visiting him or her ("The hospital sent them"). The clinician should ask if any of the other visiting clinicians have left contact information. In the absence of this information, the clinician should request the elder's permission to contact the hospital's discharge planning department or local social service agency to determine what agencies and services are involved in the elder's care. Once the agencies have been identified, the clinician should request the elder's permission to contact the agencies' staff, if this will benefit the elder's treatment and improve the coordination of the elder's care. Becoming familiar with the range of community services that are available to elders will also assist the clinician in identifying the services that might enhance the elder's function at home.

DEVELOPING THE TREATMENT PLAN

During this interview, the clinician and elder discuss the purpose of this initial visit to the elder's home. They will discuss the elder's perceptions and concerns, if any, related to the elder's home situation, ability to function within the home and community, support system and mood state. The clinician will present observations about the elder's current situation and suggestions for goals that the two could work on together. If the elder agrees, the clinician establishes a visit frequency and time and schedules the next visit. Home visits should be scheduled on a weekly basis, with the session lasting forty-five minutes to one hour in length, based on the elder's wishes and health. The discussion may also include a review of care concerns and significant persons or agencies that could be contacted to increase supports within the home or enhance the elder's functional status. Based on obtaining the elder's consent, the clinician may contact family members, friends, physicians and community agencies to obtain additional history or support services for the elder.

Subsequent sessions should include a review of progress toward the previously established treatment goals and a revision of these goals. The frequency and duration of future sessions will vary, based on the elder's observed and expressed needs. Family members, friends or professionals may be incorporated in sessions, at the mutual agreement of the clinician and the elder.

Termination from treatment should be based on the agreement of the clinician and the elder that the treatment goals have been met. The elder may continue to benefit from an in-home visitor and this option should be discussed with the elder. The clinician should assist the elder with this referral, as needed.

SUMMARY

In-home assessment and counseling of the elder is an effective treatment intervention. In-home treatment enables the clinician to obtain an accurate picture of the elder's home situation and to make counseling available to a portion of the older population that might not otherwise utilize it—the home bound elder. In the home the clinician can provide information related to changes that could be made within the home that might enhance the elder's function. The clinician can assist the elder to identify additional information or supports that would enable him or her to function more independently and safely within the home and community. Perhaps most important, the clinician provides support to the elder and the elder's family and friends to enhance their ability to adapt to and surmount the challenges that can come with aging.

REFERENCES

Buckwalter, K. C. (1988, September). *Overcoming barriers to service delivery for the mentally ill elderly.* Paper presented at the American Society on Aging Regional Seminar on Mental Health and Aging, Cleveland, OH.

Bumagin, V., & Hirn, K. (1990). *Helping the aging family.* New York: Springer Publishing Co.

Butler, R. N., Lewis, M., & Sunderland, T. (1991). *Aging and mental health: Positive psychosocial and biomedical approaches.* New York: Merrill.

Cohen, G. (1993). Comprehensive assessment: Capturing strengths, not just weaknesses. *Generations, 17*(1), 47–50.

Turner, M. (1992). Individual psychodynamic psychotherapy with older adults: Perspectives from a nurse psychotherapist. *Archives of Psychiatric Nursing, 6,* 266–274.

Index

Index